Writtle COLLEGE
LIBRARY

TEL: (01245) 424245

This book must be returned on or before the last date below, otherwise fines will be charged.
Books can normally be renewed unless reserved by another reader.

1 JUN 2005		
2 8 APR 2006		
- 4 MAY 2007		
3 1 MAY 2007		
- 5 FEB 2008		
2 2 APR 2008		
2 0 OCT 2011		
2 0 APR 2012		
- 9 NOV 2017		

To my wife Ronnie and to my daughters Lucy and Libby and their families with my love.

For Saunders:

Commissioning Editor: *Joyce Rodenhuis*
Senior Development Editor: *Zoë Youd*
Project Manager: *Jane Dingwall*
Design Direction: *Andy Chapman*

Handbook of Veterinary Obstetrics

SECOND EDITION

Peter GG Jackson

BVM&S MA DVM&S FRCVS

Department of Clinical Veterinary Medicine,
University of Cambridge, Cambridge, UK

Illustrations by John Fuller

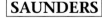

An imprint of Elsevier Limited

Edinburgh • London • New York • Oxford • Philadelphia • St Louis • Sydney • Toronto

SAUNDERS
An imprint of Elsevier Limited

First edition 1995
Second edition 2004

ISBN 0 7020 2740 5

British Library Cataloguing in Publication Data
A catalogue record for this book is available from the British Library

Library of Congress Cataloging in Publication Data
A catalog record for this book is available from the Library of Congress

Note

Veterinary medical knowledge is constantly changing. Standard safety precautions must be followed, but as new research and clinical experience broaden our knowledge, changes in treatment and drug therapy may become necessary or appropriate. Readers are advised to check the most current product information provided by the manufacturer of each drug to be administered to verify the recommended dose, the method and duration of administration, and con-traindications. It is the responsibility of the practitioner, relying on experience and knowledge of the patient, to determine dosages and the best treatment for each individual patient. Neither the Publisher nor the author assumes any liability for any injury and/or damage to persons or property arising from this publication.

The Publisher

Printed in China

 ELSEVIER your source for books, journals and multimedia in the health sciences
www.elsevierhealth.com

The publisher's policy is to use **paper manufactured from sustainable forests**

Contents

Preface to the first edition

The term 'dystocia' means difficult birth and is the opposite of 'eutocia' or normal birth. Dystocia may be defined as the inability of the dam to deliver its young through its own efforts. The diagnosis and treatment of dystocia is an important part of veterinary practice. Few tasks in practice are as pleasant and rewarding as the delivery of healthy offspring following the successful resolution of a case of dystocia. Few are more depressing than treating an obstetrical case in which the outcome is not successful.

Obstetrical work often requires attendance at antisocial hours and in difficult conditions. Cases requiring immediate attention may arise when there is other planned or pressing practice work to be done. Some cases have strong emotional overtones when a long awaited birth is about to occur or the results of a carefully planned breeding program is about to come to fruition. The owner is very anxious that all should go well. Regrettably, regular antenatal care is still relatively uncommon in animals and veterinary help may not be sought until a case of dystocia is well established. The owners of our patients vary greatly in their knowledge – from the breeder with years of experience to the owner who has never witnessed a birth before.

Our patients also vary greatly in their value, from the Thoroughbred mare worth many thousands of pounds to the elderly pet cat with little monetary but great sentimental value. All require and deserve our prompt, humane, skilful and knowledgeable attention. The veterinary obstetrician may at times require considerable physical strength, for example when delivering a calf weighing 50 kg but at all times great delicacy when working with hands unseen within the limits of the birth canal or uterus of the patient. The birth canal of all species is normally only just large enough to allow passage of the young and was not intended – although it sometimes has to – also to accommodate the obstetrician's fingers or arm.

The dividing point between dystocia and eutocia is not always clear cut. On some farms for example mild cases of dystocia pass unnoticed whilst on other farms normal cases may be unnecessarily assisted. Dystocia occurs in all the domestic species but the highest incidence is probably in cattle. The causes of dystocia are classified into maternal and fetal categories where the responsibility for dystocia is attributed to the mother or fetus respectively. In many cases both mother and fetus share responsibility for a problem and in some cases it may be difficult to pin-point the exact cause of dystocia. Within each category are many individual causes whose incidence varies greatly between the species.

Some breeds of animal within a species may be particularly prone to dystocia for example certain strains amongst the brachycephalic dog breeds. Regrettably, it has been necessary to classify some strains of bulldog as 'self-whelping', indicating the lack of need for the high incidence of cesarean section necessary in the 'non-self whelping' strains. The introduction of Continental cattle breeds into the United Kingdom thirty years ago was associated with a great increase in the incidence of dystocia due to fetopelvic disproportion. Similar problems occurred when poorly grown recipient heifers were implanted with the embryos of large beef breeds. In recent years more sensible breeding policies and legislation have reduced the incidence of some of these difficulties.

At one time, success in veterinary obstetrics was measured by the removal of the fetus(es) from the mother irrespective of the survival of either party. Now delivery of living offspring from an undamaged and healthy mother is the target of success. It is hoped that the contents of the pages of this volume will assist in the achievement of this goal.

The first chapter in this book describes normal birth in the domestic species. Veterinary surgeons may have limited experience of normal birth in some species. It is hoped that the details of normal birth will provide a useful baseline against which to measure the signs and management of dystocia. Diseases of pregnancy which may threaten the life of the fetus or mother and their management are described in the second chapter. Many aspects of the clinical approach to dystocia are the same in all species. These are dealt with together in the third chapter to avoid unnecessary repetition later when dystocia in the various species is considered.

Chapters 4–9 are devoted to the problems of dystocia in the domestic species. In each chapter the incidence, causes, investigation and treatment of dystocia are discussed in detail. In small animals, antenatal care is discussed and the advice that may be given to owners in a pre-breeding examination and consultation.

Although most obstetrical work involves the 'usual' domestic species, dystocia may occur in the small pets such as guinea pigs and the larger farmed species such as deer. Notes on some of the problems and their management encountered in these species are provided in Chapter 10. Mention is also made of the unpleasant problem of egg binding that occurs in cage and other birds.

Chapter 11 is devoted to cesarean section in all species and Chapter 12 to fetotomy, which is limited to the larger species in which manual access to the uterus is possible. Postparturient problems in large and small animals are dealt with in Chapters 13 and 14 respectively. Lastly, the important subject of the prevention of dystocia – including methods for induction of birth – is covered in Chapter 15.

Relatively few references have been included in this handbook for reasons of simplicity and ease of reading. References from which data have been directly taken have, however, been included and acknowledged. The descriptions and advice given in the handbook are based chiefly on the author's personal experiences with obstetrical work during many years in general and referral practice. The methods of treatment described are not necessarily the only ones available and for a wider discussion readers should consult the standard textbooks on veterinary obstetrics. The aim of the book has been to describe some of the problems that the veterinary obstetrician may encounter and the practical ways in which these problems may be dealt with on the farm, in the stable, in the home or in the surgery. It is hoped that the contents will be found useful and helpful to those privileged to work in this fascinating branch of veterinary science. It is hoped too that the animals we serve and their owners will also benefit.

Preface to the second edition

The second edition of *Handbook of Veterinary Obstetrics* has retained the same basic format that was used in the first edition. All 15 chapters have been revised and in most cases expanded to include new information and to ensure even greater clarity. John Fuller has drawn 30 new illustrations to complement those he drew for the first edition. The new pictures illustrate such diverse subjects as eclampsia and mastitis in the bitch, and evaluation of the cervix in cases of ringwomb in sheep. The ventrolateral approach to the uterus in bovine cesarean section is also illustrated, as is dystocia caused by the problem of bicornual pregnancy in the mare.

Although some obstetric techniques remain unchanged, there have been a number of important developments since the first edition of this book was published. The use of ultrasonographic scanning in veterinary obstetrics was considered in some detail in the first edition. A major expansion in its use has occurred since then. Ultrasonography is now an essential tool for the modern veterinary obstetrician and it is used in many different situations. It is of major importance in pregnancy diagnosis and aspects of antenatal care. In many species the fetus, parts of the placenta, and placental fluids can be monitored ultrasonographically. This is particularly important in cases where the pregnancy is thought to be at risk. Prolonged gestation can be a problem in many species and may in some cases pose a threat to fetal and even maternal life. Ultrasonography has provided an effective method of fetal monitoring in such cases. A comprehensive clinical examination and an accurate diagnosis are the cornerstones of effective treatment. Ultrasonography allows the obstetrician to obtain an immediate assessment of fetal life. The rapid biochemical and endocrine blood tests that are now available enable the obstetrician to gain an even more detailed assessment of maternal well-being, in addition to that provided by clinical examination.

A number of new, safer anesthetic agents have been introduced since the first edition was published. Analgesia should be provided routinely following cesarean section in all species and also after some manipulative obstetric techniques. Details of suitable analgesic drugs with appropriate dosages are included in the book for all species. There have also been a number of advances in our knowledge of endocrinology, especially in small animals. As a result of these advances a number of new drugs are available – although not licensed for use in all countries. Examples of new agents include aglepristone and cabergoline, which can be used to terminate canine pregnancy.

A new feature of the second edition has been the introduction of 'Obstetrician's check lists' at various points in the chapters dealing with dystocia in large and small animals. It is hoped that these check lists will provide a useful summary of the text and also rapid access to vital information in an emergency.

Owners expect and demand higher and higher obstetric skills from the veterinary profession. Students, new graduates, and more experienced colleagues may be exposed to the intense pressures that challenging obstetric cases can sometimes bring. Several readers have kindly said how helpful they have found the advice given in the first edition when dealing with obstetric cases in practice. It is hoped that this second edition will also provide safe, sensible, and practical guidance and advice to all those privileged to practice veterinary obstetrics.

Peter GG Jackson
Cambridge 2004

Acknowledgments

I would like to thank the many people who kindly contributed to the gestation and birth of the second edition of this book. My family has again provided constant support and encouragement. A number of reviewers of the first edition made helpful suggestions for improvements. Many of these have been adopted. A number of colleagues have read through and commented on sections of the book involving their specialities and have kindly offered guidance and advice. These include Rachel Bennett, Sheelagh Lloyd, Karin Mueller, Professor Sidney Ricketts, Jenny Smith, and Penny Watson. I would also like to thank Peter Cockcroft for his encouragement and support with this project and in many other ways.

Sincere thanks to Joyce Rodenhuis, Zoë Youd, Jane Dingwall and Andy Chapman of Elsevier Science for all their help and encouragement. John Fuller's artistic skills speak for themselves and he has again converted my sketches and photographs into the pictures that illustrate the work. Adrian Cornford has skilfully added color and prepared the pictures for publication.

Any errors or omissions are entirely my responsibility.

Peter GG Jackson
Cambridge 2004

Chapter 1

NORMAL BIRTH

A sound knowledge of normal birth is essential for the veterinary obstetrician to appreciate the degree of abnormality that a case of dystocia is showing. It will also provide guidance on other important facts like the prospects of fetal survival if delivery is delayed.

THE INITIATION OF BIRTH

The fetus is responsible for the initiation of birth in the domestic animal species. The endocrine pathways involved vary to an extent between species; they have not been fully elucidated in some species. A rise in the production of fetal cortisol occurs as a result of changes in and maturation of the hypothalamic–pituitary–adrenal axis of the fetus. This is thought to be caused by fetal stress, which develops as the placenta is less able to supply the needs of the growing and demanding fetus.

The *endocrine events* that precede birth, can be summarized as follows:

1. increased production of corticotropin-releasing hormone (CRH) by the fetal brain
2. increased production of adrenocorticotropic hormone (ACTH) by the fetal anterior pituitary gland
3. increased production of cortisol by the fetal adrenal glands
4. conversion of placental progesterone to estrogen
5. estrogen stimulates production of prostaglandin F2α (PGF2α) by the myometrium and also induces some cervical relaxation
6. PGF2α induces myometrial contraction, which increases intrauterine pressure and moves the fetus towards the cervix, causing further cervical dilation
7. oxytocin is released by the maternal posterior pituitary gland as the cervix is dilated by the fetus (Ferguson's reflex)
8. oxytocin induces further myometrial contractions.

The polypeptide hormone relaxin is produced by the placenta or the maternal corpus luteum quite early in pregnancy. It is involved in relaxation of the maternal cervix prior to birth and might also influence the efficiency of myometrial contractions.

THE STAGES OF BIRTH

For ease of description, parturition is divided into three stages. There is no clear demarcation between the stages, which normally merge with each other to become a continuous process. The length of each stage is quite variable. Before parturition a number of other preparatory changes such as mammary development and relaxation of the pelvic ligaments occur. The timing of these preparatory changes varies between individual animals, making them rather unreliable indicators of approaching birth.

The main *physiological events* of the three stages of labor are listed below:

- *First stage*:
  - relaxation and dilation of cervix
  - fetus adopts birth posture
  - uterine contraction commences
  - chorioallantois enters vagina
- *Second stage*:
  - uterine contraction continues
  - fetus enters birth canal
  - abdominal contraction commences
  - amnion enters vagina
  - fetus is expelled
- *Third stage*:
  - placental circulation lost
  - placental dehiscence and separation occurs
  - uterine and abdominal contractions continue
  - placenta is expelled.

In polytocous species, the first stage of labor is followed by a series of second-stage fetal deliveries. These are followed by either a third stage after each second stage or the passage of placentas after the delivery of a group of or all the offspring.

FETAL PRESENTATION, POSITION, AND POSTURE

For ease and accuracy of description the terms presentation, position, and posture are used to indicate the orientation of the fetus in normal and abnormal birth. Their definitions are as follows:

- *Presentation*: the relationship between the long axis of the fetus and the long axis of the maternal birth canal. Thus presentation can be longitudinal (anterior or posterior), transverse, or (rarely) vertical.
- *Position*: that surface of the maternal birth canal to which the fetal vertebral column is applied. Thus position can be dorsal, ventral, or lateral (right or left).
- *Posture*: the disposition of the head and limbs of the fetus.

The main features of normal birth in each of the domestic species is now described.

NORMAL BIRTH IN THE COW

Gestation length is 283 days in Holstein–Friesian cattle; 290 days is normal in some Continental beef breeds.

Preparatory changes

The most important external changes are seen in the udder, vulva, and pelvic ligaments. Towards the end of pregnancy the udder becomes enlarged and tense. Colostrum is present in the teats and becomes thicker and yellow in color as birth approaches. Leakage of milk ('running milk') prior to calving can lead to loss of the thick colostrum, leaving only normal milk. This can result in serious loss of antibodies for the calf. In heifers, substantial subcutaneous edema can develop in front of and behind the udder. The edema normally disperses within a few days of calving.

As birth approaches, the vulva normally lengthens and might become slightly tumefied and edematous. In some animals, however, no vulval changes are seen. Clear vaginal mucus – believed to be the liquefying cervical seal and resembling the estral secretion – might be seen 24–48 hours before calving. Although body temperature drops before calving, the variation in timing and extent of the change make it an unreliable parameter.

Relaxation of the pelvic ligaments is seen in late pregnancy, becoming more pronounced as birth approaches. It is the most reliable sign of impending parturition in cattle. As a result of this, the cow's tail head might appear to be raised and the gluteal muscles sunken. These changes can be less obvious in fat cows but ligamentous relaxation can be detected internally in such animals by rectal examination. The muscular tone of the tail is reduced 24 hours before calving.

On rectal examination the fetal limbs or head are palpable in the maternal pelvis or immediately in front of it. Evidence of fetal life can be detected by spontaneous movement or by response to applying gentle pressure to the fetus. A uterus containing a very large, oversized fetus can slip down under the maternal rumen, where it is less easily palpated. Although some slight softening of the cervix can occur and be detected on vaginal examination in late pregnancy, full relaxation does not occur until the first stage of labor.

Many stockpersons are extremely good at predicting the prospective time of birth in their animals. Veterinary surgeons, aware of the unreliability of the prepartum physical changes, are advised to refrain from predicting the exact time of impending parturition in their patients.

First stage of labor

The duration of the first stage of labor in cattle is in the range 4–24 hours. The difficulty of identifying the commencement of the first stage in all species makes accurate measurement of its length unreliable. External signs of the first stage include apparent discomfort, cessation of eating, pawing the ground, paddling, circling, lying down and then fairly quickly rising again. The tail may be raised, there may be muscle tremors and occasional straining. The cervix begins to soften and dilate. When fully dilated it is not recognizable on vaginal examination. The onset of cervical dilation and uterine contractions cause the chorioallantois to be pushed into the vagina. The extent of its movement depends on its elasticity and the tightness of its attachment. If its movement is restricted it may rupture in situ but otherwise it may appear at the vulva as a bluish, vascular semitransparent membrane. It may be termed the 'first water bag' although the term 'water bag' is generally confined to the amnion. Rupture of the chorioallantois causes the release of a quantity of allantoic fluid and dampness around the maternal perineum.

Second stage of labor

The duration of this stage is in the range ½–3 hours. Cattle normally give birth in a recumbent position but occasionally, and especially if disturbed, may calve standing up. The calf is normally preceded by its amnion as it enters the birth canal and unless prior rupture occurs, the amnion appears as a gray–white avascular sac at the vulva. Fetal parts may be visible through the amnion, which ruptures during delivery in 80% of cases. Once amniotic rupture has occurred the intensity of straining may increase. Abdominal straining supplements the uterine contractions and as the second stage of labor proceeds the intensity and frequency of abdominal straining increases (Fig. 1.1).

The cow may bellow loudly with effort and may roll from sternal recumbency into lateral recumbency. The greatest maternal effort is apparently associated with the passage of the fetal head through the vulva but at this point the fetal thorax is also entering the maternal pelvis. Once the head is delivered the rest of the body mostly follows with ease, although in beef cattle considerable effort may be required to deliver the thorax and hips of the calf. During delivery the position of the calf may rotate approximately 45° to the right or left allowing it to take advantage of the greatest pelvic diameter of the mother (Fig. 1.2).

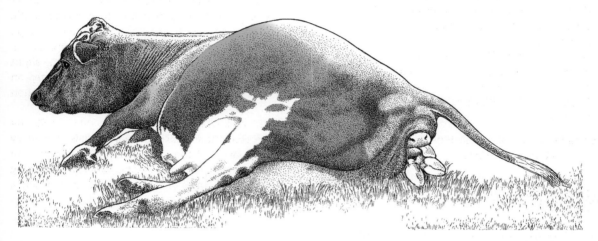

Figure 1.1 Early second-stage labor in the cow. The calf's muzzle is level with the fetlock joints of the forelimb. The amnion has ruptured and the calf's tongue is protruding. The calf's position has rotated about 45° from the dorsal position.

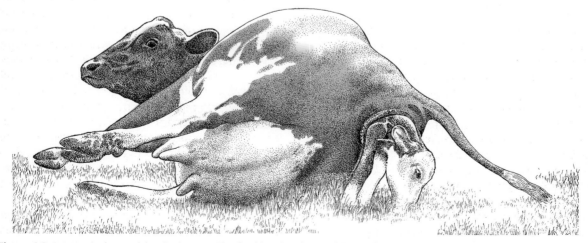

Figure 1.2 Late second-stage labor in the cow. The fetal head and part of the shoulders have been delivered.

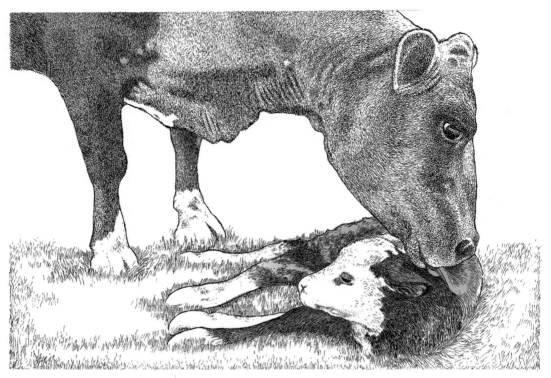

Figure 1.3 Second-stage labor is complete. The cow has risen and is licking the calf, which is attempting to assume sternal recumbency.

The majority of calves are in a dorsal position in late pregnancy and during birth the calf is in anterior (95% of calves) longitudinal presentation, dorsal position, and in a posture with the head and forelimbs extended. The fetal nose is level with and rests on the fetlock joints of the forelimbs. The umbilical cord usually remains intact following delivery in the recumbent cow and may not rupture until the cow stands after calving. Unless exhausted, the cow stands up within 10 minutes of the birth of her calf and licks it. The calf lies still immediately after birth and often shakes its head before gasping and taking its first breath. If healthy, the calf should attempt to assume sternal recumbency within 5 minutes of delivery encouraged by licks from its mother (Fig. 1.3).

Third stage of labor

The fetal membranes are normally expelled within 12 hours of birth. Retention beyond 12 hours is often followed by a further period of retention lasting from 3 to 10 days unless the membranes are removed manually.

Interference in normal calving

Whenever possible, the cow should be left to calve unaided. Supervision should be close but unobtrusive. Vaginal examination should be performed if there is any departure from the normal. The calf should be born within 2 hours of the first appearance of the amnion at the vulva. Delivery time may be longer for larger calves and in some breeds, including the Charolais. Although the bovine fetus can survive for up to 8 hours during second-stage labor, this is not always the case and any delay should be investigated.

NORMAL BIRTH IN THE MARE

Gestation length is 330 days.

Preparatory changes

Premonitory signs of parturition in the mare can be very misleading. As birth approaches, mammary development, lengthening of the vulva, and relaxation of the pelvic ligaments are seen. In some mares bead-like deposits of wax appear on the ends of the teats within 48 hours of parturition but in many mares foaling occurs without waxing. Predicting the time of birth in mares can be difficult. If milk is present in the udder a small quantity can be analyzed daily to determine the concentrations of calcium, sodium, and potassium ions. The use of these to predict the approximate time of birth is discussed under induction of birth in the mare in Chapter 15. The whole birth process is much quicker and more violent than in cattle. Any disturbance, including excessive and obtrusive observation, can cause the mare to inhibit the onset of parturition. Once any disturbance is over, foaling may follow rapidly and be completed in less than an hour. The foal is in a ventral position until the first stage of labor, when it rotates into a dorsal position and adopts the foaling posture. The cervix is much softer than in the cow and can normally be manually dilated with ease just before foaling begins. The majority of mares foal between 6.00 p.m. and midnight.

First stage of labor

The duration of this stage is very variable, lasting on average 1–2 hours. The mare is restless, uncomfortable, may kick at her abdomen and shows signs of patchy sweating. The tail is raised and periodically swished vigorously downwards and sideways. The mare postures frequently and may occasionally strain as if attempting to urinate. The stage normally ends with the passage of a small quantity of fluid from the ruptured chorioallantois.

Second stage of labor

This stage, lasting on average not more than 30 minutes, is signaled by the onset of intense straining. The mare normally lies down to foal flat on her side with her legs extended, if room allows. Straining continues with grunting, groaning, and often profuse sweating as the fetus enters the birth canal. During birth the foal, which is normally in anterior longitudinal presentation and dorsal position, has one of its extended forelegs about 8 cm in front of the other. The head may be longitudinally rotated during delivery. Passage of head and thorax appear to require additional straining effort. Once the foal is delivered – often still enclosed in the amnion – it lies with its hindlegs still in the birth canal.

The mare lies still, temporarily exhausted for up to 30 minutes after delivery. The umbilical cord is normally unbroken when the foal is born but ruptures when the mare rises or the foal moves vigorously. Premature rupture may occur if the mare foals in the standing position.

Third stage of labor

The placenta is normally passed allantoic side out within 3 hours of foaling. It is mainly pushed out by myometrial contractions supplemented by occasional straining. Portions of placenta hanging behind them upset some mares and there may be some low-grade colicky pain associated with uterine contractions during the third stage. If the placenta is retained beyond 3 hours of foaling assistance may be required with its removal.

Interference in normal foaling

The early failure of placental support that occurs during foaling means that unless the foal is delivered within a maximum of 60 minutes after the commencement of the second stage of labor there is a grave risk of fetal death. For this reason, foaling should be supervised carefully and unobtrusively. If both forelegs are equally advanced in the birth canal the risk of impaction of the fetal elbows on the pelvic brim is greatly increased. If this occurs, or if there is any other delay, assistance should be rendered. The foal should be delivered within 40 minutes of the rupture of the chorioallantois and, if it is not, the case should be investigated for dystocia.

Occasionally the chorioallantois fails to rupture at the cervical star, possibly as a result of premature separation of the membrane from the endometrium. The velvety red surface of the chorion appears at the vulva in what is sometimes termed a 'red bag birth'. This is a sign that the foal may be at risk and the chorioallantois should be opened immediately using scissors to release the foal. Assistance with delivery should be given following the opening of the membrane.

Foals born within their amnions can free themselves by vigorous movement but should be released by breaking the membrane around the head. Avoid disturbing the mare in the immediate postpartum phase in case premature rupture of the cord occurs with the risk of neonatal maladjustment and other problems. Careful management of the placenta is necessary, especially in heavy mares where severe metritis with laminitis may follow retention.

NORMAL BIRTH IN THE EWE

Gestation length is 147 days.

Preparatory changes

Relaxation of the pelvic ligaments occurs as birth approaches but is not visible in heavily fleeced ewes, where manual palpation is necessary to detect the changes. Lengthening and relaxation of the vulva is seen in some animals. Mammary growth with separation of the two teats occurs throughout the second half of pregnancy and colostrum is normally present in the teats within 24 hours of lambing. External signs of approaching birth can readily be overlooked in large flocks. Signs of first-stage labor are more obvious and the shepherd should watch carefully for these and monitor the subsequent birth process.

First stage of labor

This stage is believed to last 6–12 hours. The ewe separates herself from the flock and may appear restless and paw the ground. A few ewes show no signs of being in first-stage labor.

Second stage of labor

This stage lasts ½–1 hour and may be slightly longer in ewes lambing for the first time. The majority of lambs enter the birth canal in anterior longitudinal presentation, in the same posture as the calf. Some lambs are born in posterior presentation with the extended hindlimbs entering the birth canal first. Small lambs in anterior presentation may occasionally be born with one forelimb in shoulder flexion. The ewe normally lies down to lamb, straining vigorously and throwing her head up with effort and grunting as she does so (Fig. 1.4). Many ewes like to lie with their back against a wall or fence during lambing. The second stage is repeated as further lambs are born.

Figure 1.4 Second-stage labor in the ewe. The ewe throws her head dorsally upwards as she strains.

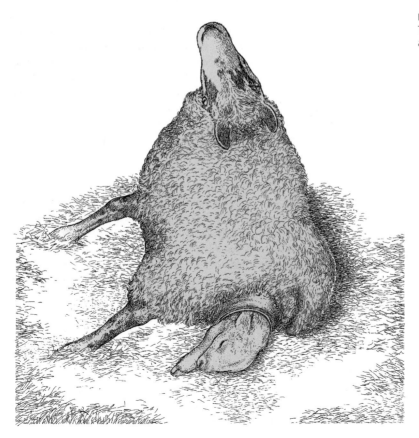

Approximately 50% of lambs are born with an intact amnion.

Third stage of labor

The placenta is normally passed within 3–4 hours of delivery of the last lamb.

Interference in normal lambing

Close observation of parturient ewes is essential and a vaginal examination should be carried out in cases where there are signs of any delay in the birth process. Multiple birth should always be suspected and the ewe examined internally in cases of doubt. Litter size in ewes can be determined by ultrasonographic scan at 60–90 days of pregnancy. Ewes may be batched for management and lambing on the basis of their prospective litter size. Although a useful guide, errors in estimating fetal numbers can occur. Individual animals should always be examined carefully per vaginam if there is any doubt that parturition is complete.

NORMAL BIRTH IN THE DOE

The birth process and timing of the stages is broadly similar to the ewe. Gestation length is approximately 150 days. The doe may vocalize loudly as if in great distress during normal delivery. Multiple births are very common and the possibility of further kids in utero must always be suspected.

NORMAL BIRTH IN THE SOW

Gestation length is 115 days.

Preparatory changes

Mammary development is evident in gilts in the last third of pregnancy and becomes more obvious as parturition approaches. Milk is present in the teats within 24 hours of farrowing. Immediately before birth, probably associated with oxytocin release, squeezing the teats will cause release of jets of milk. The vulva swells and softens in the last few days of pregnancy. In older sows these changes, and relaxation of the pelvic ligaments, may occasionally appear to be excessive resulting in a tendency to vaginal and rectal prolapse.

First stage of labor

During first-stage labor, which can extend from 12 to 24 hours, the sow shows signs of bed making – chewing and heaping up any bedding within reach. Intervals of activity are interspersed with periods of rest and the sow usually settles down in lateral recumbency just before farrowing commences.

Second stage of labor

Mild abdominal straining heralds the onset of second-stage labor. Vigorous tail swishing and the passage of a small quantity of allantoic fluid precede the arrival of each piglet. Each piglet is normally expelled quite forcibly through the vulva. Approximately half the piglets are still enclosed within their amnion and those born early in the litter have intact umbilical cords. Fifty five per cent of piglets are born in anterior longitudinal presentation with their forelimbs held by their sides; 45% are in posterior presentation with their hindlimbs extended backwards or less commonly in a hip flexion posture.

Usually, 3–6% of piglets are stillborn in normal litters and a small number of mummified fetuses are commonly seen. The stillbirth rate rises rapidly with increasing duration of labor and dystocia.

The mean farrowing time is $2\frac{1}{2}$ hours (range 30 minutes–4 hours), with piglets born at intervals of approximately 15 minutes. The sow may rise at intervals during farrowing but mostly remains recumbent until delivery of the last piglet.

Third stage of labor

Portions of placenta may be passed after each piglet, after a number of piglets, or at the end of farrowing. The chorionic surface of the last pieces of placenta from each horn may be a darker red color than the remainder of this tissue. After farrowing is complete the sow may rise, pass urine, and then lie down to continue feeding her piglets. However, these signs are not reliable indicators that farrowing is complete.

Interference in normal farrowing

Piglets may need assistance to escape from their amniotic sacs and be protected from injury if the sow stands during parturition or shows signs of aggression. Any delay in parturition must be investigated to ensure early diagnosis and treatment of dystocia and to avoid high levels of stillbirth. On many pig farms, birth is induced by intramuscular injection of prostaglandin F2α or a synthetic analog. Healthy sows within 48 hours of their prospective farrowing date are induced and normally farrow 20–30 hours later. Treatment is given in the early to late morning and staff are able to supervise farrowings during working hours the following day. A reduction of stillbirth rate and a reduced preweaning mortality should result. On some farms, once farrowing is underway its conclusion is hastened by an intramuscular injection of oxytocin. This should only be done in animals in which it is known that cervical dilation is complete and in which there is no obstructive dystocia.

NORMAL BIRTH IN THE BITCH

Gestation length is 63 days.

Preparatory changes

In maiden pregnant bitches, mammary development may occur as early as 3–4 weeks into gestation. In late pregnancy mammary development becomes more pronounced but the onset of lactation is extremely variable. In some bitches milk may be found in the teats 2 weeks, and occasionally even earlier, before whelping. In others there may be no sign of milk in the teats until whelping is actually under way.

In the last week of pregnancy the vulva becomes enlarged, elongated, and rather flabby, and there may be a little clear vaginal discharge. In some bitches, however, this discharge is present throughout pregnancy. Relaxation of the pelvic ligaments and abdominal musculature occurs in the last few days of pregnancy. The most reliable sign of impending parturition in bitches is the fall in body temperature of up to 1°C that occurs within 24 hours of whelping.

First stage of labor

The signs of this stage are very variable both in intensity and duration. They may extend over 4–24 hours. The bitch is restless and may show a strong desire to make a nest under tree roots, under furniture, or on the owner's bed. Pawing, shivering, panting, flank watching, and occasionally vomiting and mild straining may be seen. The signs normally show a steady and progressive increase in intensity as second-stage labor approaches. Nervous bitches often experience a more stormy first stage than their more placid counterparts and may refuse to settle down or be separated from their owners. Familiarization with the whelping quarters well before birth may help reduce the problem. Mild sedation may be necessary. Very occasionally no external signs of first stage are seen.

Second stage of labor

The bitch usually lies in lateral recumbency during delivery but occasionally walks around pausing to strain in a squatting position. The chorioallantois of each puppy normally ruptures at the pelvic inlet allowing the amniotic sac to enter the pelvic canal. A small quantity of allantoic fluid may pass out through the vulva at this stage before delivery of the puppy. The puppies rotate through 180° to assume the dorsal position of birth. Sixty per cent are born in the anterior longitudinal presentation and 40% in the posterior presentation (Fig. 1.5). Posterior presentation is often erroneously referred to by dog breeders as a 'breech birth'. In a true breech birth, the tail and hindquarters of the puppy are presented with both hindlegs in hip flexion.

Once the presenting part of the fetus has engaged in the pelvis, reflex abdominal straining commences and the puppy is usually delivered with relative ease after two or three expulsive efforts. Straining may be particularly intense in small breeds with small litters where there is a degree of fetopelvic disproportion. The first puppy should be born within 6 hours of the commencement of second-stage labor. The interval between puppies is 5–60 minutes (average 30 minutes), tending to be longer near the end of the delivery of the litter. The interval between puppies can be as long as 4 hours without it necessarily being abnormal. Ideally, the intervals should be shorter and of even length. Some bitches regularly take up to 24 hours to complete whelping successfully but they must be closely supervised. During delivery a dark green discharge accompanies the puppies and arises from the breakdown of the marginal hematomata of the zonary placenta. During delivery the bitch's respiratory rate may become very shallow and rapid (150/minute) and may be exacerbated by excessive heat or poor ventilation in the whelping quarters. Inexperienced bitches may stand during delivery of one or more of their litter and there is a small risk that they may accidentally tread on other members of their litter.

As soon as each puppy is delivered the bitch normally licks its head and opens the amniotic vesicle if this has not occurred spontaneously. The bitch severs

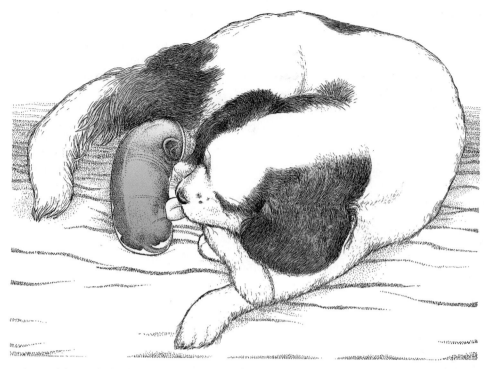

Figure 1.5 Second-stage labor in the bitch. Approximately 40% of puppies are born in posterior presentation.

the umbilical cord with her teeth about 2 cm from the puppy. Between puppies, the bitch may lapse into a somnolent state until the next puppy enters her pelvis. She will often rouse herself at intervals from her resting position to lick and clean the pups or her vulva. Muscle fasciculations resembling shivering are sometimes seen in the hindlimbs but there is normally no sign of hypothermia.

Third stage of labor

The chorioallantois may be delivered after each puppy, after a group of puppies or at the end of whelping. The bitch will often eat each placenta as it is passed but this may cause vomiting. Owners frequently suspect that one or more placentas have been retained having failed to observe the bitch eating them. The duration of the third stage is very variable but should be completed within 2 hours of the delivery of the last puppy.

Interference in normal whelping

As in other species, observation should be careful but discreet. Steady progress in whelping is anticipated and

care taken to ensure survival of the puppies by ensuring their release from the amniotic vesicle and avoiding accidental or careless damage by the bitch. Excessive interference must be avoided.

NORMAL BIRTH IN THE QUEEN CAT

Gestation length is 63 days.

Preparatory changes

Activity is often reduced in the last week of pregnancy and the cat seeks a quiet, dark, warm area in which to give birth. Normal activity is maintained in some cats, which happily climb trees within hours of giving birth. Some change in temperament may be seen with the cat, either seeking or shunning human company. Appetite may be reduced in late pregnancy. Sudden intra-abdominal fetal movements may appear to cause her alarm. Relaxation of the pelvic ligaments and the abdominal musculature occurs as kittening approaches. Mammary development intensifies, the teats become pink, and milk is present within 24 hours of birth.

Body temperature in the queen falls by 0.5–1°C within 12 hours of birth.

First stage of labor

During this stage the cat appears restless and may vocalize frequently. Nesting behavior becomes increasingly intense, with the cat tearing up or rearranging her bedding. She may visit her litter tray frequently and strain unproductively. Many domestic cats choose to give birth away from home. Duration of the first stage is variable at 2–12 hours.

Second stage of labor

The first kitten is normally born within 5–60 minutes of the commencement of abdominal straining – the longer period being seen in some primiparous cats. A series of loud cries may accompany fetal delivery, especially the first kitten, and may alarm the inexperienced owner. Subsequent kittens are born at 5 to 60 minute intervals and the second stage is normally complete within 6 hours. Great variation in the duration of second-stage labor is seen and long pauses – sometimes lasting several hours – may occur, extending the birth process to 24 hours without loss of fetal life. During kittening the cat may rise suddenly from her recumbent position to lick her vulva and move around in her quarters. It has been suggested that these sudden movements may increase intra-abdominal pressure and hasten fetal delivery. During delivery, a dark brown discharge is normally seen, which arises from the breakdown of the marginal hematomata of the zonary placenta. Once each kitten is delivered the queen licks it and removes any residual portions of the amnion (Fig. 1.6).

Third stage of labor

The placenta may be passed after each kitten, after one or two kittens or at the end of the second stage. The process is normally completed within 2 hours of kittening. If unattended, the cat will consume the placentas which may cause vomiting.

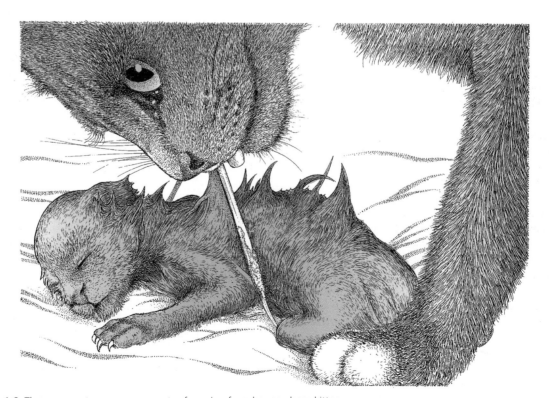

Figure 1.6 The queen cat removes remnants of amnion from her newborn kitten.

Interference in normal kittening

As many cats give birth away from home, close supervision is often not possible and problems may not be discovered until the cat returns home with or without her kittens. The great variation in normal behavior can make monitoring progress difficult but any sign of maternal distress or unexpected delay should be investigated. Some kittens may require assistance in breaking free from their amniotic sacs. Inexperienced cats may fail to sever the umbilical cords of their kittens, which may become entangled with each other's cords. Careful dissection with scissors is required to free them.

THE FATE OF THE FETAL MEMBRANES

The fetal membranes are usually consumed by the mother (with the exception of the mare) if she has access to them shortly after the completion of second-stage labor. The herbivorous ruminant species rarely suffer any adverse after effects if they eat their placenta. On many farms, however, they are collected and disposed of as soon as possible after birth has occurred. Small animals normally eat their placentas but many breeders do not encourage this, preferring to collect and dispose of them.

CHANGES IN THE FETUS DURING THE PERINATAL PERIOD

The fetus that has been protected and nourished within the maternal uterus throughout pregnancy has to undergo major changes at the time of its birth. Once contact with the placenta is severed by rupture or compression of the umbilical cord, the fetus must breath or it will die. During delivery the fetus may have become hypoxic as it passed through the confines of the birth canal. Less well-developed fetuses, such as those of the dog, may be able to withstand a degree of hypoxia for a longer period than more highly developed fetuses, such as those of the large ruminants. The fetus has practiced breathing movements during pregnancy. Increasing levels of fetal cortisol will have encouraged surfactant production in the lungs to reduce surface tension and facilitate postnatal breathing and gaseous exchange. The developing hypoxia during its birth, exposure to air, and a lower ambient temperature after its birth cause the fetus to gasp and expand its lungs for the first time.

Application of mild pain, such as pinching the nose or feet or splashing cold water on the head, will also encourage the fetus to gasp. After the first gasp, other gasping movements may be made before normal breathing commences. Fluids within the fetal lungs are absorbed and may be drained away or coughed up from the trachea. Removal of fluids can be aided by raising the hind end of the fetus to facilitate drainage or by application of suction.

Shortly after birth, closure of the ductus arteriosus and the foramen ovale increases the blood supply to and from the lungs. Retraction of the severed umbilical blood vessels occurs shortly after birth. The ductus venosus, which allowed the umbilical vein bringing oxygenated blood back from the placenta to bypass the liver during pregnancy, closes and the hepatic portal circulation becomes fully functional. The urachus is sealed and all urine is now voided through the urethra. Fetal hemoglobin is replaced by adult hemoglobin.

During its intrauterine life, fetal body temperature is maintained by contact with maternal tissues. After birth the fetus is vulnerable to hypothermia. Although there is some variation between the species, most fetuses have deposits of mitochondria-rich brown fat; piglets are born with very small reserves of brown fat. Metabolization of brown fat releases heat and energy in the first few hours of life, helping the neonate to maintain body warmth and survive. Licking by its mother helps to dry the fetal coat and in many species the fetus also seeks warmth and shelter from its mother. Shivering can occur in some neonates, such as calves, within a few hours of birth. Puppies are unable to shiver effectively to generate body heat until they are 2 weeks old, making them particularly susceptible to hypothermia in the neonatal period.

The newborn fetus must seek maternal milk and access to this is helped by a caring and experienced mother. Colostral transfer and nourishment are vital postnatal events. Rising levels of fetal cortisol in late pregnancy are thought to cause maturation of thyroid and pancreatic function, enabling glucose homeostasis to be maintained.

CHANGES IN THE MOTHER IN THE POSTPARTURIENT PERIOD

Following fetal birth a number of important changes occur, especially in the maternal reproductive system. These include involution of the uterus, removal of placental and other debris from the uterus, closure of the cervix, restoration of the endometrium, and resumption of sexual activity. There is great variation between the domestic species in the timing of these events. In the mare, for example, overt ovarian activity is evident at the foal heat 5–10 days after foaling. In the seasonally monestrous bitch, overt ovarian activity might not be seen until 4–6 months after whelping.

Postparturient events have been particularly well documented in the cow. Involution of the uterus commences immediately after calving and is complete by 25–50 days. Uterine fluids have disappeared by 7–10 days. The cervix closes within 24 hours of normal calving. The caruncles slough from the endometrium by 10 days after calving and are restored by 25 days. Ovarian activity commences at 10–14 days after calving and breeding can occur at 40–80 days.

In addition to these events, the maternal body has to respond to the demands of lactation and restore the antibodies lost through colostral transfer.

Chapter 2

PROBLEMS OF PREGNANCY

SUPERFECUNDATION

Superfecundation occurs without causing problems when offspring from more than one sire are conceived at the same estrus period. It is seen chiefly in promiscuous dogs and cats, but also in cows served by more than one bull. Owners may seek help to establish the parentage of the offspring in relation to particular sires. This can be done by genetic profile. On many pig farms, sows are routinely served by more than one boar and hence superfecundation is widespread but not obvious if boars are of the same breed.

SUPERFETATION

Superfetation occurs when an animal that is already pregnant comes into estrus, is served, and conceives a second litter. This occurs in wild species such as the kangaroo and there are periodic reports of the phenomenon occurring in the sow. Evidence presented suggests the sow produces two separate litters 2 weeks or so apart. Some doubts remain about the validity of this and it is thought that embryonic diapause is a more likely explanation. Superfetation may appear to occur and the veterinary obstetrician may be consulted in certain circumstances, for example:

- Equine twin abortion – the mare may produce two foals of very different size, one having died some weeks earlier, and the owner may incorrectly suspect that they had been conceived at different times and that superfetation had occurred.
- A pregnant cow may adopt the calf of a herdmate and suckle it. The owner thinks she has calved but her own calf is then born a few days later, and again the owner may incorrectly suspect superfetation.

TELEGONY

Telegony is the misconception that a pure bred animal mated accidentally by a mongrel may never breed true again. Believed occasionally by some dog and horse breeders.

INTERSPECIES BREEDING

Breeding between species may occur successfully in some cases, e.g. horse × donkey in which mule or hinney is produced. It also occurs following matings between cow and bison. The hybrids produced from these matings are normally sterile. Successful goat × sheep mating can occur. The conceptus normally develops to about 6 weeks and is then aborted. Very occasionally, the pregnancy goes further and later abortion occurs. Interspecies breeding should not be confused with engineered crosses, for example the 'shoat' in which hybridization is achieved by cell manipulation. The tabloid press occasionally claims erroneously that kittens have been born to bitches or puppies to queen cats.

ECTOPIC PREGNANCY

The condition of fetal development outside the uterus is common in humans. The human placenta is discoid, hemochorial, and very invasive and a fetus may become established in the oviduct (tubal pregnancy) or attached to abdominal organs, including the ovary. Urgent surgery is necessary to terminate the problem. The placentation of the domestic animals makes true ectopic pregnancy extremely unlikely, although periodic claims with no scientific basis that it has occurred are made in the literature. Such apparent ectopic pregnancy is seen in the following circumstances:

- 'Abdominal pregnancy': the fetus(es) starts life in the uterus. The uterus may be ruptured in a road or other accident. The fetus(es) passes into the abdomen. They may survive initially but only if the placenta is not compromised. If the fetus(es) survive to term they cannot re-enter the uterus and surgical delivery would be necessary. The fetuses mostly die and may become mummified or adherent to abdominal viscera and may be discovered at laparotomy during the investigation of an abdominal mass or other abnormality.
- 'Vaginal pregnancy': the fetus is found in the vagina and was thought by some to have been conceived there. The fetus mostly lodges there as a result of an incomplete abortion. This may also happen after treatment of bovine mummified fetus (see below) with prostaglandin injection, which results in the fetus being expelled from the uterus into the vagina, from where it has to be manually removed.

DEATH OF THE CONCEPTUS

The conceptus is vulnerable, especially in its early life, to various adverse factors that might kill it, inflict serious damage, or cause minor but non-life-threatening injury. There is evidence that, following service, 98% of cows actually conceive and yet few herds achieve a conception rate (evidenced by positive pregnancy diagnosis at 6 weeks) of greater than 50%. The remaining embryos do not survive.

Adverse factors affecting the conceptus

- Genetic abnormalities involving either the autosomes or the sex chromosomes.
- Failure of hormonal support – especially progesterone.
- Failure of the maternal body to recognize the presence of the embryo.
- Environmental stress, for example extremes of temperature, starvation, radiation.
- Infection affecting the conceptus, its placenta or the uterus.
- Chemical factors, for example poisons and drugs (e.g. methallibure).
- Immunologic factors.

Note

The incidence of all these adverse factors in animals has not been fully investigated. In humans, fetal loss is believed to be caused by genetic abnormalities in 75% of cases. In animals, the incidence of genetic problems has received relatively little attention. The incidence of infectious abortion in the farm animals is documented in the reports of the Veterinary Laboratory Agency. In sheep, for example, approximately 55% of abortion cases are caused by infection.

The fate of the conceptus when exposed to adverse factors (Fig. 2.1) depends on the severity and nature of the challenge and on the age of the conceptus.

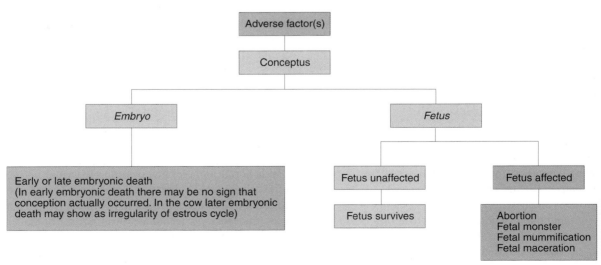

Figure 2.1 Adverse factors affecting the conceptus.

Abortion

The fetus and its environment are so damaged that survival is impossible and the contents of the uterus pass out through the cervix. In the larger species, some assistance may be needed to help the dam deliver the aborted fetus and normal obstetric methods are used for this. In the case of the dog and cat, abortion may occasionally pass unnoticed and the dam consumes the small conceptuses.

Once the process of abortion commences little can be done to stop it. In women, threatened miscarriage can be halted in some cases by bed rest, but this is not possible in animals.

All cases of abortion should be investigated to ensure that there is not an infectious cause that could be transmitted to other animals. The cause should be assumed to be infectious and hygienic precautions taken immediately until a definitive diagnosis is available.

Note

Not all the litter are necessarily affected by adverse factors and some of the litter will die whereas the rest survive. If the majority of a polytocous litter die, actual abortion will probably occur. In other cases, the minority are affected and become mummified and are eventually delivered at the time the rest of the litter are born at term. The management of cases of late, partial abortion in the bitch is discussed in Chapter 9.

In dogs (and possibly pigs and cats) the phenomenon of *fetal resorption* can occur. Cases in which pregnancy has been confirmed are later found to be non-pregnant and yet no evidence of abortion has been observed. In other cases, the number of fetuses born is less than the number of fetuses clearly demonstrated by ultrasonography earlier in pregnancy. In such cases fetal tissues are believed to become autolyzed and 'digested' by scavenger cells in the blood. Resorption of part of the litter may occur in subsequent litters in some dogs and cats. Sequential ultrasonographic scans of such patients may demonstrate the death and eventual disappearance of individual fetuses, often at 4–5 weeks of pregnancy. The reason for such fetal deaths is not known but may be caused by lack of space for individual placentas. Plasma progesterone profiles of such patients usually remain at normal levels.

Fetal anomalies

Fetal anomalies can involve minor or major abnormalities in the fetus. They are usually not incompatible with fetal life. The term 'fetal monster' or 'monstrosity' is used to describe a fetus that has suffered severe physical damage usually affecting its appearance but not causing its death in the uterus. In some cases the damage is caused by inherited genetic abnormality but in many cases the exact cause is unclear. Our predecessors thought that monsters were caused by supernatural forces. They paid great attention to the physical abnormality demonstrated and gave each type of monster a scientific name and placed it in a class, order, and species.

In cattle breeding, where artificial insemination can produce thousands of calves from one bull, any evidence of monsters sired by a bull should be reported to the owner of the bull in case hereditary factors are involved.

Some monsters result in dystocia and examples of these and methods for their delivery will be discussed in subsequent chapters.

Minor abnormalities – like polydactyly in cats – are relatively unimportant and are not life threatening. A large number of anomalies have been described and some of the more common ones are listed below:

- *Achondroplasia*: short-limbed 'dwarf' offspring, for example bulldog calves in Dexter cattle. Assistance with delivery is often required.
- *Anasarca*: fetal skin and subcutis are edematous. Serious problems at birth may be encountered.
- *Cleft palate*: seen in all species, especially puppies and calves.
- *Conjoined fetuses*: usually monozygotic twins ('Siamese twins') that have partially or completely failed to separate. The fetus may have two faces (diprosopus) or two heads (dicephalus). Many other partial divisions have been described. One of the worst in terms of dystocia is when the fetuses are joined at their hindquarters (pygodidymus). The fetus in anterior presentation may appear normal but cannot be delivered because the co-twin is attached behind. An abnormal monozygotic twin is the fetal mole (*Amorphus globosus*), which has an umbilical cord supplying a small structure of mixed fetal tissue surrounded by skin. It is usually an incidental finding at the birth of its normal co-twin and does not cause dystocia.
- *Entropion*: especially lambs. This is not life threatening but causes severe eye damage.
- *Imperforate anus*: especially piglets.
- *Muscular hypertrophy*: 'double muscling', for example in Belgian Blue cattle. This abnormality is selected on purpose in some countries because of the high value of such calves, which also have a very high rate of dystocia.

- *Perosomus elumbis*: this unpleasant monster has been recorded in most of the larger species. The affected fetus has a shortened spinal cord, which terminates in the thoracic region. As a result the hind limbs have no nerve supply, cannot be moved in the uterus and develop ankylosed joints. These can cause dystocia at delivery and the fetus is non-viable.
- *Schistosomus reflexus*: quite rare but still one of the most common forms of anomaly in farm animals, especially calves. The spinal cord is severely deviated so that the anterior and posterior ends are close together. The fetus has an abnormal body wall and the thoracic and abdominal contents may be uncovered. The fetus can survive during pregnancy but causes dystocia and is non-viable at birth. If alive it must be euthanized (see Fig. 4.6).

Specific chromosome abnormalities

A number of specific chromosome defects have been reported in animals. Autosomal defects include trisomy, which causes Down syndrome in humans and has also been found in cattle. Translocation (a form of genetic depletion) has been seen in various breeds of cattle. The Robertsonian 1/29 translocation has been identified in many breeds; it results in reduced fertility in both male and female affected animals.

Aging of the sperm or ovum can also predispose to genetic abnormalities.

Sex chromosome defects, including XXY karyotype (also known as Klinefelter's syndrome), occurs very rarely in bulls that have testicular hypoplasia and a reduced sperm count.

Intersex animals are quite commonly encountered. True hermaphrodites, which have both ovarian and testicular tissue, are extremely rare. Pseudohermaphrodites are often seen in pigs. Many are male pseudohermaphrodites, which are genetically female but with a partially male phenotype. They have a uterus and testes that may be scrotal or abdominal. They may have a vulva and clitoris or a penis.

An extremely common type of intersex is the freemartin heifer calf born as co-twin to a male. Placental fusion occurs early in bovine twin pregnancy. Mullerian inhibiting substance and hormones cross the placentae to influence the sexual development of both fetuses. XX and XY cell populations are seen. The infertile female calf has a grossly abnormal genital tract – the cervix and anterior vagina are absent. The vaginal length of a normal 4-week-old heifer calf, measured by careful insertion of a smooth plastic rod, is 12–15 cm in length. In a freemartin of the same age the vaginal length is only 5–6 cm. The male twin to the freemartin mostly has normal fertility. Freemartinism also occurs less commonly (or is seldom recognized) in the small ruminants and may be found to be present in ewes thought to be infertile.

Intersexes in goats are quite common. The intersexuality gene is linked to the autosomal dominant polling gene. Most intersexes are male pseudohermaphrodites. They are genetically female, have a wide range of phenotype appearances, and have an internal uterus. Some are phenotypically female often with an enlarged clitoris. Others have testis-like gonads in a scrotal or ovarian position.

Sex-linked abnormalities are also seen, for example 'white heifer disease' (so-named because of the high incidence in, but not confined to, white and roan Shorthorn heifers) in which parts of the Mullerian duct are missing. Such animals are normally infertile.

Fetal mummification

One possible fate of the fetus that dies in utero is that it will remain in the closed uterus. Its fetal and body fluids will be resorbed and it will become mummified. The corpus luteum normally remains active and the dam does not return to estrus. In most cases the mummified fetus becomes dry and paper-like (papyraceous mummification). In cattle, another form of mummification, possibly of genetic origin, has been seen in Channel Island breeds. Hemorrhage occurs between the chorion and the endometrium, possibly as a consequence of fetal death and the dead fetus becomes surrounded by sticky fluid. This is sometimes known as hematic mummification.

Fetal mummification occurs in all species. In the polytocous dog, cat, and pig a number of fetuses may become mummified but the rest of the litter remains normal. A number of small mummified fetuses may be delivered along with the normal living fetuses at term. In the mare, one member of a pair of (undesirable) twins may die and become mummified as the fetuses compete for uterine space. Eventually – often at 7 months into pregnancy – both twins may be aborted, one alive but unviable through prematurity and the other mummified. In the ewe, mummified fetuses are occasionally diagnosed when those members of the flock that have not lambed are checked after lambing. Treatment is as in the cow (see below) but in many cases such animals are culled.

Fetal mummification in the cow

Clinical signs   Fetal mummification is mostly detected on rectal examination of the cow that has either passed her prospective calving date or does not look as heavily pregnant as her dates suggest. The uterus feels tight and the fetus hard to the touch. There are no cotyledons and no fremitus in the uterine arteries. A corpus luteum may be palpable in an ovary and blood progesterone levels are elevated. The obstetrician should beware of possible confusion with other intra-abdominal masses, for example fat necrosis. Ultrasonographic scan through the rectal wall will be helpful in confirming the diagnosis. The fetus will normally remain in the uterus for as long as the corpus luteum persists. Occasionally, spontaneous regression of the corpus luteum occurs and the mummified fetus may pass into the vagina and the cow returns to heat. Mummified fetuses are occasionally seen during routine meat inspection.

Treatment   An injection of prostaglandin F2α analog (for example 500 μg cloprostenol) is given to lyze the corpus luteum. It regresses, the cow comes into estrus, the cervix opens and the fetus passes into and lodges in the vagina usually within 2–3 days. It must be removed with care from the vagina by gentle traction using plenty of lubrication. Other treatments have included the use of estradiol injections or cesarean section. Access for the latter would be difficult and prostaglandin F2α or its analogs remain the treatment of choice.

Prognosis   The prognosis for recovery and future fertility is good.

Fetal maceration

This occurs if fetal death is accompanied by loss of the corpus luteum, opening of the cervix and entry of autolytic and other bacteria into the uterus. The fetus decays in the uterus and its soft tissues break down and are passed as a foul vaginal discharge. In many cases the bones are too large to pass through the cervix and are left in the uterus normally preventing subsequent conception. Sharp fragments of bone may become embedded in the endometrium and endometritis occurs in some cases. Fetal maceration can also occur in full term fetuses that fail to leave the uterus, for example in sows.

Clinical signs   There is a foul-smelling vaginal discharge in an animal thought to be pregnant. In cattle it may be possible to palpate sharp bony fragments within the uterus during rectal examination. Fragments of bone may also be detected protruding from the cervix into the vagina. They can also be detected by ultrasonography. In small animals bony fragments can be detected by X-ray.

Treatment   This is often unsatisfactory because it is difficult to remove bony fragments from the uterus. If access by the fingers through the cervix is possible in the larger species, bony fragments may be removed and uterine lavage performed. Some success has been achieved dilating the cervix in valuable cattle by daily local application of prostaglandin E. In sheep, hysterotomy has been employed but is seldom economically justified. In the smaller species hysterectomy may be required and this has also been attempted in gilts suffering from the toxic form of primary uterine inertia (see Chapter 8).

Prognosis   The prognosis for complete resolution and future fertility is guarded.

HYDROPS UTERI

The term implies excessive amounts of fetal fluids within the pregnant uterus. The fetus itself may or may not be edematous and may show anasarca, hydrothorax or ascites. Two forms of hydrops uteri have been described (depending on the site of excessive fluids): hydrops amnion and hydrops allantois. In some cases it is not possible to be sure which of the fetal sacs is involved. Hydrops uteri is estimated to occur in 1 in 7500 bovine pregnancies. The incidence appears to be falling although the reasons for this are not clear.

Hydrops has been reported in most of the domestic species but is most common in the cow and has been well documented in this species and in the mare.

Hydrops amnion and hydrops allantois in cattle

A summary of findings is given in Table 2.1.

Hydrops amnion

Incidence   The condition is mostly sporadic but there may be groups of several cases in a herd.

Etiology   The condition is often associated with an abnormality of the fetus, especially cleft palate (the calf may fail to swallow its amniotic fluid). Other

Table 2.1 Characteristics of hydrops amnion and hydrops allantois		
	Hydrops amnion	**Hydrops allantois**
Incidence	n	$15n$
Onset	Insidious	Rapid
	5–6 months gestation	7–8 months gestation
Calf	Abnormal	Normal
Placenta	Normal	Abnormal
Prognosis	Guarded	Poor
Fluid	Mucoidal	Watery
Specific gravity	1.08	1.02
Na^+ (mmol/L)	120	50
Cl^- (mmol/L)	90	20

coincidental abnormalities include pituitary hypoplasia in Guernsey cattle and bulldog calves in Dexters.

Clinical signs   Nothing might be seen until calving when there appears to be more amniotic fluid (syrupy consistency) than normal. If the uterus is very distended contractions may be weak and assistance is required with delivery. Other cases may have excessive abdominal enlargement and the owner may suspect twins. The cow may show some difficulty getting up due to increased weight as pregnancy progresses.

Diagnosis   Rectal examination may assist in evaluation of signs. The uterus is large and it may be possible to palpate the fetus and the cotyledons are normal to the touch. Ultrasonographic scan of the uterus may indicate that relatively large amounts of amniotic fluid are present but this may be difficult to visualize or interpret with certainty at the stage of pregnancy at which hydrops amnion is seen. Excessive quantities of amniotic fluid are noted at birth. The calf may be deformed and placenta may be retained (as happens with other forms of uterine distension and inertia). Differential diagnosis: other causes of abdominal enlargement.

Treatment   If the cow is bright and active she may need no specific treatment but assistance may be required at calving. If the cow is distressed it may be necessary to terminate her pregnancy by an injection of prostaglandin F2α (see the further discussion of treatment under hydrops allantois).

Hydrops allantois

Incidence   The condition is mostly sporadic but there are occasional reports of the same cow being affected twice. The overall incidence of the condition may be falling.

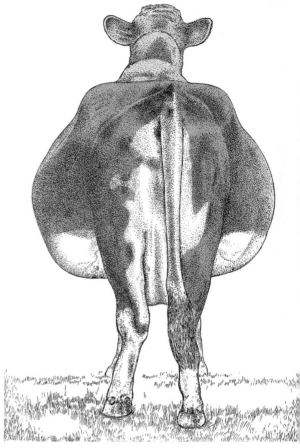

Figure 2.2 Hydrops allantois in the cow, showing gross abdominal distension.

Etiology   This is not clear. Placental abnormalities have been blamed and possible interference with sodium metabolism at cell level suggested.

Clinical signs   The onset is often rapid and the condition may be life-threatening. The abdomen is enlarged and tense but the cow herself looks ill and is often in poor bodily condition despite her large size (Fig. 2.2). The uterus is massively enlarged and may contain >200 L of fluid with a resultant enormous increase in body weight. Abdominal pressure is greatly increased: Breathing may be labored, appetite depressed, and complications such as rectal or vaginal prolapse, hip dislocation, rupture of the prepubic tendon, and recumbency may follow. On rectal examination the uterus is grossly enlarged and apparently filling the entire abdomen and pushing backwards and upwards into the pelvic cavity. Numerous very small accessory cotyledons are palpable but the fetus is mostly inaccessible to touch.

Ultrasonographic scan of the uterus per rectum reveals excessive quantities of allantoic fluid and the numerous small cotyledons, which are features of the disease.

Diagnosis   The clinical signs, a sudden severe onset and specific rectal findings are usually diagnostic. Differential diagnosis: normal twin pregnancy, hydrops amnion, rumenal tympany, abomasal disorders, peritonitis, ascites. Abdominal paracentesis – aspiration of fluid that can be identified as allantoic fluid – is present (see Table 2.1 for composition).

Prognosis   The prognosis is extremely guarded.

Treatment

Considerations   (1) prospective calving date; (2) condition of the dam, especially her ability to rise and eat; (3) viability of the calf (if known); (4) relative value of the cow and calf; (5) the availability of nursing care.

Methods   (1) conservative (await developments), possibly the best course if the cow is in reasonable health and her calving date near; (2) diuresis – not very effective; (3) uterine drainage – temporary relief but the uterus rapidly refills and there is a risk of infection; (4) induction of birth – risk of losing a premature calf and the obstetrician will probably have to deal with uterine inertia if birth is induced. Induction may be achieved by administration of 20 mg dexamethasone by intramuscular injection. This is followed with an intravenous drip of oxytocin (Long 2001) given over a period of 30 minutes. Manual assistance with delivery may also be necessary; (5) elective cesarean section, possibly with partial drainage of the uterus before surgery. There is a risk of shock when the uterus is emptied but this is not a serious problem because the fluid is extracirculatory. Sudden loss of abdominal pressure could however lead to splanchnic complications. The fetus is usually very small and poorly developed but sometimes survives.

Hydrops allantois in the mare

The condition is quite rare. Most cases have a sudden onset at approximately 7 months gestation. Massive abdominal distension and colicky signs are seen. Rectal examination reveals gross uterine enlargement and tension; the fetus is seldom palpable. A transabdominal ultrasonographic scan reveals the presence of excessive quantities of uterine fluids. Fetal viability can be ascertained by ultrasonography if the fetus can be located.

Treatment   Abortion is induced as a life-saving treatment: prostaglandin F2α is used to induce birth. In early cases no other treatment may be necessary. In later cases the obstetrician may manually dilate the cervix, puncture the chorioallantois, and deliver the foal. Allantoic fluid is drained from the uterus via the cervix, before and after fetal delivery. Intravenous fluid therapy is administered if the mare shows signs of shock. Uterine involution and delivery of the placenta are assisted by administration of 20–30 IU oxytocin. The foal is often deformed – a cerebellar or a cerebral abnormality are often present – unlike the cow where the calf is usually normal. In some cases the uterus may contain nearly 100 L of allantoic fluid with the foal. Mares may breed again normally the next year.

Hydrops uteri in other species

Occasional reports in other species include the sheep and dog. The condition is not well documented and may be hydrops amnion. It is seldom life threatening but may need relief in the form of cesarean section or treatment of associated uterine inertia at term.

RUPTURE OF THE UTERUS DURING PREGNANCY

This may be less serious than rupture during or after fetal delivery. The event may pass unnoticed as the uterine contents are normally sterile and not likely to induce peritonitis. The consequences may be serious if hemorrhage or a crushing injury occurs at time of uterine rupture. In a road accident a dog may sustain multiple injuries including a ruptured uterus, which may be discovered at a laparotomy carried out to investigate serious abdominal bleeding.

If the fetus passes into the peritoneal cavity (see Ectopic pregnancy, above) it will be unable to be delivered normally and will require surgical removal at term.

The uterus of sheep and goats is particularly fragile and great care must be exercised whenever heavily pregnant animals are handled. This is necessary to avoid damage which could be fatal as a result of shock and/or hemorrhage.

RUPTURE OF THE VAGINA

Seen chiefly in sheep, this condition may be encountered as a series of cases in a flock. In one study (Knottenbelt 1988) 17 cases were reported. Of these 10 were found dead, six had to be destroyed, and one died after surgery. All had a tear in the dorsal vaginal wall

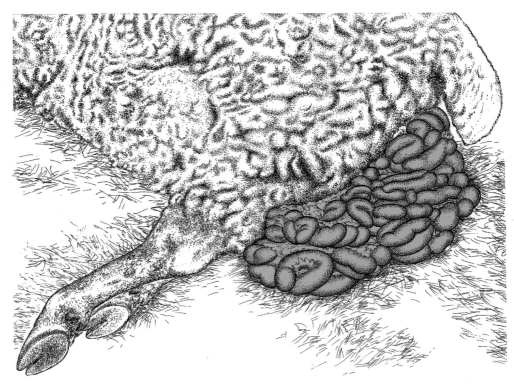

Figure 2.3 Vaginal rupture in a pregnant ewe, showing prolapse of the small intestine.

and had suffered partial evisceration through the defect (Fig. 2.3). The ewes shared a number of common features: Most were in poor condition, all carried more than one lamb, all had elevated blood urea and betahydroxybutyrate, most were aged 3–6 years, and all had low calcium levels. Blood estrogen and progesterone levels were normal. Some had suffered prior vaginal prolapse. The prognosis in living patients should be very guarded.

Treatment　If spotted early, surgical repair may be possible but vital tissues might be already compromised. Euthanasia is indicated in moribund animals.

Prevention　This is difficult because the cause is unknown. Exercise during pregnancy and careful feeding with suitable mineral supplementation may help prevent the condition.

HERNIATION OF THE PREGNANT UTERUS

In this condition the uterus passes into an existing hernia or an acquired rupture. Any abdominal hernia may be involved. The uterus can be trapped in the hernia by the fetus growing too big to pass back into the abdomen. In the case of large hernias the efficiency of abdominal straining at term may be compromised and assistance in both circumstances will be required.

Inguinal hernia

This hernia is seen chiefly but rarely in the bitch. The original hernia may be acquired or congenital. It may pass unnoticed until pregnancy. A swelling is seen in the inguinal region and may be reducible at an early stage. In most cases the uterus enters the hernial sac but as the fetus(es) grows its size exceeds that of the neck of the hernia. The fetus may die if the blood supply is compromised but if it is diagnosed promptly the hernia can be explored surgically, the trapped uterus released and the hernia repaired. If problems occur at parturition the hernia may be emptied during cesarean section.

Diaphragmatic hernia

This rarely contains the pregnant uterus and is repaired in the standard way. If the patient attempted to give birth while suffering from this hernia the efficiency of straining would be compromised.

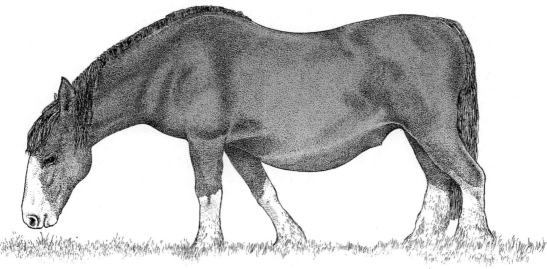

Figure 2.4 Rupture of the prepubic tendon in the mare. Note the gross ventral edema and the displacement of the left teat from its normal site between the hind legs of the mare.

Ventral hernia

This is chiefly a problem in heavily pregnant large animals but is occasionally seen in old cats or dogs with weak abdominal muscles. The weight of a multiple pregnancy may predispose as – rarely – may excessive straining at parturition. (A massive subcutaneous hematoma in the udder of a sow may give the false appearance of a hernia.) Abdominal muscles give way under the increasing weight of the uterus, which is then only supported by skin and subcutis. Total rupture of abdominal floor and evisceration is fortunately extremely rare. The efficiency of straining is greatly compromised and uterus may 'hang down' at an abnormal angle in the hernial sac. Surgical repair is seldom possible and it may be necessary to supervise and assist with fetal delivery and possibly with feeding of the newborn. Affected animals are normally not retained for breeding.

Perineal hernia

This is occasionally seen in pregnant sheep close to term. The hernia seldom contains the uterus but may interfere with the efficiency of delivery and assistance with this is required. Repair is not normally attempted in large animals.

RUPTURE OF THE PREPUBIC TENDON

This is seen chiefly in the heavy horse but occasionally in other farm species. The prepubic tendon ruptures as a result of the great increase in tension that accompanies advancing pregnancy. The condition and threatened condition are mostly accompanied by gross edema just anterior to the udder (Fig. 2.4). The edema is characteristically painful, unlike the 'normal edema' that often accompanies approaching parturition in horses (and to a lesser extent other animals). The obstetrician may be able to palpate the compromised tendon per rectum in smaller mares. Little can be done in large animals once the tendon has actually ruptured but if it is believed to be at risk of rupture the ventral abdomen may be supported with a canvas sling attached to the animal's back supporting the ventral area. Parturition in such cases must be supervised and aided to avoid excessive straining. In some cases it may be possible to terminate pregnancy and risk to the tendon by induction of birth.

Damage to the pubic attachment of the abdominal muscles has been reported in cats, mostly as the result of road traffic accidents. Abdominal straining may be compromised in affected animals but surgical repair is often possible.

PROLAPSE OF THE VAGINA DURING PREGNANCY

Prolapse of the vagina is an important and common condition requiring careful management. It is seen chiefly in cow, ewe, and sow; less commonly in mare, doe, bitch, and queen.

Etiology   Excess antepartum relaxation of pelvic tissues and increased intra-abdominal pressure.

Predisposing factors   These include: breed in cattle (there is a high incidence in Hereford cows); high levels of estrogen in the diet (for example in some clovers); possible high endogenous production of estrogen; sloping environment; rumenal tympany; overfeeding with bulky food. Other factors include aging – the pelvic muscles and ligaments become less elastic with successive pregnancies.

Clinical signs   Eversion of the vagina with exposure of the mucosal surface (Fig. 2.5). In the early stages the appearance of the prolapse may be intermittent. The prolapse may be partial or complete and in the latter case the cervix may also be visible. The exposed organ is vulnerable to damage and possibly infection. Small animals may cause additional damage by licking the prolapsed organ. The sow may rub her hindquarters against the bars of her farrowing crate. In all cases the obstetrician must ensure that it is the vagina, and not the rectum, that is involved – sometimes both are affected.

Treatment

1   Aims   To prevent further damage to the organ, replace it after appropriate cleaning, supervise birth, and be prepared for possible postpartum recurrence.

2   Considerations   Severity of prolapse, species involved, proximity of parturition, extent of damage sustained.

3   Methods

- *Conservative*: if the prolapse is intermittent or slight the obstetrician or attendant may simply clean, lubricate, and replace the prolapse periodically while awaiting birth. Parturition is then carefully supervised to avoid further damage to the prolapsed organ. In the cat and dog it may help to put a protective collar round the patient's neck to prevent licking. A cow may be placed in a stall with an elevated rear end so that her hindquarters are higher than her head. The forces of gravity may assist in keeping a small prolapse in place. In other cases repeated injections of epidural anesthetic combined with xylazine have been used to prevent straining, with varying degrees of success.

- *Suturing methods/trusses*: numerous suture patterns are available including a simple mattress suture and Buhner's purse-string suture (Fig. 2.6). In each case, careful cleaning of the prolapse and administration of epidural anesthetic is required. In sheep, a plastic vaginal truss or prolapse replacer ('Moffat' replacer) is very effective and is usually tied onto the fleece on either side of the perineum (Fig. 2.7). The ewe is able

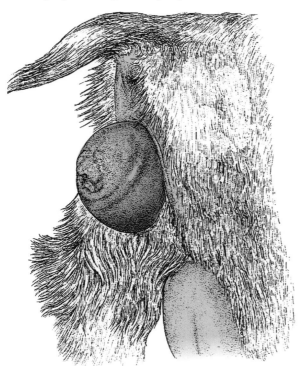

Figure 2.5 Vaginal prolapse in a doe goat.

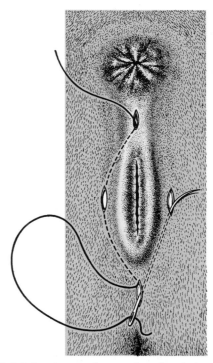

Figure 2.6 Buhner's suture for retention of vaginal prolapse.

to lamb without removal of the replacer. Lambing can be delayed or the vagina severely lacerated if sutures are in place and the ewe is unsupervised. At one time heavy metal trusses and clamps were used to hold the vagina closed often with poor results. With any suture pattern the obstetrician must ensure that the patient is able to pass urine. This can be achieved by suturing only the dorsal two-thirds of the vaginal lips.

- *Surgical techniques*: these are used for difficult chronic cases and especially when parturition is a long way ahead. The techniques available include: (i) Caslick's operation, in which the upper portion of the vulval lips is sutured as is used to prevent vaginal wind sucking in mares; (ii) Farquarson's operation – essentially a submucous resection of the prolapsed part of the vagina; (iii) Winkler's operation – in which the cervix is fixed to the prepubic tendon to

prevent the genital tract including the vagina from slipping backwards and predisposing a prolapse.

Vaginal hypertrophy in the bitch

Hypertrophy of the vaginal mucosa may look like a vaginal prolapse but is not and is mentioned here as an important differential diagnosis only. It is usually seen at estrus when a fold of the ventral vaginal wall just in front of the external urethral orifice becomes enlarged and edematous. Careful vaginal examination will reveal its origin well forward from the vulva. It then passes back and out through the vulval lips. Licking by the bitch may further damage the structure. The mucosa will usually disappear when the estrogen influence of estrus regresses. If the hypertrophy does not regress, surgical removal via an episiotomy wound may become necessary. If the bitch is not required for breeding she

Figure 2.7 Replacement of vaginal prolapse in the ewe with a plastic Moffat prolapse replacer.

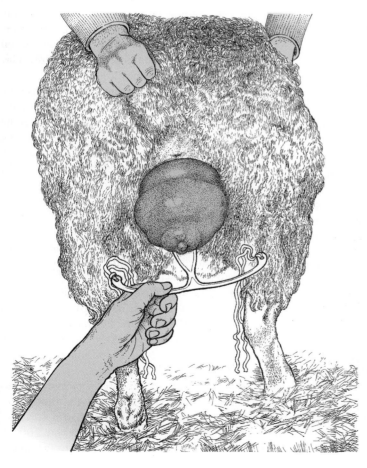

may be spayed after the end of metestrus. Alternatively, estrus may be controlled by progestagen therapy.

METABOLIC DISEASES ASSOCIATED WITH PREGNANCY

Incidence   Most metabolic diseases are seen in ruminants and in some cases have no direct association with pregnancy. Hypomagnesemia, for example, may occur in a group of animals (especially cattle and sheep) and affects both the pregnant and non-pregnant. Pregnant animals may be under greater stress and therefore more likely to fall victim to magnesium deficiency. Hypocalcemia occurs especially in the cow around the time of parturition and may be responsible for primary uterine inertia in this species (see Chapter 4). The incidence of hypocalcemia is in many cases related to the management of the animal during pregnancy and also to the heavy demands for calcium in the lactation that follows parturition. Detailed consideration of these diseases is beyond the scope of this book although further brief mention is made of them in Chapters 13 and 14.

PREGNANCY TOXEMIA

This is a condition that is directly related to pregnancy and may threaten the continuation of pregnancy and the life of the animal and its offspring. The condition and its management are very important to the obstetrician and will be considered in summary form here. For full discussion of the biochemical pathways involved in its etiology and a more detailed consideration of its medical treatment appropriate textbooks should be consulted. Hyperlipidemia in ponies and donkeys is also frequently related to pregnancy and early lactation and is discussed below.

Pregnancy toxemia in cattle

Incidence   The condition is quite uncommon but may affect both beef and dairy cattle. It is seen in beef heifers, especially those carrying twins, and may follow a sudden deterioration in the quality of their diet in late pregnancy. Bad weather may also predispose to the disease. It is also occasionally seen in the form of an outbreak in dairy cows, which develop fatty liver disease in late gestation. The condition has also been seen in overweight beef cows.

Etiology   An energy deficit: the energy demands of the mother and offspring are not being met by the dietary energy intake. A sudden deterioration in the quality or quantity of the food in late gestation can predispose to the disease. In dairy cows, attempts to reduce the incidence of milk fever by drastically reducing their diet in late pregnancy may actually predispose to pregnancy toxemia. This is likely to occur if the cows are overweight and prone to fatty liver disease. In beef heifers the presence of a second fetus doubles the fetal energy demand.

Clinical signs   The condition is seen in the last 2 months of pregnancy and especially in the last few weeks. The animal is often dull, anorexic, and loses weight quite rapidly. The feces are scant and covered in mucus but later on in untreated cases a severe diarrhea may be seen. Rumenal activity is reduced or absent and an acetone-like odor is detected on the breath. If the condition is unrecognized the animal may attempt to calve at term. She may be too weak to do so and may die during or after calving. When a case of pregnancy toxemia is seen the unborn calf should be examined to check (as far as possible) its health by rectal examination and by ultrasonography if necessary.

Clinical pathology   The patient is hypoglycemia, hyperketonemic, and ketonuric. Blood β-hydroxybutyrate and volatile fatty acid levels are elevated. In some cases fatty liver disease is present and liver enzyme assays, bile salt assays, and liver function tests may suggest dysfunction of that organ. A liver biopsy can be taken to confirm the diagnosis.

Diagnosis   Although rare, the condition must not be forgotten in animals showing signs of dullness and anorexia in late gestation. Ketosis can also readily occur in animals that are anorexic for other reasons and hence a full clinical examination and evaluation of the patient is always necessary.

Prognosis   This must always be guarded as the outlook for both cow and calf may be uncertain. Untreated cases may die within 7–14 days. The prognosis is especially poor in those animals that are not eating at all. If the animal is eating, even a little, the prognosis is still guarded but more favorable.

Treatment   Early diagnosis and aggressive treatment are required if the patient's life and that of her calf (or calves) are to be saved: 400 mL of a 40% glucose solution is given by intravenous injection; 200 mL propylene glycol is given as an oral drench. Treatment with the latter may be required for up to 5 days if the patient is not eating. Steroid therapy can be used but it should be remembered that it may induce birth, although this may in fact be desirable.

Induction of birth is required if the patient does not show a rapid response to medical treatment: 20–30 mg of betamethasone and 500 μg of cloprostenol are given by intramuscular injection. Birth of the calf should follow 24–30 hours later. Assistance at birth may be required and the possibility of twins must be remembered. (For further details on induction of birth and alternative treatment regimens, see Chapter 15). If the patient is gravely ill and inappetant it may be necessary to remove the calf (or calves) by an elective cesarean section. The calf should survive even if the delivery is up to 2 weeks before the prospective calving date.

Treatment of the ketosis and its underlying cause must continue after natural, induced or surgical delivery of the calf. Nursing care must be of the highest standard and the animal must be tempted with very good quality food.

Pregnancy toxemia in sheep and goats

Incidence   Very high in sheep, where it may be a flock problem, and sporadic cases also occur in goats. In sheep the condition is seen in ewes in poor condition that are receiving an inadequate diet. Bad weather conditions and lack of shelter are also important predisposing factors. The condition is seen mostly in animals that are carrying twins or triplets and in which the demand for energy by the lambs is particularly high. It is also seen in fat ewes or does in which fatty infiltration of the liver may have occurred as a result of an energy deficit. In such animals the liver pathology may itself both predispose to pregnancy toxemia and the continuation of ketosis.

Etiology   An energy deficit through inadequate diet in late pregnancy when the demand for energy by the litter is very high.

Clinical signs   Affected animals may initially have difficulty in keeping up with the rest of the flock. Apparent blindness may follow and if housed signs of head pressing and other neurological signs may be seen. Within 24–48 hours the animal is unable to rise unaided. Coma and death follow. Close examination of a case reveals a low body temperature, rumenal stasis, and the distinct smell of acetone on the patient's breath. In sheep flocks, a number of ewes are normally affected with individuals often showing a spectrum of

stages of the disease. In doe goats, anorexia and lethargy in late gestation should raise suspicions of pregnancy toxemia. Later signs are like those seen in sheep.

Diagnosis   This is based on the history of the flock, the clinical signs and clinical pathology.

Clinical pathology   Hypoglycemia, hyperketonemia and ketonuria are present. Calcium and magnesium levels should also be determined to ensure that they are normal. Renal failure may occur in advanced cases and in these patients blood urea nitrogen and creatinine levels may be raised.

Prognosis   Must be very guarded. The further from lambing or kidding the animal is the poorer the prognosis. Loss of appetite which is often present is another poor sign as is biochemical evidence of renal failure. Euthanasia should be considered in moribund animals.

Treatment   An intravenous injection of 80 mL of 40% glucose is given immediately and 120 mL of propylene glycol is given orally as a drench. Oral or intravenous fluid is given in cases where there is evidence of dehydration or renal failure. *If the patient is within 48 hours of parturition, consideration should be given to induction of birth.* Full recovery is highly unlikely until the litter has been born and the drain on energy supplies has ceased. The exact lambing date of individual ewes is rarely available but an approximate (although sometimes inaccurate) estimate of how close to lambing she is can be determined by the state of relaxation of the pelvic ligaments and the presence or absence of milk in the udder. Relaxation of the cervix is also a sign of approaching birth and may be viewed by speculum or palpated manually. In goats, the owner usually has an accurate kidding date.

Lambs and kids are very unlikely to survive if they are born more than 48 hours early. If their state of maturity has been wrongly estimated they may die within the first 24 hours of their birth even if they look well when they are born. If the ewe or doe is in a comatose condition, immediate delivery of the lambs by elective cesarean section may be the only alternative to euthanasia. If possible, 10 mg dexamethasone should be given by intramuscular injection to the mother 2–3 hours before surgery. This may help fetal survival by encouraging surfactant production in the lungs and maturing other neonatal body systems.

Birth in ewes can be induced in less severe cases by giving an intramuscular injection of 16 mg of betamethasone or dexamethasone; 125 μg of cloprostenol can be given at the same time. Birth normally follows 24–72 hours later. In the doe, 5–10 mg of dinoprost or 62.5–125 µg of cloprostenol may be given by intramuscular injection. Induction of birth is further discussed in Chapter 15.

After fetal delivery, in all cases medical and nursing treatment of the pregnancy toxemia must continue until appetite and metabolic pathways have returned to normal.

In mild cases of pregnancy toxemia, medical care may allow pregnancy to continue until term when some assistance with delivery may be required. Recently, bovine somatotropic hormone (BST) has been found useful to treat both pregnancy toxemia and fatty liver disease. It is not licensed for use in some countries, including the UK.

Prevention   The difficulty in treating pregnancy toxemia and the poor results obtained mean that every effort must be made to prevent the disease. When cases occur in a flock the management of the ewes must immediately be investigated to ensure that food supplies, including trough space, are adequate especially for those animals carrying more than one lamb. Such animals should in any case have been identified by ultrasonography in early pregnancy. A steadily rising plane of nutrition is essential in the last few weeks of pregnancy. Suitable precautions should also be taken in subsequent years.

HYPERLIPIDEMIA IN PONY AND DONKEY MARES

Incidence   Hyperlipidemia is seen much more commonly in ponies (especially Shetlands) and in donkeys than in horses. It occurs mostly in late pregnancy and early lactation. Overweight animals may be particularly prone to the disease.

Etiology   Caused by fat mobilization in response to a sudden energy deficiency. Fatty acids are released and then converted to triglyceride in the liver. Fat is deposited in the liver, kidneys, and other tissues leading to organ failure. Poor nutrition, transportation, or a heavy parasite burden are predisposing factors.

Clinical signs   Dullness, anorexia, and muscle fasciculations are early signs and may lead to coma, terminal intractable diarrhea, and death. Weight loss and ventral edema are seen in some patients. The mare often appears thirsty but is unable to swallow. Fetal death and abortion are occasionally seen.

Clinical pathology   Blood glucose levels are normal or reduced and ketones are not found in the urine.

Blood samples show a thick layer of cloudy fat floating on their surface. Free fatty acid and triglyceride levels are elevated and there may be specific changes associated with renal and hepatic failure.

Prognosis   Must always be very guarded especially if nervous signs are seen. At least 65% of cases do not survive. If abortion occurs the prognosis for recovery is better as the disease can be diagnosed and treated early in its course.

Treatment   Intravenous glucose may help if given early and attempts should be made to deal with underlying problems such as parasitism. Oral glucose therapy (1 g/kg body weight given as a 5% solution by stomach tube every 5 hours) with subcutaneous insulin therapy (0.1–0.3 IU/kg every 12–24 hours) may aid recovery; 40–100 IU heparin/kg given subcutaneously every 6 hours has also been used. Fluid therapy is necessary in dehydrated animals or those unable to drink.

Prevention   Is much better than cure. Ponies and donkeys should not be allowed to become too fat in pregnancy. Sudden changes in diet or other stresses should be avoided.

ANOREXIA IN THE BITCH AND QUEEN DURING PREGNANCY

In a very small proportion of bitches a period of anorexia with occasional vomiting occurs at about 3 weeks and occasionally up to 5 weeks into pregnancy. The cause of the condition, which may be mistaken for pyometra, is unknown. It is discussed further in Chapter 9 but in every case the bitch must be carefully examined to ensure that no disease is present. A similar condition has been reported as occurring very rarely in early or late pregnancy in the queen.

METABOLIC DISEASES IN SMALL ANIMALS DURING LATE PREGNANCY

A severe pregnancy toxemia-like condition has been reported in malnourished bitches in late pregnancy. Affected animals are lethargic and anorexic. Hypoglycemia, ketonemia, and ketonuria are present. Diagnosis is based on clinical signs and plasma biochemistry. Eclampsia associated with calcium deficiency occurs occasionally in late pregnancy in both dogs and cats. Eclampsia may be complicated by hypoglycemia and other metabolic abnormalities. Immediate intravenous glucose therapy is necessary with further treatment depending on biochemical findings and the condition of the patient. These conditions are further discussed in Chapters 9 and 14.

Pregnancy toxemia has also been reported in pregnant guinea pigs and is discussed in Chapter 10.

PREPARTURIENT RECUMBENCY IN ANIMALS

This problem has a wide range of possible causes and must be dealt with by very careful clinical examination of the patient. A wide list of differential diagnoses both related and unrelated to pregnancy must be considered. The obstetrician is chiefly concerned with diseases of the reproductive system but *all* surgical, medical and management possibilities must be considered. It is very easy and regrettable for example to overlook a fractured leg in a heavily pregnant recumbent cow.

Some of the more common species problems are listed below:

- *Mare*: general weakness in an old mare in poor condition. Cast in her stable. Spasmodic colic is very common in late pregnancy but a full colic examination is required. Colicky signs are also seen in cases of uterine torsion during pregnancy (see Chapter 5). Accidental injury.
- *Cow*: hypocalcemia may occur in late pregnancy, as may hypomagnesemia. Acute mastitis can be seen, especially coliform. Acute metritis with fetal death and emphysema. Other acute infections such as blackquarter. Rumenal acidosis/carbohydrate engorgement. Injury to legs, pelvis, and nerves. Starvation. Hydrops uteri. Colicky signs may be seen in the uncommon condition (during pregnancy) of uterine torsion.
- *Ewe*: pregnancy toxemia, hypocalcemia, hypomagnesemia, injury, starvation.
- *Sow*: very heavily pregnant sows may 'do the splits' with resultant bony and soft tissue damage. Acute infection in udder or uterus. Simple overweight and 'laziness' exacerbated by being confined in a crate for too long before farrowing.
- *Small animals*: eclampsia and hypoglycemia before whelping are very rare but can occur. A possible road traffic accident should always be considered.

Prognosis   Must always be guarded – it depends on the cause, the condition of the mother, and the patient's environment. It is also influenced by the availability, practicality, and willingness of nursing care and on the time to expected parturition. If the patient is bright and can be well looked after by careful nursing until parturition this may be all that is required. In some cases induction of birth may be necessary. Inappetance and deterioration in the patient's general condition, with pressure sores and other consequences of prolonged recumbency, indicate a poor long-term prognosis.

Treatment   Depends on specific diagnosis of the cause of recumbency. Highest standards of nursing and management are essential to bring about a successful conclusion.

PROLONGED GESTATION

Some variation in gestation length is to be expected but any case of prolonged gestation must be carefully monitored. It is advisable not to predict time of parturition – owners are often good at this but veterinary surgeons less so. Clients are often very anxious at this time. It is very important in all species to check that the patient is still pregnant in case an unseen abortion has occurred. The date of service should be checked and also the estimated time of parturition that the owner has calculated to ensure that no mistake has been made. Brief mention of the problem is made below. For a full discussion of assessment and management of a particular species, see the appropriate chapter on dystocia. For methods of induction of birth in each species, see Chapter 15.

Mare

It is not at all uncommon for a mare to go 'over her time' and in some breeding seasons a number of mares may do so. Prolonged gestation is mostly a sign of fetal dysmaturity and occasionally a mare may carry the foal to 13 months before delivering quite a small fetus. The mare is quite unlike the cow in this respect.

Cow

Prolonged gestation often leads to dystocia due to fetopelvic disproportion. Numerous factors influence gestation length, for example breed – in continental breeds gestation length is 290 days compared with 283 days for indigenous breeds. Male calves may have a longer gestation than heifer calves. Calves from certain sires may be predisposed to longer gestation. Induction of birth or elective cesarean section is necessary in some cases. An apparent prolonged gestation is sometimes suspected in cases of fetal mummification – a condition that is discussed above.

A less common cause of prolonged gestation is the rare condition of pituitary aplasia. Genetic causes have been identified in Ayrshire, Guernsey, and Jersey cattle. Bovine virus diarrhea virus can cause severe damage to the fetal brain and pituitary in early pregnancy. Other viruses that can cause brain damage and prolonged gestation include Akabane and Blue tongue viruses. The condition has also been associated with the consumption of toxic plants such as skunk cabbage (*Veratrum californicum)* in some countries. The absence of a pituitary gland prevents the release of fetal adrenocorticotropic hormone (ACTH) at the end of normal gestation and hence parturition cannot be initiated in the normal way. Gestation in such cases may extend well beyond 1 year. Affected calves may also suffer from hydrocephalus. Abnormal cranial shape may be detected in some cases by rectal palpation or ultrasonographic scan. Parturition may be induced using corticosteroids.

Sow

Prolonged gestation may indicate fetal death, for example in toxic primary uterine inertia. For details of treatment and management of this condition, see Chapter 8.

Ewe and doe

Although seldom a problem the condition may be caused by exposure of the fetus to Border disease virus, which may compromise pituitary function. Consumption of toxic plants such as cauliflower saltwort (*Salsola tuberculatiformis*) during pregnancy has also caused prolonged gestation in some countries.

Dog

The single pup syndrome may predispose to the condition. For further discussion on this and the management of prolonged gestation in the bitch, see Chapter 9.

Cat

Prolonged gestation is seldom a problem but may be associated with the presence of a single kitten.

VAGINAL DISCHARGE DURING PREGNANCY

This may occur in all species and is of considerable concern to owners. The problem is seen most frequently in sows and bitches. In all species a vaginal discharge may indicate a pathological process in the vagina or uterus but it may also be present during a normal pregnancy. The obstetrician should always carry out a full investigation whenever possible to ensure that all is well with the pregnancy and to reassure the owner.

A vaginal discharge may indicate a threatened or a progressing abortion. The discharge in such cases may be blood stained and may contain fresh or macerated fetal tissues together with placental remnants. The dam may show signs of general illness including pyrexia in cases where the abortion has been caused by infectious agents. The discharge in such cases may be purulent and foul smelling. Vaginal smears reveal large numbers of neutrophils. Bacterial cultures and viral isolation techniques can be used to identify causal organisms. The discharge may arise from the vagina and in all cases the uterus should be examined to determine whether a normal pregnancy is present or not. Manual palpation – per rectum in horses and cattle – may be used in the large animals. Ultrasonographic techniques are used in all species and radiographic appraisal of the small animal uterus may also be helpful. Ultrasonographic scanning will enable the well-being of the fetus to be evaluated in terms of movement, size, heart rate, etc. The thickness and attachment of the placenta and the clarity of the amniotic fluid can also be evaluated in some cases. The stage of pregnancy may sometimes be too early for a firm diagnosis of pregnancy to be made.

A bloody discharge during pregnancy in the mare may arise from varicose veins in the vaginal wall. If blood loss is heavy the veins may be cauterized or ligated. The pregnancy is usually unaffected.

Mares occasionally develop a purulent vaginal discharge during pregnancy. This may be associated with a vaginitis or urinary tract infection. Placentitis can also give rise to these symptoms – the placenta may appear thickened when scanned and purulent material may be seen passing through the cervix when viewed through a speculum. The well-being of the fetus must be assessed – it may not yet be compromised – and immediate parenteral antibiotic therapy should be administered. A swab should be taken for culture and sensitivity tests.

Many sows show evidence of a white mucopurulent vaginal discharge a few days to a few weeks after service. Such discharges are normally non-pathological and in such cases the sow is well. Vaginal discharges can also be associated with bacterial abortion and endometritis and affected animals may be anorexic and pyrexic. If the problem of vaginal discharge affects many sows in the herd bacterial cultures should be taken from a number of affected animals to identify the organism involved. Early ultrasonographic pregnancy diagnosis will determine whether fetal life is affected, or indeed if it is present. A blood-stained vaginal discharge within a few days of service may be seen in some cases of pyelonephritis. Affected animals may show hematuria, pyuria and, if untreated, rapidly become toxemic.

Some bitches produce small quantities of a clear mucoidal discharge throughout pregnancy; this is non-pathological. A foul discharge may indicate a complete or partial abortion and must be fully investigated (see above and also Chapter 9).

A mucopurulent discharge in older pregnant bitches may occasionally be caused by local vaginal infection associated with crops of leimyomata in the anterior vagina. Such infection is normally harmless but the pregnancy should be monitored ultrasonographically to ensure that fetal life is normal and the surrounding amniotic fluid is clear. Similar discharges may also be seen in cases of pyometra and the possibility of this developing about 3 weeks post service should be investigated. Ultrasonographic evaluation of the uterus will clearly distinguish whether the uterus contains pus as in pyometra or a normal pregnancy.

A dark green vaginal discharge in pregnant bitches or a brown discharge in the queen cat may suggest fetal death and must be investigated urgently. In late pregnancy such a discharge often indicates fetal compromise following placental separation from the endometrium. Such animals must be submitted to a full obstetric examination as described in Chapter 9. Very occasionally only one puppy – that situated nearest to the cervix – has died and ultrasonographic scanning reveals that the rest are normal. Careful monitoring of such cases including regular checking of blood progesterone levels is mandatory.

REFERENCES

Knottenbelt DC 1988 Vaginal rupture associated with herniation of the abdominal viscera in pregnant ewes. Veterinary Record 122:453–456

Long SE 2001 Abnormal development of the fetus and its consequences. Arthur's Veterinary Reproduction and Obstetrics, 8th edn. WB Saunders, London, p 139–140

Chapter 3

CLINICAL MANAGEMENT OF CASES OF DYSTOCIA

SPEED OF ATTENDANCE

All obstetric cases should be treated as potential emergencies and seen without delay. Although some experienced clients may be able to give reliable information over the telephone there can be no substitute for a veterinary clinical examination to ascertain all aspects of the case. On occasion this approach may lead to a case being seen unnecessarily early in its course but arrangements can then be made for a strategic follow-up consultation later. It is much better to be too early than too late with an obstetric case. Clients should be encouraged to report potential problems at an early stage, and also to be aware of their own limitations as obstetricians.

The larger farm animals and horses are normally seen on their own premises but in sheep breeding areas ewes suffering from dystocia are often brought in to the surgery for treatment. Although owners of small animals may fear that a car journey to the surgery may interrupt the birth process this does not seem to be a major problem. In some cases such a journey may actually speed-up delivery. It is generally agreed that the facilities available make a surgery consultation preferable for examining obstetric cases in small animals provided the owner has suitable transport.

ANTENATAL EXAMINATION

Although widely practiced in human obstetrics, antenatal care including fetal monitoring is not the norm in veterinary obstetrics. The majority of obstetric cases are not seen until a problem actually exists. In some cases this might have been anticipated had the patient been examined during or even before pregnancy. In small animal and in equine practice antenatal care is fortunately becoming more common and the subject will be discussed more fully in the chapters devoted to dystocia in the mare (Chapter 5), dog and cat (Chapter 9), and the prevention of dystocia (Chapter 15).

CASE HISTORY

In cases of serious emergency, time may not permit the taking of a full case history but whenever possible this should be done. Much information can be quickly obtained even in emergency cases. The following points should be ascertained:

- Is the birth premature or overdue? If there is any doubt, check the service dates personally.
- Has the patient given birth before? Is this her first litter (i.e. primiparous) or has she had several previous litters (i.e. pluriparous)?
- Were there any previous problems at birth? If so what were they, how were they resolved and what was the outcome?
- What is known about the sire of the present litter? Was he used last time? Is there a large disparity in body size between sire and dam? Have any other animals pregnant to the same sire suffered dystocia recently?
- Has the patient suffered any illness or accident during pregnancy? If so what were the details?
- Has the animal been off color during the past few days?
- Has the patient been straining and if so when did it start and how vigorous has the straining been?
- Has there been any vaginal discharge and what was its nature?
- Have any fetal membranes, fetal fluids, or fetal parts been seen at the vulva?
- Has anyone already attempted to assist with the patient? The possibility of lay interference and resultant damage must always be borne in mind.

- In the case of the normally polytocous species (dog, cat, pig, sheep, and goat) have any of the litter been born and were they living or dead? Was any difficulty noticed during their delivery?

GENERAL EXAMINATION OF THE MOTHER

This should be performed whenever possible. In an emergency the examination may initially have to be cursory but if there is any reason to believe the mother is unwell a full clinical examination must be carried out. Failure to perform this examination may have very serious consequences. In cattle, for example, acute life-threatening environmental mastitis may already be present and possibly contributing to the causes of a case of dystocia. Failure to diagnose and treat this problem may result in the death of the patient despite successful fetal delivery. The examination may influence the program of treatment.

The clinical examination should include the following:

- General appearance and condition of the patient. Is she bright and well or dull and dejected? Does she appear ready to give birth – are the normal preparatory signs of the species present?
- What is her bodily condition? Is she overweight, in good condition or emaciated?
- Is she able to stand and walk? Is she recumbent and immobile? This latter observation should be made with care since some animals already in their second stage of labor may be unwilling to rise even though they are otherwise well.
- What are the parameters of temperature, pulse, and respiration? These may be elevated in a case in which prolonged, vigorous straining has occurred and may also be altered by concurrent disease or environmental factors. Parturient sows may suffer heat stroke in warm weather or if adjacent to powerful heat lamps provided for their piglets.
- Can any fetal parts be seen at the vulva? Are they exposed or covered by chorioallantois and amnion or only by amnion? Are the parts moist (possibly indicating recent exposure) or are they dry (possibly suggesting a protracted case).
- What is the identity and condition of any visible fetal membranes? Moist fresh membranes may have appeared recently but dry or foul-smelling membranes may indicate prolonged exposure or possibly fetal death.

- Is there any vaginal discharge? Some discharge including a little blood is normally present during birth. A foul-smelling or abnormally discolored discharge may indicate fetal death. In the dog a green, or in the cat a brown, vaginal discharge normally accompany second-stage labor. The presence of such discharges *before* any fetal delivery may indicate an existing threat to fetal life.
- What is the degree of abdominal distension? Such distension may indicate the presence of a large number of unborn offspring in the polytocous species but is not a reliable parameter.
- Is there any evidence of fetal life? Can any exposed fetal parts be seen to be moving spontaneously or can unborn fetuses be seen or felt moving through the flanks of the mother? Such observations may also be unreliable although excessive movements may indicate fetal stress including hypoxia. Normal maternal straining efforts may cause deceptive passive movements of exposed fetal parts. Later obstetrical investigation should determine the validity of these preliminary observations.

The case history and the general clinical examination may influence the treatment of the case and its prognosis.

OBSTETRIC EXAMINATION

Wherever possible, veterinary obstetricians should seek to deal with their patient in the most suitable environment for both parties. In many cases when the animal cannot be moved there may be no choice other than to deal with the animal where it is. If possible, obstetric cases should be examined, diagnosed and treated in a clean, warm and well-lit environment.

Restraint of the patient

The restraint and detailed description of the internal examination of each species will be dealt with in chapters devoted to the individual species. A number of general points may be dealt with here. Animals may be particularly aggressive and potentially very dangerous at parturition and obstetricians must ensure their own safety and that of the owners, attendants, and assistants while the patient is being examined and treated. The larger species are usually secured either by a halter or head collar or (in the case of cattle) in a crush or similar mechanical head restraint. Sows are currently normally restrained in farrowing crates but if loose the obstetrician should be protected by an attendant with a pig board standing by the sow's head. The other species are usually held manually by their owners or attendants. In all cases at least one but preferably two helpers are required but, especially on farms, assistance is often very limited.

In the case of violent or particularly aggressive animals possibly being handled or restrained for the first time, sedation may be required and for some manipulations in the mare general anesthesia may be advantageous.

Vaginal examination

Vaginal examination must be performed with gentleness, care, and with the strictest cleanliness. It is essential that veterinarians set a good example for others to follow in these matters. The perineum and adjacent areas should be washed with soap and water to which may be added a little disinfectant such as chlorhexidine. Obstetricians must ensure that their hands have been carefully washed, their fingernails are short, and rings removed. Proper protective clothing is required and in the larger farm species waterproof trousers and a parturition overall are essential. A long overall is not suitable for use with the foaling mare. In the smaller species normal surgery clothing is suitable. Gloves may be worn (latex hand gloves for small animals and long plastic arm-length gloves for the farm species) but may in some cases reduce the sensitivity required for obstetric work. If the birth canal is believed to be infected or if there is a zoonotic risk, gloves are essential. Pregnant women should not work with sheep at lambing time, the two species share a number of common pathogens that can cause abortion.

Instrumentation should be available but the obstetrician's fingers, hands, and arms are the most important aids. Small fingers and long arms are very useful in veterinary obstetrics but not all colleagues are fortunate enough to have them. Details of specialist instrumentation will be discussed in subsequent chapters.

Before examining the birth canal and its contents the obstetrician's hands should be lubricated either by soap and water or preferably by using a proprietary obstetric lubricant. In the larger species the hand and parts of the arms may be inserted with relative ease into the dilated, parturient birth canal. In the dog the forefinger is mostly used but in the toy breeds and in cats it may only be possible to insert the lubricated little finger. In very small animals such as guinea pigs and mice digital vaginal examination is often not possible.

The aim of the vaginal examination is to explore the accessible parts of the birth canal to determine:

- Whether the caudal parts of the canal are dilated and also the diameter of the cervix. (*Note*: the cervix is not normally directly palpable in the dog or cat.)
- The state of natural lubrication or dryness of the birth canal and whether the birth canal has sustained any damage or is obstructed for any reason.
- Whether any fetuses are present, their location within the birth canal and if possible their living state. (*Note*: it may not be possible to be sure whether the fetuses are alive or dead at this stage and further tests such as ultrasonographic assessment may be required.) The obstetrician must always be careful not to predict fetal viability or survival until the case is fully assessed.
- Whether the presentation, position, and posture (see below for definitions) of such fetuses is normal and if abnormal to determine the exact nature of any palpable abnormality.
- The presence of any fetal membranes and, if possible, whether their uterine connections are intact or detached.
- The relative size of the soft tissue and bony components of the palpable parts of the birth canal, and the likelihood of fetuses being able to pass through it; the presence of any obvious bony damage such as a pelvic fracture or sacral displacement; the presence of any soft tissue damage and its likely effect upon birth.
- The tonic state of the uterus if palpable (not normally directly palpable in small animals).
- Whether dystocia is present; to diagnose its cause and enable a tentative plan of treatment to be formulated.
- Whether vaginal delivery is likely to be possible.

PRESENTATION, POSITION, AND POSTURE OF THE FETUS

These terms enable orientation of the fetus to be accurately described in cases of normal and abnormal birth. They are defined as follows:

- *Presentation*: the relationship between the long axis of the fetus and the long axis of the maternal birth

canal. Mostly longitudinal (anterior or posterior) but can occasionally be transverse or vertical.
- *Position*: that surface of the maternal birth canal to which the fetal vertebral column is applied. Mostly dorsal but may be ventral (fetus 'upside down') or lateral (right or left).
- *Posture*: the disposition of the head and limbs of the fetus.

Thus a calf during normal birth would be in anterior longitudinal presentation, dorsal position, and with a posture in which the extended head and neck were resting on the extended forelimbs. A puppy during normal birth would be in anterior longitudinal presentation and dorsal position. It has a posture in which the head and neck are extended, the forelimbs, with shoulders flexed, are held by the side. The hindlimbs are extended behind. Examples of presentation, position and posture are shown in Fig. 3.1.

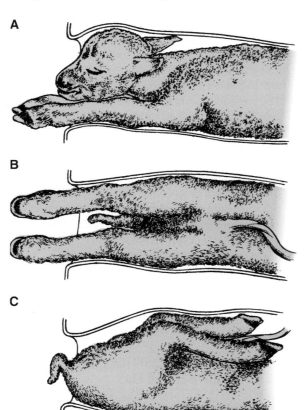

Figure 3.1 Examples of presentation, position and posture. (A) Lamb in anterior presentation, dorsal position, head resting on extended forelimbs. (B) Posterior presentation, left lateral position, hindlimbs extended. (C) Posterior presentation, ventral position, bilateral hip flexion (breech presentation).

CAUSES OF DYSTOCIA

Birth is an extremely complicated process and dystocia may arise if any part or parts of the process fail or become uncoordinated. For convenience of description, the causes of dystocia are divided into maternal or fetal causes, depending on whether the mother or her offspring were 'responsible' for the problem. In many cases both maternal and fetal factors are involved and the classification of causes becomes less exact. Our greater knowledge of the endocrine control of the birth process has shown that although in many species the fetus initiates the process, a cascade of hormone changes follows in the mother. The maternal components of birth are the provision of expulsive forces and a bony and soft tissue birth canal through which the fetus can pass. The fetal components of birth include initiation of the birth process; the assumption of correct presentation, position, and posture; and being sufficiently small to pass through the birth canal.

A summary of the causes of dystocia is set out in Table 3.1. The incidence of the various causes of dystocia varies greatly between the species and will be discussed in detail later. In general, however, the relatively small ovoid fetuses of the polytocous species are less prone to maldisposition than are the larger fetuses of the monotocous species, with their long limbs and necks. The prolonged birth pattern seen in the polytocous species may predispose to a higher proportion of uterine inertia among the causes of dystocia in these species.

DIAGNOSIS AND PLAN OF TREATMENT

As a result of the general clinical examination, the detailed obstetric examination, and any useful background information provided by the patient's history, the obstetrician will normally be able to arrive at a diagnosis of the cause of dystocia and formulate a plan for the resolution of the case. Such a plan should initially be tentative because, if the first attempt at treatment is unsuccessful, alternative treatments may have to be employed and must always be kept in mind.

The welfare of the patient must be paramount when planning and carrying out treatment. The wishes of the owner – sometimes quite forcibly expressed – must be carefully considered but the final course of action is decided by the obstetrician. In practice, economic considerations have to be taken into account to ensure

Table 3.1 Causes of dystocia

Maternal causes

Failure of expulsive forces
  Uterine
    Primary uterine inertia   *Myometrial defects*: overstretching, degeneration (senility, toxic, etc.), uterine infection, systemic illness, small litter size, heredity
    Biochemical deficiencies: estrogen/progesterone ratio, oxytocin, prostaglandin F2α, relaxin, calcium, glucose
    Hysteria/environmental disturbance
    Oligoamnion (deficiency of amniotic fluid)
    Premature birth
    Secondary uterine inertia (the consequence of another cause of dystocia)
    Uterine damage including rupture
    Uterine torsion (may also cause obstruction of birth canal)
  Abdominal
    Inability to strain (because of age, pain, debility, diaphragmatic rupture, tracheal / laryngeal damage)

Obstruction of the birth canal
  Bony pelvis: fracture, breed, diet, immaturity, neoplasia, disease
  Soft tissue:
    Vulva   congenital defect, fibrosis, immaturity
    Vagina   congenital defect, fibrosis, prolapse, neoplasia, perivaginal abscess, hymen
    Cervix   congenital defect, fibrosis, failure to dilate
    Uterus   torsion, deviation, herniation, adhesion, stenosis

Fetal causes

Hormone deficiency   ACTH/cortisol: initiation of birth
Fetopelvic disproportion   fetal oversize ⎫ ± pelvic defect
                              fetal monster ⎭
Fetal maldisposition:
    malpresentation (transverse, lateral, vertical, simultaneous)
    malposition (ventral, lateral, oblique)
    malposture (deviation of head and limbs)
Fetal death

---

that the cost of the proposed treatment can be met and is realistic.

Possible treatments are:

- *Conservative treatment*: the obstetrician may consider the case to be not quite ready for assistance and decide to allow the patient a finite period of time before taking further action.
- *Manipulative treatment*: assisted vaginal delivery after correction of any fetal maldisposition.
- *Drug therapy to increase myometrial activity*: the use of specific ecbolic drugs such as oxytocin. Calcium or glucose therapy may be required in cases where a deficiency is suspected.
- *Surgical treatment*: at cesarean section the uterus is opened surgically to allow removal of the offspring via laparotomy. On occasion the uterus may be found to be so damaged at surgery that hysterectomy is necessary.

Fetotomy (sometimes termed 'embryotomy') is the division – by the obstetrician working per vaginam – of the fetus into small portions that can more easily be delivered through the birth canal.

Regrettably, and fortunately very occasionally, the mother may be in such a poor state or its economic value is so low when presented for treatment that euthanasia is necessary.

AFTERCARE OF THE MOTHER AND YOUNG

Although the main responsibility for this rests with the patient's owner, the obstetrician must ensure that mother and young are well after delivery and advise on specific aspects of their care if appropriate.

Chapter 4

DYSTOCIA IN THE COW

INCIDENCE

The incidence of bovine dystocia is very variable and is influenced by many factors. The overall incidence is within the range 3–10% of all calvings but can be very much higher. The following factors – some of which are interrelated – have been shown to influence the incidence of dystocia in cattle.

Environmental factors

Diet   Animals that have been poorly fed and are in poor condition may suffer increased levels of dystocia, and reduced calf viability. Heavy feeding may increase calf weight, intrapelvic fat deposits, dystocia, and the risk of vaginal laceration. The efficiency of straining may also be reduced in fat animals. Drastic reduction of diet in the last few weeks of pregnancy in a vain attempt to reduce fetal size at birth should be avoided. The fetus continues to grow at the expense of the mother, who may develop pregnancy toxemia and become too weak to calve.

Supervision   Parturient cattle should be closely but unobtrusively supervised by an experienced stock person. Although overzealous supervision can lead to excessive diagnosis of dystocia, in some cases it results in a decreased stillbirth rate. Disturbance of cattle immediately prior to calving may increase the incidence of dystocia.

Disease   Hypocalcemia at calving is one cause of primary uterine inertia. Some herds with diseases such as salmonellosis and brucellosis may experience an increased incidence of dystocia, amongst other problems.

Induction of birth   Although this may reduce dystocia due to fetopelvic disproportion, the incidence of fetal maldisposition, failure of the cervix to dilate, and retention of the fetal membranes may increase.

Intrinsic factors

Age, parity, body weight, and pelvic size of dam
A higher incidence of dystocia is seen in heifers bred when young, poorly grown, and at their first calving. The incidence of dystocia may fall with increasing dam size and weight. Postponing breeding until a body weight of 400 kg is attained in Friesian–Holstein heifers has reduced the incidence of dystocia, even though calf body weight may be higher in heavier heifers. Pelvic diameters and area also increase with increasing body size and weight. It has been suggested that the external distance between the tubera coxae should be greater than 40 cm before a heifer is bred, as such animals will have a pelvic area of at least 200 cm^2.

Breed   Major differences in incidence are seen, with the highest figures being in the continental beef breeds. Gestation length in these breeds is longer and calf size in proportion to maternal size is larger. Typical survey figures for the incidence of dystocia are:

- Aberdeen Angus 3%
- Friesian–Holstein 6%
- Charolais 9%
- Simmental 10%
- Belgian Blue heifers with double-muscled calves 80%.

The Charolais breed had a poor reputation for ease of calving when bred to both Charolais and indigenous breeds. Its tendency to produce large calves and a relatively small maternal pelvic inlet were contributory factors to dystocia and a high stillbirth rate. Some success has been achieved in selecting lines of cattle for ease of calving in the Charolais and other breeds.

Calf weight, sex, and size   Many surveys have found that the incidence of dystocia increases with increasing calf weight. Heavier calves often have larger body dimensions than lighter ones. Male calves are heavier and often have a longer gestation than females. Twin calves are smaller than singletons but the incidence of dystocia in multiple births for reasons other than size is higher. Double-muscled calves are heavier and have greater body dimension, and their dams are more likely to experience dystocia. They are seen in a number of breeds including Belgian Blue, Charolais, and South Devon cattle.

Gestation length   This has already been observed to be longer in some continental breeds, where it may approach 290 days instead of the 'normal' 283 days. In late pregnancy calf weight may increase at the rate of 0.5 kg/day and fetal long-bone length also increases. Both factors can increase the incidence of dystocia.

Sire effect   Certain animals within a breed may sire calves born with a higher incidence of dystocia. In some cases, longer gestation and greater calf size may be responsible. Some studies have suggested a grandsire effect. Other surveys have suggested hereditary dam and grand-dam effects. The effects of these individual contributory factors is small but avoiding breeding animals with a poor calving reputation can be beneficial.

Calf presentation   The incidence of dystocia and stillbirth is higher in calves in posterior presentation.

CAUSES OF DYSTOCIA IN THE COW

A number of surveys of cases of bovine dystocia have indicated that the incidence of the various causes is approximately as shown in Table 4.1. The incidence of fetopelvic disproportion increased dramatically when sires of the larger continental beef breeds became popular.

Table 4.1 Causes of dystocia, and their incidence (%) in the cow	
Cause	**%**
Fetopelvic disproportion	45
Fetal malpresentation	26
Failure of cervix/vagina to dilate	9
Uterine inertia	5
Uterine torsion	3
Other maternal abnormalities	7
Other fetal abnormalities	5

Data from Jackson PGG 1985 Bovine dystocia. DVM&S Thesis. University of Edinburgh.

SPECIFIC CAUSES OF BOVINE DYSTOCIA

Details of the more important causes of bovine dystocia are described below, with information concerning their recognition and treatment. Manual delivery of the fetus is discussed in the section called Manipulative delivery (p. 64).

FAILURE OF THE EXPULSIVE FORCES

Uterine inertia

Primary uterine inertia

Etiology   The most common cause is hypocalcemia, with the cow showing signs of milk fever as calving is about to begin. Other causes include distension of the uterus caused by hydrops uteri, general debility with reduced tone and responsiveness in the myometrium, and environmental disturbance. The presence of twins may cause such stretching of the myometrium that effective contractions cannot occur. Primary uterine inertia has also been seen in overweight beef cows that fail to go into labor. Some such animals may be mildly ketotic and possibly on the verge of pregnancy toxemia.

Clinical signs   Preparations for birth begin but do not continue into second-stage labor. The fetus is normally in the correct presentation, position, and posture. The cervix is dilated or easily dilatable with manual pressure but there is no evidence of uterine contractions. The fetal membranes, especially the amnion, are often still intact. In cases of hypocalcemia the patient will be dull, reluctant or unable to rise, and have a low temperature, dilated pupils, and reduced rumenal activity. The head is turned back to the flank and, if untreated, the cow may become comatose with death ensuing. In cases of hydrops uteri there will probably have been a history during pregnancy of increasing abdominal size and debility. If accessible the uterine wall is found to lack muscle tone when palpated.

Treatment   If hypocalcemia is suspected, intravenous treatment with 400 mL of either 20% or 40% calcium borogluconate solution should be given. A further 400 mL of the drug is given by subcutaneous injection. If the farm has a history of coincidental magnesium deficiency, an injection of 400 mL calcium:magnesium: phosphorus:dextrose solution should be given intravenously. In many cases, parturition will resume but delivery should be assisted with moderate traction, as it should be in cases of uterine inertia resulting from other causes. Failure to deliver the calf promptly may result in its death if placental separation occurs. Following removal of the fetus, an injection of 20 IU oxytocin should be given by intramuscular injection to encourage uterine involution and placental expulsion.

Secondary uterine inertia

Etiology　The consequence of another cause of dystocia, for example fetal maldisposition, with resultant tiring of the myometrium.

Clinical signs　The uterine wall is felt to be flabby and lacking in tone often after the fetus has been delivered.

Treatment　The primary cause of dystocia is treated and the fetus delivered. Uterine involution is encouraged after delivery by injection of oxytocin as in primary uterine inertia.

Premature birth

May be accompanied by failure of normal uterine contractions and, if unobserved or early in gestation, by fetal death.

Etiology　May be caused by any factors that compromise fetal life and/or placental function.

Clinical signs　There may be an unexpected vaginal discharge during pregnancy. An abnormal and sometimes foul-smelling placenta may be visible or is passed by the patient. The fetus, often small and hairless, is palpable in the anterior vagina or uterus. If the fetus has been delivered and not observed, only placental remnants may be left in utero.

Treatment　The fetus and birth canal may both be very dry. The fetus is delivered by gentle traction applied by hand to its head and limbs after thoroughly lubricating all the structures involved.

All cases of premature birth in cattle (a pregnancy of less than 271 days of gestation) must be notified in the UK to the local Divisional Veterinary Manager (DVM) of the Department for Environment, Food and Rural Affairs (DEFRA). The DVM may require the fetus or its stomach contents, a vaginal swab, maternal milk and blood samples to be submitted to the Veterinary Laboratories Agency (VLA) and examined for evidence of brucellosis. Other infectious causes should also be investigated and for this a piece of placenta, including a cotyledon, may be of additional diagnostic value.

Failure of abdominal expulsive forces

Etiology　The abdominal musculature – so important during the second stage of labor – is either incapable of contracting or it is too painful for the animal to strain. In very old cows, or those suffering from hydrops, the abdominal muscles may have been stretched beyond the capacity of their natural elasticity. Tears in the muscles occur in cases of ventral hernia and as a result attempts to strain are compromised, as they are in cases of rupture of the prepubic tendon (see Chapter 2). Painful conditions involving the abdomen, diaphragm, or chest such as traumatic reticulitis/pericarditis may cause voluntary inhibition of attempts to strain. Laryngeal and diaphragmatic damage are rare in adult cattle but anything that compromises closure of glottis to enable straining to occur such as a tracheostomy wound could also compromise birth.

Clinical signs　Birth fails to occur despite the presence of normal preparatory signs and first-stage labor. Difficulty should be anticipated following recognition of the primary problem. Vaginal examination reveals a dilated cervix with the fetus in normal presentation at the pelvic inlet. In cases of ventral hernia the fetus may be only just palpable or even beyond reach. Its position can be ascertained by external ballottement.

Treatment　In cases of abdominal distension the fetus is delivered manually. If beyond reach it may be raised by assistants lifting the abdominal floor externally and is also aided by the patient lying down. In cases of diagnosed traumatic reticulitis or pericarditis where maternal health is deteriorating, or in cases of laryngeal or diaphragmatic disease, an elective cesarean should be considered.

Uterine rupture

Etiology　Tearing of the uterus may occur as a result of traumatic injury to the cow, for example following collision with a vehicle. It may also occasionally occur spontaneously through an unsuspected weak point in the uterine wall. The fate of the fetus in such cases depends on whether it passes into the peritoneal cavity and the degree of compromise sustained by the fetal membranes. Small tears may be symptomless and the fetus remains in the uterus, where it develops normally and is born without difficulty. Larger tears may allow passage of the fetus into the peritoneal cavity. Maternal death may follow rupture with severe uterine hemorrhage. In cases where the placenta is compressed and its circulation is compromised, fetal death can occur. Sterile peritonitis may result in the fetus becoming adherent to the mesentery or other abdominal organs. Signs of pregnancy fail to develop and the intra-abdominal abnormalities may be detected by investigative clinical examination and possibly by exploratory laparotomy. If the placenta is unaffected by uterine rupture the fetus may survive until the end of gestation but its extrauterine location means that normal vaginal delivery is impossible.

Clinical signs   These will depend on the degree of damage sustained and the fate of the fetus. External signs of hemorrhage following a road accident may suggest uterine damage, among other problems. Fetal death following uterine rupture may produce few signs other than failure of an established pregnancy to progress. If the fetus survives and develops within the peritoneal cavity, pregnancy may progress normally to term. Signs of imminent birth and even cervical relaxation may occur but birth does not follow. Transient colic may occasionally be seen. Vaginal examination may reveal a small empty uterus and the placenta disappearing through a defect in the uterine wall. The site of rupture – often on the dorsal curvature of the uterus or ventrally just beyond the pelvic brim – may be palpable or may be beyond reach. Occasionally, loops of maternal small intestine may be palpable. These must not be confused with the exposed intestinal loops often palpable with a schistosomus reflexus fetus (see p. 48). The uterus feels smaller than normal on rectal examination and occasionally the intraperitoneal fetus may be palpable. It may be possible to locate the fetus in an abnormal position – such as underneath the rumen – by external ballottement or a transabdominal ultrasonographic scan.

Treatment   The fetus should be delivered from the peritoneal cavity by laparotomy. If the presence of a uterine rupture is anticipated an elective laparotomy/cesarean section just prior to the end of gestation will increase the chance of delivering a living fetus. The extent of any peritonitis should be noted. If this is severe, or if it involves the ovaries or oviducts, future breeding may have a poor prognosis and the cow should be salvaged at an appropriate time.

Uterine torsion

This is discussed in the section on obstruction of the birth canal (see p. 43).

OBSTRUCTION OF THE BIRTH CANAL

The bony pelvis

The dimensions of the bony pelvis are too small to allow passage of the fetus.

Etiology   *Maternal immaturity* is the most common cause and often occurs as a result of heifers being served at too young an age. This is a particular problem when the stock bull is allowed to run with the herd after the heifer calves have reached puberty at 6 or 7 months of age and misalliance takes place. Small pelvic size is seen in poorly grown heifers and may very occasionally occur as a result of pelvic fracture. A small pelvis is a component in dystocia due to fetopelvic disproportion and is exacerbated in cases where the fetus is larger than normal. In most heifers who suffer misalliance, fetal size is within the normal range for the breed.

A less common cause of a small bony pelvis is *sacral displacement*, in which the fused sacral bones and the first few coccygeal vertebrae are set at an abnormal angle to the lumbar vertebrae. As a result of the problem – which may have a hereditary etiology – the dorsoventral diameter of the maternal pelvis is severely reduced, allowing less room for passage of the fetus.

Lumbosacral subluxation may be caused by a cow or heifer being mounted by a very heavy bull. The downward displacement of the vertebral column that results at the lumbosacral junction may also reduce the size of the pelvic inlet.

Clinical signs   There is lack of progress in the second stage of labor. If the fetus is able to partially enter the pelvis, severe unproductive straining may occur. A single large fetal foot may be seen at the vulva. If the fetus is too large to enter the pelvis, no progress is made after the completion of first-stage labor and the heifer looks uncomfortable, strains occasionally, and may stand with her back arched and tail raised. Vaginal examination reveals the presence of a small bony pelvis of insufficient size for the fetus to pass through.

Treatment   The obstetrician must decide – by comparing fetal and pelvic dimensions – if the fetus is likely to be able to pass through the maternal pelvis. In many cases of misalliance involving young heifers vaginal examination reveals that the calf will clearly *not* pass through the pelvis. In cases of doubt, moderate traction may be applied but if this is unsuccessful cesarean section is indicated (for further discussion on decision-making in such cases see the section on Fetopelvic disproportion, p. 46). The technique of 'pubic symphysiotomy', in which the unfused pubic symphysis of heifers is prized open with an obstetric chisel, has no place in modern bovine obstetrics.

Prevention   Prompt removal of the bull from the breeding herd should avoid exposure of heifer calves to service. Suspected or confirmed pregnancy in calves served by mistake should be terminated as soon as possible by injection with prostaglandin F2α. If misalliance is observed the pregnancy may be terminated 10 days later by use of prostaglandin F2α, which causes luteolysis of the supporting corpus luteum.

Termination after 5 or 6 months of pregnancy should be used with care. Fetal maldisposition and other problems may complicate delivery and corrective manipulation through the small maternal pelvis may be very difficult. In such cases it may be wiser to allow the heifer to proceed to term supported by good feeding and to deliver the calf by elective cesarean section either just before birth is due or following signs of first-stage labor (see also Chapter 15).

The soft tissues

The vulva

Etiology   Relaxation of the vulva is part of the normal preparations for birth but occasionally – especially in heifers – full relaxation of this part of the birth canal does not occur. In older animals damage sustained at an earlier calving or a horning injury with the formation of scar tissue and fibrosis may occur preventing normal relaxation.

Clinical signs   Although relaxation of the pelvic ligaments has occurred, the vulva may not appear to be relaxed or there may be evidence on close examination of an earlier injury. Some difficulty may be experienced in inserting the lubricated hand, and the lips of the vulva may have a hard and fibrous consistency. Beyond the confines of the vulva, vaginal dimensions are normal.

Treatment   In poorly relaxed heifers, gentle manipulation and stretching of the vulva with a clean lubricated hand may cause the vulva to relax sufficiently to allow calving without damage being sustained. If relaxation does not occur within a few minutes, or if scar tissue is present, there is a risk that the dorsal commissure of the vulva will tear upwards into the rectum. This must be prevented by performing an *episiotomy*. An incision is made about one-third down the lateral wall of the vulva through the skin mucosal junction (Fig. 4.1) to allow the vulva to stretch in a

controlled fashion during the passage of the fetus. The episiotomy wound should be repaired by suturing the skin and mucosa immediately after delivery to re-establish the normal morphology of the vulval lips.

The vagina

Etiology   The vagina also relaxes in preparation for birth but the presence of scar tissue from a previous calving injury may cause a loss of elasticity. Less commonly, congenital stenosis of the vagina may be present. The lumen of the vagina may be obstructed by embryonic remnants, a hymen, perivaginal abscesses, and also by tumor or cyst formation. Vaginal prolapse seldom causes obstruction to birth but may require careful protection during fetal delivery.

Clinical signs   Lack of progress during early second-stage labor may be observed but vaginal abnormality might not be detected until the obstetrician performs an internal examination. Scar tissue and perivaginal hematoma formation may have been detected at the routine postnatal check following a previous calving. In normal parturient cattle the vaginal wall is soft, gently elastic to manual pressure, and capable of expanding to accommodate fetal passage. The vagina is occasionally partially obstructed by a vertical pillar of mucosa-covered tissue just caudal to the cervix. Hymenal remnants are unusual in cattle but if present are located immediately anterior to the external urethral orifice. Usually thin and easily broken down, they extend laterally from the vaginal walls to occlude part or almost all of the lumen. Perivaginal abscesses or hematomas may press on the vaginal walls, through which they may be felt as smooth fluctuating or firm masses. The contents of masses in the vaginal wall can be investigated by needle aspiration or a direct ultrasonographic scan. Vaginal tumors are uncommon in cattle but occasionally one or more leiomyomas may be palpable attached to the vaginal wall and, more seriously, a large invasive squamous cell carcinoma may obstruct the caudal vagina.

Treatment   The extent and consistency of the obstruction is palpated and if possible the fetus is guided past it assisted by gentle stretching of surrounding tissues. This may be done with one hand initially. Further dilation may be achieved by inserting both hands with the fingers intertwined into the vagina and gradually separating the arms as they are advanced in an anterior direction. It may also be possible to guide the fetus past one side of a vertical pillar in the vagina, but if this is not possible the structure can be removed with scissors

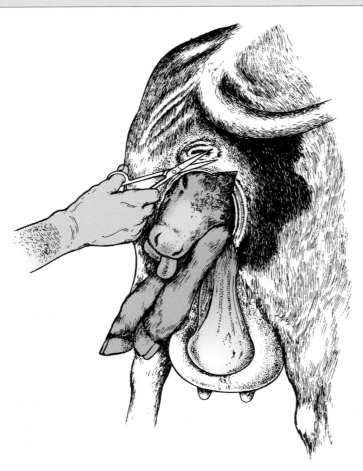

Figure 4.1 Technique of episiotomy.

after clamping both extremities with artery forceps to control hemorrhage. Hymenal remnants can usually be broken down by the obstetrician's fingers. It is unwise to attempt to drain perivaginal abscesses or deal with hematomas immediately before fetal delivery and if they or other structures present a serious obstruction, the fetus should be delivered by cesarean section.

The cervix

Failure of cervical dilation is the third most common cause of bovine dystocia and its management requires careful clinical judgment.

Etiology The mechanism of cervical dilation in cattle is poorly understood. Hormonal factors together with physical dilation caused by the approaching calf and its fetal sacs are involved. Failure of these and other factors to exert their influence may result in the cervix remaining closed or only partially dilated.

Cervical obstruction can also result from the presence of scar tissue arising from previous injury, possibly at an earlier calving.

Clinical signs Signs of first-stage labor are prolonged and do not proceed to the second stage. Cervical obstruction is detected on vaginal examination when the case is investigated. When fully dilated the cervix is flattened into the vaginal wall and is not palpable. When fully closed, the obstetrician's finger may be inserted into but not passed through the external os. During pregnancy the os is sealed with a thick mucous plug, which is passed out through the vagina a few hours before fetal delivery. The partially dilated cervix is palpable as a circular rim extending into the lumen of the vagina at the junction of the vaginal and uterine walls. Partial dilation may allow passage of parts of the fetus such as a foot or the nose but not wider parts such as the thorax, to which the edges of the cervical rim are tightly applied. If only slightly dilated the obstetrician may insert a finger through the external os and touch part of the fetus within the uterus. It may be possible to detect signs of fetal life such as spontaneous movement, and also to determine whether the fetal membranes are intact or have ruptured. In the latter case the fetus can be directly palpated and there may also be evidence of loss of fetal fluids into the vagina. Some assessment of fetal health may also be made by rectal palpation.

Treatment   The patient is examined to ensure that signs of imminent birth including ligamentous relaxation and colostrum in the udder are present. An attempt is made to dilate the cervix manually by inserting one or two fingers (or the hand with the fingers pointed in a conical shape) into the external os. Expansion of the fingers may be accompanied by dilation of the cervix, which can be felt to give way laterally under gentle digital or manual pressure. The hand is then inserted through the cervix and lateral pressure continued by circular and outward movements of the hand and forearm. If the cervix remains closed and it is considered that the fetal membranes are intact and the fetus is in good condition, the patient may be left for 30 minutes and then re-examined. Some clinicians have found spasmolytic drugs effective in producing cervical relaxation. Vetrabutine hydrochloride (Monzaldon; Boehringer Ingelheim) given by intramuscular injection at a dose of 2.5 mg/kg may help in some cases. Cesarean section should follow if no progress has been made after 30 minutes. Surgical delivery is also indicated if there is evidence that scar tissue is obstructing the cervix or that fetal life is at risk.

The technique of cervical section or vaginal hysterotomy has been described for treatment of non-dilation of the cervix. In this technique the rim of the cervix is incised in one or more places to allow dilation of the birth canal at that point. There is a considerable risk, especially in the ventral quadrant, of severe hemorrhage, and uncontrolled tearing may also occur as the fetus passes through. The technique has no place in modern bovine obstetrics; cesarean section is a much safer procedure.

Torsion of the uterus

Uterine torsion has been found to be the cause of up to 7% of all bovine dystocia cases in some surveys. The pregnant uterus rotates about its long axis with the point of torsion being the anterior vagina just caudal to the cervix. Less commonly, the point of torsion is cranial to the cervix. In the majority of cases torsion is in an anticlockwise direction as the obstetrician stands behind the cow. The degree of torsion varies from 45 to 360°. A few cases of uterine torsion during pregnancy have been reported.

Torsion of the uterus during pregnancy

This a rare condition seen much less frequently than torsion of the uterus as a cause of dystocia at term (see below).

Etiology   Unknown, but possibly associated with uterine instability and episodes of excited exercise.

Clinical signs   The condition has been reported in animals from mid-pregnancy onwards. Affected animals may show signs of discomfort, some straining, and the tail head may be raised. Death may occur in untreated cases. The torsion is palpable on rectal examination as a rope-like structure involving the anterior vagina, cervix, and uterine body. The uterus may feel tenser than normal.

Treatment   Surgical correction is necessary in most cases. The uterus is approached by a left flank laparotomy. The uterus (which may have some vascular compromise and is fragile) is carefully untwisted. Antibiotic and non-steroidal anti-inflammatory therapy is provided. The fetus and placenta can be monitored after treatment by ultrasonographic scan. Separation of the placenta from the endometrium and abortion may be complications.

Torsion of the uterus as a cause of dystocia at term

Etiology   The bovine uterus has been said to be basically unstable for a number of reasons. These include: (1) the caudal parts of the uterus are attached to the lateral walls of the pelvis by the broad ligaments; (2) as pregnancy advances the cranial parts of the uterine horns lie on the abdominal floor with no stabilizing ligamentous attachment; (3) a single-calf pregnancy chiefly occupies one horn of the uterus, making the organ heavier and more bulky on one side than the other; (4) the instability may be increased by the cow lowering her front end first when lying down. Torsion occurs when the cow – or the fetus – makes a sudden movement causing the unstable uterus to rotate about its long axis. The bovine amnion is fused in places to the surrounding allantois, which is attached through the chorion to the uterine wall. If the fetus rotates

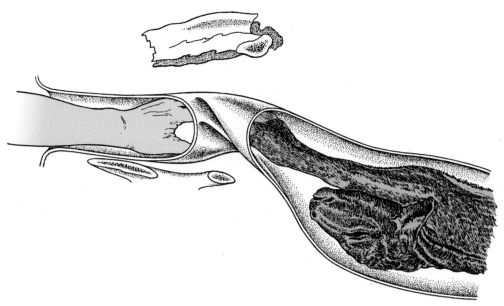

Figure 4.2 Torsion of the uterus – vaginal examination.

about its long axis in late gestation the uterus may be rotated with it. Reduced exercise may increase the incidence of torsion.

Clinical signs   The first signs may be noted towards the end of first-stage labor, which is prolonged, and the cow may show signs of mild discomfort. The patient may adopt a 'rocking-horse' stance so that the dorsal surface of her spine is concave and the fore- and hindlimbs are held respectively further forward and backwards than normal. Torsion of the birth canal may cause one or both lips of the vulva to be pulled in. Vaginal examination reveals an abnormal disposition of the birth canal (Fig. 4.2). The hand cannot immediately be passed anteriorly towards the cervix. The vagina narrows conically and folds of vaginal mucosa may be felt going into an oblique spiral. The direction of the vaginal folds may indicate the direction of the torsion – either clockwise or anticlockwise.

If the torsion is less than 180° the obstetrician's hand may be passed through the constriction to palpate the fetus. In such cases care must be taken to avoid mistakenly thinking a dead fetus is alive. When palpated through the twisted anterior vagina the fetus may appear to float away from the obstetrician's hand and then spontaneously return as if alive. The cervix is normally dilated.

If the torsion is greater than 180° the birth canal may be totally occluded, with the vagina coming to a conical end with no recognizable cervix being palpable. Rectal examination will confirm the displacement, with the broad ligaments being abnormally palpable as taught bands in the caudal abdomen.

Prognosis   This is quite good in cases that are recognized and dealt with promptly. In cases that have not been treated for some time after they occurred severe compromise of the blood supply to the uterus may occur. In such cases the calf may die and the uterine wall may become necrotic and friable. Uterine rupture may occur spontaneously or at attempted treatment by rolling, and peritonitis, toxemia, and death may occur. The possibility of unseen uterine damage should always be remembered in cases in which treatment has been delayed or which do not do well after treatment.

Treatment   A number of methods are available:

Rotation of the fetus and uterus per vaginam back into their correct position   This is possible if the obstetrician's hand can pass into the uterus and touch the fetus and if fetal fluids remain within the uterus. The fetus is grasped by a convenient prominence such as the elbow, sternum, or thigh and is rocked from side to side before being pushed right over in the opposite direction to the torsion (Fig. 4.3). If the maneuver has been successful the torsion will have disappeared and the vagina regains its normal morphology.

Rolling the cow   The principle of this method is to roll the cow around its uterus while that organ remains

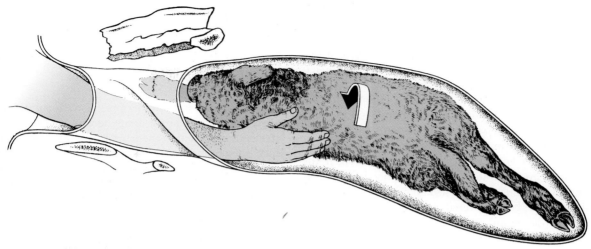

Figure 4.3 Torsion of the uterus – rotation of the fetus and uterus per vaginam.

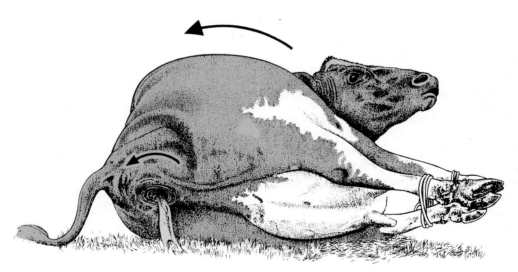

Figure 4.4 Torsion of the uterus – rolling the cow.

still. Three assistants are required. The cow is cast on the side to which the torsion is directed (Fig. 4.4). Thus in an anticlockwise torsion she is cast on her left side. The two forelegs and the two hindlegs are tied together and the head is restrained with a halter or head collar. The cow is rolled sharply over onto her other (right) side. The patency of the vagina is checked and if the torsion persists the cow is gently rolled back onto her other (left) side and the process is repeated. The cow may have to be rolled two or three times before the torsion is corrected.

The efficiency of rolling can be improved by putting external pressure on the cow's abdomen in an attempt to 'hold the uterus still' while the cow's body is rolled. Manual pressure over the uterus can be used or a board rested against the caudal abdomen and downward pressure exerted by a person standing on it.

The calf should always be delivered by the obstetrician as soon as the torsion has been corrected. The cervix may close within 30 minutes of resolution of the torsion preventing fetal delivery by the vaginal route and necessitating cesarean section.

Surgical correction   This may be necessary if fetal rotation is impossible and rolling the cow is unsuccessful. A left flank laparotomy is performed on the standing cow under local anesthetic (see also Chapter 11). The uterus is located and the direction of the torsion confirmed by palpating and examining the cervical region. The uterine wall or a fetal limb within the uterus is grasped firmly and an attempt made to rotate the uterus back into its correct position.

Once the uterus is correctly in place the calf may be delivered per vaginam or by cesarean section. If the uterus cannot be rotated cesarean section must be performed with the uterus in its abnormal position. Once the fetus has been delivered the uterus can normally be readily rotated into its correct position after repair of the uterine wall. The condition of the uterine wall should be carefully checked before abdominal closure. If the uterus is discolored, its blood supply may have been compromised. If normal color is not restored after correction of the torsion the prospects for survival are not good. Antibiotic cover and the administration of a non-steroidal anti-inflammatory drug such as flunixin may aid recovery and provide analgesia.

Downward deviation of the uterus

Etiology   This uncommon cause of dystocia may occur in animals suffering from a ventral hernia or rupture of the prepubic tendon. In such cases the pregnant uterus is unsupported and passes partially into the hernia. The caudal uterus and cervix are under tension and deviate sharply downwards just in front of the pelvic brim.

Clinical signs   The condition should be anticipated in cases of ventral hernia or prepubic tendon rupture when spontaneous delivery is unlikely to occur. First-stage labor is not followed by fetal delivery and vaginal examination is performed. The birth canal may be partially or completely occluded but the oblique vaginal wall folds found in cases of uterine torsion are absent.

Treatment   The obstetrician's hand can usually be passed through the constriction of the birth canal by application of gentle pressure. The fetus may be beyond reach in the standing animal and casting the cow may assist the obstetrician to locate the fetus and deliver it by traction. Alternatively, the abdominal floor can be raised by using a sack under the abdomen held and lifted by two assistants. Cesarean section is performed if vaginal delivery is impossible. Postparturient repair of the ventral hernia or prepubic tendon are not normally practical. The udder may hang close to the ground increasing the risk that it might be damaged and making access for the calf difficult.

FETOPELVIC DISPROPORTION

Etiology   This important cause of dystocia occurs when the fetus is larger than normal, the pelvis is smaller than normal, or there is a disproportion between them. Factors affecting pelvic and fetal size are discussed above (see p. 40). In summary, pelvic size is influenced by the age, breed, weight, and pelvic dimensions of the dam. Fetal size is influenced by many factors including breed, parental and grandparental factors, gestation length, sex of the calf, litter size, parity of the dam, double-muscling of the fetus, and the nutritional state of the dam.

Clinical signs   The cow is unable to complete, or has great difficulty in completing, the second stage of labor. Straining of varying intensity is seen and the fetal feet and possibly the nose (in cases of anterior presentation) may be visible at the vulva. In a normal birth the calf is usually delivered within 2 hours of the fetal nose being seen at the vulva – in cases of fetopelvic disproportion this does not occur. If the case is untreated the calf will die, with serious consequences for the cow.

Treatment   Vaginal examination is often difficult as the disproportion between calf and pelvis may leave little room for the obstetrician's hands. In some cases a severe degree of disproportion may be immediately obvious and it is clear that successful vaginal delivery is highly unlikely. In such cases, if the calf is alive immediate cesarean section should be carried out. If the calf is dead and access to it within the uterus is possible, delivery after fetotomy may be considered. If access per vaginam is likely to be difficult, cesarean section is advisable. In other cases where vaginal delivery is considered possible an attempt to deliver the calf by trial traction should be made.

The important decision-making process of deciding whether a fetus is likely to pass through the birth canal is discussed in the section Manipulative delivery (p. 64).

DYSTOCIA CAUSED BY FETAL MONSTERS

Etiology   Fetal monsters arise from adverse factors affecting the fetus in the early stages of its development. The adverse factors are mostly of genetic origin but may also include physical, chemical, and viral factors. These adverse factors are particularly likely to affect the fetus before day 42, when organogenesis is complete in cattle. Fetal monsters are relatively uncommon and mostly occur sporadically but the incidence in cattle is higher than in other species. Occasionally a series of monsters may be encountered on one farm or a series of farms, which may have been sired by one bull. A large number of monsters have been recorded and only the more common ones are described here. A review of the literature suggests that 33.2% of bovine fetal monsters are conjoined twins, 31.8% are schistosomes, and 8.4% bulldog calves. Other monsters account for 26.6% of cases with none exceeding 8% of the total. Fetal monsters pose problems for the obstetrician as it is often impossible to palpate the whole structure per vaginam. The monetary value of a monster calf is clearly low and where vaginal delivery seems likely to be complicated it is often better to proceed immediately to cesarean section if the fetus is alive or fetotomy if the fetus is dead. When cesarean section is employed problems may be experienced in removing the abnormal fetus from the uterus and, before this can be done, some fetotomy may be necessary.

Conjoined twins

Sometimes known as 'double monsters', these are the most common group of monsters and arise from incomplete division of a fertilized ovum and show great variation from partial duplication to almost complete separation of the two individuals. Their presence, although rare, should always be suspected when an apparently normal birth cannot be delivered as anticipated.

Great variation on the degree of separation is seen but the following are amongst the most common conjoined twins:

- *Diprosopus*: the monster has two faces, including mouths with cleft palates, but not two complete heads. The wide double face will normally prevent the fetus from entering the maternal pelvis and cesarean section or fetotomy is required to permit delivery.
- *Dicephalus*: two heads and necks that join at the shoulder (Fig. 4.5). The divergence of the necks again prevents normal entry into the pelvis. Treatment is by removal of one head by fetotomy followed by vaginal delivery of the rest of the fetus or by cesarean section.
- *Dipygus*: duplication of the trunk and some of the limbs. Delivery is normally by cesarean section.
- *'Siamese twins'* (the somatodidymi): separation of the twins is almost complete with points of attachment being along the sternum or elsewhere. One of the more common of these rare monsters is *pygodidymus*, in which the two calves are joined at the rump and are facing in opposite directions. It is seldom possible to detect the point of attachment on vaginal examination. The first calf is often in normal presentation, seems quite small, but cannot be moved by traction. Delivery is by cesarean section

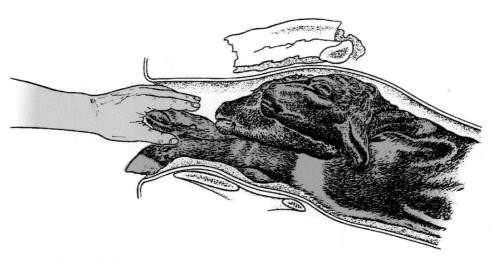

Figure 4.5 Fetal monster – dicephalus.

with fetotomy required in most cases to permit removal from the uterus.

The *fetal mole* or acardiac monster *amorphus globosus* is occasionally seen as co-twin to a normal calf. It consists of a collection of mixed fetal tissues, is mostly quite small, and is not normally associated with dystocia.

Schistosomus reflexus

The monster most frequently described in the literature, this is also known as a 'celosomian monster' or 'moon calf'. In this monster the spinal column has undergone dorsiflexion and the head and tail approximate. The limbs are ankylosed and deformed (Fig. 4.6). The vertebrae and ribs form a discoid plate of bony tissue. The grossly abnormal shape makes unaided passage through the birth canal unlikely. The deformed calf may be a singleton fetus or co-twin to a normal calf.

The calf may be presented with either its head and extremities or its exposed viscera towards the pelvis. When the head and extremities are presented they may be mistaken for twin calves presenting simultaneously but careful examination should reveal that they all belong to the same abnormal fetus. When the viscera are presented they may be covered by a thin membrane or be fully exposed to direct touch. The intestines, heart (beating if alive), and the liver may all be palpated. The size of the small intestine should indicate that it is of fetal rather than maternal origin. (Maternal small intestine may appear at the vulva in cows with uterine rupture.) The fetal intestines could, however, have arisen from a calf with a simple umbilical defect and not from a schistosome. Occasionally an additional fetal abnormality may be present. Cases have been recorded in which the monster also had hydrocephalus (see below) and the cow was suffering from hydrops amnion.

Treatment It is occasionally possible to carefully deliver a small schistosome monster by traction following generous lubrication but in most cases this is not possible. In head and extremities presentations, cesarean section, with fetotomy at surgery, is mostly necessary. If the fetus is alive it must be euthanized before fetotomy with an intracardiac injection of pentobarbitone sodium. When the viscera are presented they may be removed from the dead or euthanized fetus manually followed by fetotomy if it is possible to pass the wire around the monster. In other cases cesarean section is required.

Bulldog calf

This monster is seen chiefly in Dexter and Kerry cattle (and occasionally in Holstein–Friesians and other breeds). The abnormality is a very severe form of achondroplasia, possibly associated with a single autosomal gene, and in purebred Dexters approximately one in five calves may be affected. The abnormal fetus has

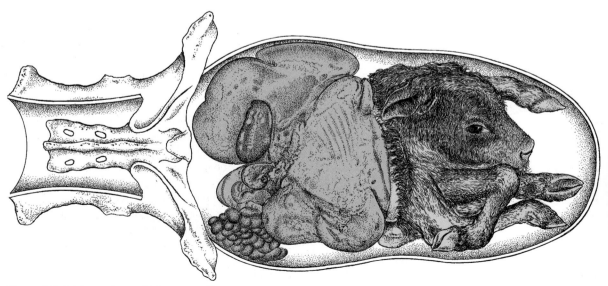

Figure 4.6 Fetal monster – schistosomus reflexus.

a very large bulldog-like head with very short legs. There may be an additional complication of either fetal ascites or, less commonly, anasarca. Affected fetuses are occasionally expelled without assistance but dystocia may arise if the head is unable to enter or pass through the birth canal. Manual delivery by the obstetrician is usually possible aided by generous lubrication.

Perosomus elumbis

This monster has a deceptively normal anterior end but rudimentary lumbar vertebrae and spinal cord, and hindlimbs that are contorted and ankylosed, possibly as a result of lack of movement by the developing fetus. In anterior presentation the monster may initially be mistaken for a normal calf but attempts at assisted delivery are resisted by the rigid hind parts, which may not permit passage through the pelvis. In posterior presentation the abnormal fetus can be more readily recognized. Delivery is by fetotomy or cesarean section possibly accompanied by fetotomy.

Hydrocephalus

Affected animals have a gross enlargement of the cranium that can prevent the fetus from entering and passing through the maternal pelvis. In some cases when the calf is dead it may be possible to break down the cranial swelling manually or to separate it from the cranium using the embryotome. In other cases cesarean section may be required. Cranial enlargement is also occasionally seen in calves with pituitary hypoplasia in which prolonged gestation has occurred.

Fetal anasarca

Generalized subcutaneous edema is present in this abnormality. Affected calves often have no hair and uterine fluids appear to be deficient leaving little natural lubrication. Generous application of obstetrical lubricant and instillation of fluids into the uterus will normally allow delivery of the fetus by traction. Some reduction in body size may be achieved in the dead calf by making numerous incisions into the skin, which allow some release of subcutaneous fluid with resultant reduction of body dimension.

Fetal ascites

This may be seen in calves at term or in cases of premature fetal death. The head, neck, and thorax of the calf will readily enter and pass through the maternal pelvis but the distended abdomen will not. If there is mild disproportion the calf may be delivered by traction after generous use of lubricant. If access to the fetal abdomen is possible through the cow's vagina it may be drained using a scalpel blade or catheter to release the abnormal fluid, with resultant reduction of fetal abdominal bulk. In the occasional case cesarean section may be required.

FETAL MALDISPOSITION

The term 'maldisposition' includes abnormalities of presentation, position, and posture that render it difficult or impossible for the fetus to enter or pass through the birth canal.

Etiology It is not clear why the fetus adopts its normal birth posture but it has been suggested that the mammalian fetus may 'practice' assuming this posture during the later stages of pregnancy. Mild or severe fetal ill health and fetal death may predispose to fetal maldisposition, as may maternal ill health or abnormal hormone levels. A mild fetal maldisposition may be made worse as it fails to engage correctly at the pelvic inlet and expulsive forces compound the difficulty. Self-correction of a maldisposition is extremely unlikely.

Clinical signs A delay in fetal delivery with unproductive straining may be seen if part of the fetus has entered the maternal pelvis. In normal birth the fetal forelimbs and nose are seen at the vulva. In some maldisposition cases these normal findings are absent. In cases of lateral deviation of the head the fetal forelimbs alone may be seen at the vulva whereas in bilateral shoulder flexion the fetal head may protrude from the vulva. In breech presentation (bilateral hip flexion) only the fetal tail may be seen. The abnormality is confirmed by careful vaginal examination.

Treatment In many cases uterine and abdominal contraction will force the abnormally disposed fetus tightly into or against the pelvic inlet, making it difficult for the obstetrician to diagnose the abnormality or take corrective action. To provide more space the fetus must be repelled (i.e. pushed back) from the pelvic inlet. The hand is placed against a solid fetal part such as the head, brisket, or (in posterior presentation) the hindquarters. The fetus is repelled from the pelvic inlet by gentle but firm pressure exerted by the obstetrician. The maneuver is aided by generous lubrication and also, if necessary in cases where little uterine fluid remains, by instilling some warm water into the uterus. In cases where the maldisposition has been present for some time, repulsion and manipulation of the fetus is restricted by loss of fetal fluids and by the uterine walls contracting tightly around the fetus. Maternal straining is often increased by attempts at fetal repulsion and in some cases an epidural anesthetic is required. An injection of $300 \, \mu g$ clenbuterol can be given to reduce the tone of the myometrium. Although facilitating fetal repulsion, the epidural anesthetic will also result in reduced maternal straining assistance during the subsequent delivery.

Once the nature of the maldisposition is clearly identified the obstetrician should attempt to replace any abnormality into its correct position. Although it is occasionally possible to deliver a very small fetus in an uncorrected maldisposition, such delivery should not normally be attempted in cattle. There is a considerable risk that damage to the soft tissues of the birth canal will occur, unless great care is exercised, as the fetus is replaced in its correct disposition.

Sharp, pointed, or hard extremities of the fetus, such as the hooves, teeth, or poll of the head, should be covered by the obstetrician's hand to avoid damage to or penetration of the uterine wall. Once the fetus has been returned to its normal birth posture it should be delivered by traction in the normal way. If the maldisposition cannot be corrected or if, after correction, a degree of fetopelvic disproportion is discovered the fetus must be delivered by cesarean section or by fetotomy.

The common maldispositions seen in cattle are discussed in greater detail below.

Malpresentation

Posterior presentation

Although calves 'coming backwards' may be delivered spontaneously, posterior presentation is not normal in cattle. Assistance during delivery may be required, especially when fetopelvic disproportion is also present. Despite anecdotal accounts by farmers it is not normally possible to convert a posterior presentation into an anterior one. In an uncomplicated posterior presentation the fetal hindlimbs may be seen at the vulva with the soles of the hooves showing dorsally. This orientation of the hooves can also occur in very rare cases with the fetus in anterior presentation, ventral position, and with a deviation of the head, and care must be taken to ensure that the exact nature of the maldisposition is known.

Vaginal examination will permit the limbs to be followed up towards the hocks, hips, and tail. The relative sizes of the fetal hindquarters and the maternal pelvis need to be compared and a decision taken as to whether traction is likely to be successful.

Whenever delivery of the fetus by traction in posterior presentation is planned, the obstetrician must ensure that sufficient help is available *before* delivery is attempted.

The umbilical cord may break or become compromised at an early stage during the delivery of a fetus in posterior presentation. When this occurs the fetus may attempt to breathe while its head is immersed in amniotic fluid and death by drowning can occur if there is even the slightest delay during delivery.

Transverse presentation

This may be dorsotransverse, ventrotransverse, or laterotransverse, depending on whether the dorsal, ventral, or lateral surface of the fetal body is facing the pelvic inlet. In some cases the fetus may lie obliquely across the pelvic inlet. Careful palpation per vaginam will confirm the orientation of the fetus. An attempt is made to place the fetus in a longitudinal presentation by obstetrical version – repelling one end of the body and applying gentle traction to the other. Ideally the caudal end of the body is brought towards the pelvic inlet because the two hindlimbs may be more easily manipulated into the pelvis than the forelimbs and head. Once in a longitudinal presentation the fetus must be rotated from its lateral position into a dorsal position. Delivery by traction follows correction of the malpresentation. If the malpresentation cannot be corrected the fetus must be delivered by cesarean section or fetotomy.

Vertical presentation

An extremely unusual malpresentation in which the fetal body is found lying vertically across the pelvic inlet. The fetus may be in dorsovertical, ventrovertical, or laterovertical presentation, depending on which body surface is facing the pelvic inlet. An attempt is made to place the fetus in a longitudinal presentation by repelling one end of the fetus and applying gentle traction to the other. If manipulative delivery is impossible the fetus must be delivered by cesarean section or fetotomy.

The 'dog sitting position' form of vertical presentation, which has been described in the mare, is rarely encountered in cattle. However, this abnormality should be suspected if the head and shoulders of the calf have been delivered but no further progress is possible, even when modest traction is applied to the fetus.

The situation is somewhat similar to the problem of stifle lock (see the section Manipulative delivery, p. 69). In the dog sitting position only the head and shoulders pass through the vulva; in stifle lock the head, shoulders, and thorax pass through the vulva.

Careful examination may reveal that the fetal hindfeet are resting on the pelvic floor, thus preventing caudal extension of the hindlimbs to allow fetal delivery. If the presence of a dog sitting position is confirmed, an attempt should initially be made to repel the fetal hindlimbs from the pelvic brim back into the uterus. If this can be accomplished, the fetus can be delivered by traction. Repulsion of the whole calf is seldom possible. In cases where this cannot be achieved, euthanasia of the calf and fetotomy may be necessary. Removal of the head and thorax of the calf will allow repulsion of the caudal parts of the calf and after locating the hind limbs, delivery in posterior presentation.

Malposition

In normal delivery the calf is in dorsal position with its spinal column beneath that of the dam. Abnormalities of position include *ventral position*, in which the calf is 'upside down', or *lateral position*, when the calf is 'lying on its side'. These abnormalities of position may also be seen when the fetus is in posterior presentation. Although very small calves can occasionally be delivered in an abnormal position it is unwise to attempt to do so and the fetus should be manipulated into a dorsal position by the technique of obstetric rotation. An attempt is made to rotate the calf around its long axis by applying lateral pressure to the shoulders (or the hindquarters in a posterior presentation). This may be done by direct pressure or by rocking the calf from side to side around its long axis before pushing it firmly back into dorsal position.

In cases where little fetal fluid remains or the uterus has contracted tightly down onto the fetus, rotation prior to delivery may be difficult or impossible. In such cases, after generous application of obstetric lubrication, rotation may be attempted as traction is applied. Downward pressure is exerted on one extended limb and upward pressure on the other as traction is applied. If no progress is made, delivery by cesarean section may be necessary. If there is good access to the uterus and the calf is dead, delivery by fetotomy may be attempted.

It should be remembered that in some cases of apparent malposition the cause of the problem may be torsion of the uterus, in which case a degree of vaginal narrowing may be detected. For details of diagnosis and treatment of uterine torsion, see the section Obstruction of the birth canal (p. 43).

Malposture

Abnormality of posture may involve the head, forelimbs, hindlimbs, or a combination of these. In some surveys lateral deviation of the head and carpal flexion have been recorded as the most common malpostures in cattle.

Lateral deviation of the head

Clinical signs   The fetal forelegs are normally found within the vagina and the feet may protrude through the vulva. The head may not be immediately palpable but as the forelegs are traced upwards the base of the neck is palpable and further examination will indicate the position of the head. Occasionally the fetal neck is rotated axially and the fetal mandibles are uppermost. The head is usually found lying against the rib cage and in more extreme cases – especially when fetal size is small – may be almost beyond reach near the fetal rump.

Treatment   The fetus is repelled, the muzzle is located and covered by the obstetrician's hand before being guided round in the arc of a circle and up into the pelvis (Fig. 4.7). If the muzzle is just beyond reach the fetal head can be safely grasped using the eye sockets. A calving rope may be looped around the lower jaw, tightened, and used to pull the head round with one hand while the obstetrician's other hand protects the uterus from damage by the calf's muzzle and teeth. The rope should not be used thus attached to apply traction to the calf. If the head is even further forward traction may be applied to the bend in the neck in an attempt to bring the head within reach. If it is impossible to correct the malpresentation it may be necessary to perform cesarean section or fetotomy.

Downward deviation of the head

Clinical signs   Varying degrees of this condition are seen. In mild cases the fetal nose rests on the pelvic brim in the *vertex posture* (Fig. 5.5). In more severely abnormal cases the head may be deviated downwards between the forelimbs and adjacent to the sternum in the *breast–head posture*.

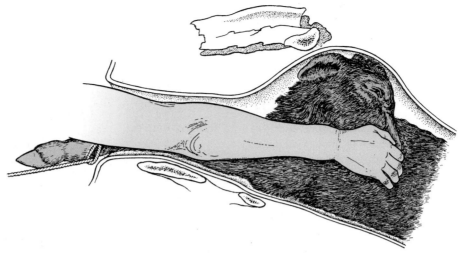

Figure 4.7 Correction of fetal malposture – lateral deviation of the head.

Treatment Having located the forelimbs in the vagina, a search for the head is made. The vertex posture is corrected by repelling the fetus and lifting the muzzle up into the pelvis. If the head is displaced below the forelimbs there may be insufficient room to bring it up into the pelvis unless one of the forelimbs is flexed and pushed back into the uterus. Once the head has been retrieved, the forelimb is relocated and the calf delivered by traction. In cases where great difficulty is encountered in attempting to bring the head up the cow may be cast, rolled on her back, and her legs secured. Gravitational forces may then assist in bringing the fetal head down into the pelvis. If manipulative delivery proves impossible, delivery must be performed by cesarean section or fetotomy.

Retention of a forelimb

This may involve carpal flexion or shoulder flexion affecting one or both forelimbs. Incomplete extension of the elbow, which causes dystocia in mares, is seldom encountered in the cow.

1. Carpal flexion

Clinical signs If only one leg is involved, the normal leg and the head are found within or protruding from the vagina. The flexed carpus of the other foreleg is found at the pelvic inlet or impacted in the vagina.
Treatment The fetus is repelled and the flexed carpus pushed upwards and forwards from the obstetrician so

that the missing foot can be found more readily. The foot is cupped in the hand and brought carefully up into the pelvis (Figs 4.8 and 4.9). Occasionally, maternal straining or lack of space can make this maneuver difficult because the obstetrician is trying to raise the carpus and retrieve the fetal foot at the same time. In this case a calving rope can be placed around the fetlock and is used to bring the foot within reach while the obstetrician repels the carpus. Once the foot is within reach it must be cupped in the hand and brought into the pelvis as before. In rare cases where manipulation is impossible and the calf is dead fetotomy may be required.

2. Shoulder flexion

Clinical signs If both legs are involved the fetal head alone may be found in the vagina or protrude from the vulva, where it may become swollen and edematous. If only one limb is affected the other limb often protrudes from the vulva with the head.
Treatment The fetus is repelled to allow the retained limb to be found and manipulated into its correct position (Fig. 4.10). If the head is grossly swollen, generous lubrication and firm pressure are needed to push it back into the vulva and towards the uterus. If the calf is dead and repulsion difficult, the head may be amputated using a scalpel or the embryotome. Once the calf has been repelled the missing limb or limbs are located by searching the uterus methodically. The calf's neck is followed down to the shoulder.

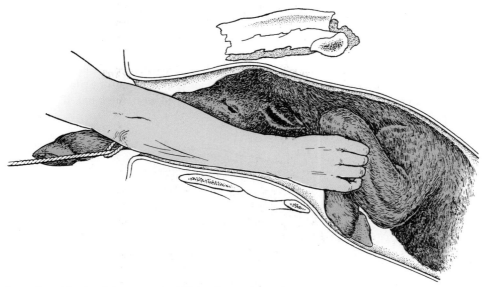

Figure 4.8 Correction of fetal malposture – carpal flexion (stage 1); see the text.

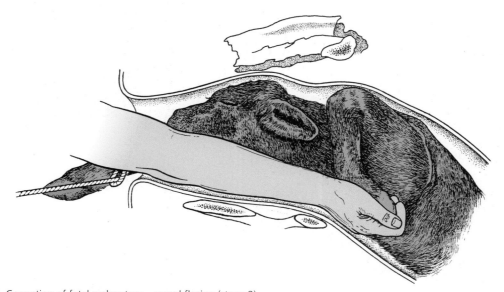

Figure 4.9 Correction of fetal malposture – carpal flexion (stage 2).

The obstetrician's hand is advanced down the limb towards the carpal joint. The limb is grasped and brought up into the carpal flexion position, and then the foot is brought into the pelvis as described above. In some cases it may help to loop a calving rope around the retained limb and slip it down towards the carpus. Gentle traction on the rope will bring the carpal joint within reach of the fingers. If correction of the malpresentation is impossible delivery is by cesarean section or fetotomy.

Retention of a hindlimb

This occurs in some cases of posterior presentation and may involve hock flexion or hip flexion of one or both hind limbs.

1. Hock flexion

Clinical signs The tip of the fetal tail may protrude from the vulva and the flexed hocks are palpable either at the pelvic inlet or impacted within the pelvis. If only one limb is flexed at the hock the other may extend through the vulva.

Treatment   This is aimed at extending the flexed limb and bringing the foot up into the pelvis. Great care must be taken to ensure that the uterus is not damaged in this manipulation. Plenty of lubrication is essential and the fetus is carefully repelled by pressure on its perineal region. One of the fetal hindfeet is located and cupped in the obstetrician's hand. The foot is drawn backwards and upwards in the arc of a circle into the pelvis (Fig. 4.11). Upward pressure is exerted on the hock. In some cases both movements (raising the foot and exerting pressure on the hock) can be accomplished with one hand. If this is impossible the

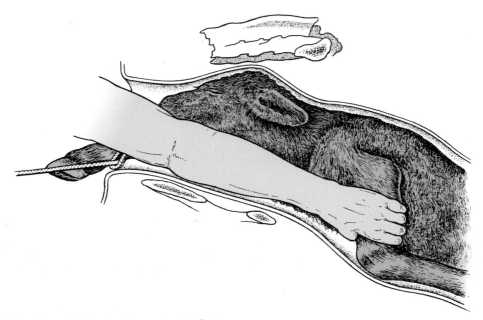

Figure 4.10 Correction of fetal malposture – shoulder flexion.

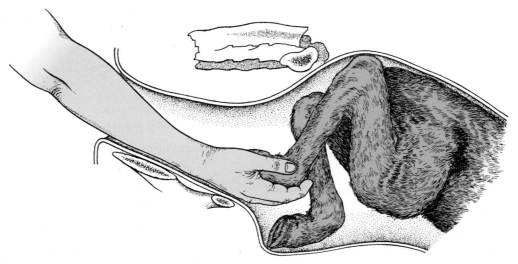

Figure 4.11 Correction of fetal malposture – hock flexion.

obstetrician may have to transfer from one position to the other. Alternatively, an assistant can be asked to push the hock upwards while the obstetrician deals with the foot. (A small obstetrician may be able to insert both hands into the uterus and carry out both procedures at once.) A calving rope can be looped round the pastern joint and then taken between the hooves and used to gently lift the foot backwards and upwards while the obstetrician pushes up on the hock joint. Care must still be taken to protect the uterus from damage by the fetal hoof. The second leg is dealt with in a similar fashion. Lack of space may make the manipulation more difficult with the second limb and further repulsion may be required to provide room in which to extend this limb.

If the hock joint is ankylosed and the fetus is dead the lower limb is sawn through just below the hock with the embryotome.

2. Hip flexion (breech presentation)

Clinical signs   The tail may protrude from the vulva or be held against the fetal flank. The fetal hindquarters are palpable on vaginal examination (see Fig. 12.8). The hindquarters may be level with the pelvic inlet or lying in front of and below the level of the pelvic floor. Occasionally, only one limb is retained and the other is in the normal extended position.

Treatment   The aim of treatment is to convert the hip flexion into hock flexion and then extend the limb(s) into an uncomplicated posterior presentation. The fetus is repelled by exerting pressure on the rump and the obstetrician reaches down one of the limbs to locate the hock joint, which is pulled backwards and upwards into the flexed position. It may help to pass a calving rope round the limb and slide it down to the hock. Gentle traction on the rope may help bring the hock joint within reach. With the hoof cupped in the hand, the flexed hock is extended into the pelvis (as described above in the section Hock flexion). The second limb is dealt with in a similar manner. These manipulations may be aided by the administration of epidural anesthesia and clenbuterol. It is not possible to deliver a calf in an uncorrected hip flexion malposture. This should not be attempted in cattle as severe damage may be sustained by the birth canal.

If manual correction of the malposture is impossible the limbs may be removed by fetotomy (see Fig 12.8) in the dead fetus while in the living calf cesarean section may be required.

Simultaneous presentation

Twinning and multiple birth

Twinning occurs in about 3% of all calvings. Triplets are much less common and higher numbers of calves, up to 11, have been recorded on rare occasions in the literature. Whenever a calf has been delivered the obstetrician should always search the uterus to ensure that no further fetus remains.

The cow is not well equipped to deal with multiple birth and a number of problems may occur during pregnancy and at parturition. Attempts to induce twin pregnancy either by superovulation or by implantation of twin embryos have not always met with good results. The incidence of both uterine inertia and of retention of the fetal membranes is higher than with a normal singleton birth.

Dystocia in twinning and multiple birth can arise in a number of ways:

- Uterine inertia: caused especially by overstretching of the myometrium.
- Simultaneous presentation of two or more fetuses: the fetuses may be in the same presentation (usually anterior or posterior) or one may be in anterior and the other in posterior presentation.
- Maldisposition of the first, the second, or subsequent fetuses.

Clinical signs   Twins may be suspected or anticipated as a result of a larger than normal abdominal size during pregnancy, by recognition of twins on ultrasonographic pregnancy diagnosis, or following implantation of twin embryos. Signs of dystocia vary with the exact nature of the problem. Careful vaginal examination will indicate the presence of more than one calf. Great care should always be taken in any delivery to determine if the fetal parts presented belong to one or more than one fetus. This is achieved by methodically following all the palpable extremities back to the body to ascertain their origin. If two heads or two sets of forelegs are palpable they probably belong to two calves but the remote possibility of a double-headed monster or an additional pair of limbs should be borne in mind. The obstetrician should try to build up a mental picture of the position of the extremities and their origin (Fig. 4.12). Gentle repulsion of one calf may help identify which limbs belong to that calf, as they will go back into the uterus with the repelled body.

Treatment   After carefully sorting out the disposition of the fetuses an attempt should be made to deliver

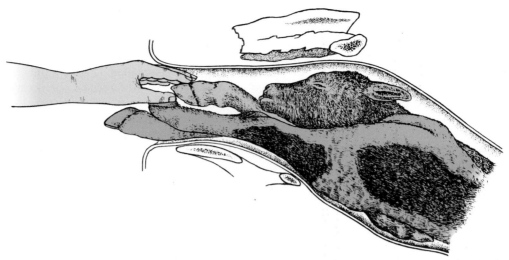

Figure 4.12 Dystocia caused by simultaneous presentation of twins. The twin in anterior presentation has a flexed left shoulder.

one after it has been placed, if necessary, into the correct presentation. If one calf is closer to the pelvic inlet or birth canal than the other this calf should be delivered first, followed by the second. If one calf is in posterior presentation this should be delivered first because only two extremities – the hindlimbs – have to be manipulated into the pelvis. After delivery of the second calf the uterus must be carefully checked to ensure that another calf is not present. Following the delivery of multiple calves uterine involution and placental passage may be encouraged by administration of 20 IU oxytocin by intramuscular injection.

DYSTOCIA CAUSED BY FETAL DEATH

Death of the fetus in late pregnancy or in the early stages of parturition may result in dystocia, which may arise in a number of ways:

- The fetus may have suffered from chronic hypoxia during pregnancy, possibly as a result of an ineffective placenta. This situation may arise especially in first-calf heifers, which show little preparation for calving and in which the fetus is found to be dead when signs of impending delivery eventually occur.
- The fetus may fail to release sufficient quantities of those hormones, including ACTH and cortisol, that initiate parturition.
- The fetus is unable to adopt the normal birth posture and thus maldisposition may occur, preventing birth.

- The cervix may fail to dilate fully – thus not allowing the fetus to pass.
- Uterine fluids may be lost and fetal delivery may be impeded by absence of natural lubrication.

When numbers of cases of stillbirth and dystocia caused by fetal death are encountered in a herd, further investigations are advisable. The management of the cattle during late pregnancy and at calving should be reviewed. Could the farm staff be missing early signs of dystocia and not seeking help until too late? The role of iodine deficiency in the etiology of fetal death in late pregnancy is unclear but there is some evidence that *Leptospira hardjo* or *Neospora caninum* may be involved in some cases. Low-grade pregnancy toxemia may reduce the responses of the maternal body to the initiation of parturition by the fetus.

Clinical signs The first sign of fetal death may be a foul-smelling vaginal discharge at the time that birth is anticipated. Investigation will reveal a partially or fully dilated cervix through which may protrude necrotic fetal membranes and parts of the fetus. If infection has gained access to the fetus through the cervix the fetus may be bloated and emphysematous. Pockets of gas are palpable beneath the fetal skin and the hair is readily pulled out. The loss of fetal fluids makes it difficult for the obstetrician's hand to move around in the uterus, the walls of which are tightly applied to the dead fetus. There is no sign of fetal life. If the fetus has been ill before death it may have developed fetal ascites with gross abdominal enlargement. In the early stages the cow may be quite unaffected but in a proportion of cases severe life-threatening metritis with toxemia ensues. Fetal death earlier in pregnancy may result in abortion, fetal mummification, or fetal maceration (described in Chapter 2).

Treatment   If the cervix is dilated an attempt is made to deliver the fetus by traction per vaginam. The obstetrician's hands and arms should be protected in such cases by arm-length plastic gloves. Obstetric lubricant is introduced by hand into the uterus and applied to the presenting parts of the fetus. If conditions in the uterus are very dry, warm water may be carefully introduced into the uterus using a stomach pump and tube. Traction is applied to the fetus either directly by hand or through calving ropes attached in the normal way. If the fetus is decayed traction may result in one or more of the extremities being pulled off. In such cases the remainder of the fetus is delivered manually, aided if necessary by fetotomy.

The emphysematous fetus may seem much too large to pass through even a fully dilated cervix. With ample, frequently applied lubrication resistance can usually be overcome without the cow sustaining damage. In some cases fetal volume may be reduced by incising into some emphysematous parts of the skin to release the gas. The abdominal size of the ascitic calf can be reduced by draining the fetal abdomen if access can be gained.

If manual delivery of the dead fetus is not possible it may be delivered by fetotomy or cesarean section. Both procedures in these circumstances carry a severe risk to maternal health but may be the only course available.

SIGNS OF DYSTOCIA IN THE COW

Identifying the exact point at which normal birth ceases and dystocia occurs is not easy. Although the overall duration of calving varies considerably there should be evidence of continuous progress during fetal delivery. Birth may be slower in certain breeds, such as the Charolais, or if the calf is relatively large. The calf can survive for up to 8 hours during second-stage labor but delivery time is normally much shorter than this. Any apparent or suspected departure from the normal should be investigated. Specific signs of dystocia include:

- Prolonged, non-progressive, first-stage labor.
- The cow standing in an abnormal posture during first-stage labor – in cases of uterine torsion the cow may stand with a dipped back in the 'saw horse' posture.

- Straining vigorously for 30 minutes without the appearance of a calf.
- Failure of the calf to be delivered within 2 hours of the amnion appearing at the vulva.
- Obvious malpresentation, malposture, or maldisposition – for example the appearance of the fetal head but no forelimbs, the tail but no hindlimbs, the head and a single forelimb.
- The appearance of detached chorioallantois, fetal meconium, or blood-stained amniotic fluid at the vulva. These signs suggest that fetal hypoxia may be present and that fetal death may have occurred.

APPROACH TO A CASE OF DYSTOCIA IN THE COW

Cases of bovine dystocia should be attended without delay. The history of the case should be taken and a general clinical assessment and examination should be carried out as discussed in the chapter on the Clinical Management of Cases of Dystocia (Chapter 3).

OBSTETRICIAN'S CHECK LIST

Call received

- Brief history taken
- Check drugs and equipment
- Attend case as quickly as possible

Assistance required

Ideally, the obstetrician should have the help of three assistants: one to manage the head of the patient and two to assist with fetal delivery at her rear end. They also help prevent the cow from swinging her rear end around during examination and treatment. On many occasions this number of helpers is not available on a farm. If severe problems are anticipated or encountered treatment may have to be delayed until sufficient help has been assembled.

Restraint of the patient

If possible, the patient should be examined in a clean, well-lit, and sheltered area. If necessary and practical she should be moved to such a place before treatment is commenced. The cow's head should be restrained in quick-release fashion with a halter or – initially – in a crush. The head should be tied low to allow the cow to lie down with ease during delivery if she wishes. She must also be able to arch her back with ease to allow the tilting of her pelvis, which facilitates fetal passage. Once secured, however, the confines of a standard crush allow insufficient room for assisted delivery – a problem avoided by having swinging side gates. Where facilities are less sophisticated the cow can be secured behind a gate.

Sedation

In some cases – especially with nervous, unhandled heifers – sedation with xylazine may be required before an internal examination can be performed with safety. Sufficient sedation is normally achieved by giving the patient 5 mg of xylazine per 100 kg body weight by intramuscular injection. Although currently not licensed in some countries for administration by this route, 10–15 mg of xylazine given by intravenous injection into a vein of a 450 kg cow has been found useful. Xylazine may increase the strength of myometrial contractions but this normally presents no problem. Heavy sedation may produce recumbency, which may make some procedures such as fetal manipulation more difficult.

Uterine relaxation

This may occasionally be required if strong myometrial contractions are obstructing an obstetrical maneuver such as correction of a malposture. Clenbuterol at a dose of 300 μg for the average cow given by intramuscular injection will cause uterine relaxation in such circumstances or reduce the strength of uterine contractions that were increased by the use of xylazine.

Epidural anesthesia

This is only required at calving if intense maternal straining makes procedures such as fetal repulsion very difficult. Frequent maternal defecation is suppressed by epidural anesthesia but so is any maternal assistance with delivery. Myometrial activity is unaffected. In the average cow, 7 mL of 2% lidocaine (lignocaine) given via the space between the first and second coccygeal vertebrae is effective in controlling straining while maintaining the patient's ability to stand.

Equipment

- A clean, waterproof parturition gown and overtrousers with Wellington boots are advised. Unless infection is suspected or the obstetrician's arms are sensitive to bovine vaginal secretions, protective sleeves and gloves are not normally worn.
- Three nylon calving ropes of different colors with short wooden cylindrical handles to which they may be attached. Calving chains with detachable handles may be substituted for two of the ropes if preferred, but at least one rope is required as chains are unsuitable for attachment to the fetal head. Ropes and chains should be sterilized after use and maintained until needed in sterile containers.
- A calf puller such as the HK or the Vink model is extremely useful in careful professional hands when little help is available.
- A sterile surgical kit for cesarean section (see Chapter 11) and also suture material for general use. Two pairs of artery forceps in case of vaginal or other hemorrhage. Electric clippers and skin dressing for skin preparation in case of surgery. An extension lead and portable halogen light.
- A fetotomy set – if available.
- Obstetric lubricant – synthetic colloidal gels are very useful and at least 750 mL should be available for a calving. Some obstetric lubricants are available in powdered form and are mixed with clean warm water before use. Soap and water can be used as a lubricant but tends to disperse natural lubricants. In emergency lard, liquid paraffin, etc. may be used.
- Drugs – oxytocin, calcium borogluconate/calcium: magnesium:phosphorus:dextrose solutions, injectable antibiotics, uterine pessaries, a non-steroidal anti-inflammatory drug such as flunixin or ketoprofen, tetanus antitoxin, local anesthesia, clenbuterol. An antiseptic such as chlorhexidene.
- Warm water – at least 5 liters in a plastic container should be taken to cases where no supply is known to be available.
- Equipment for resuscitation of the calf should this be necessary. In particular, doxapram hydrochloride should always be available to stimulate respiration.

Case history

A case history is taken on arrival (see Chapter 3).

General clinical examination of cow

This is also discussed in the Chapter 3. Special attention must be paid to the cow's udder to ensure that there is no evidence of developing coliform mastitis. Fetal movement may be noticed at the cow's left flank and, if this is vigorous, it may indicate that placental separation is causing fetal hypoxia and hypermotility.

Signs of placental separation may be seen at the vulva if parts of the chorioallantois with detached cotyledons are visible (Fig. 4.13). An unpleasant fetid odor may suggest that the fetus is dead. A light yellowish-green vaginal discharge may indicate fetal hypoxia with associated expulsion of meconium. The presence of visible fetal parts and their relative position may give a preliminary indication that fetal presentation is normal or abnormal. If the fetal head has been within the birth canal for some time the fetal tongue may have become swollen and slightly cyanotic in appearance.

Vaginal examination

The whole perineal region around the vulva is carefully washed with warm water containing a mild antiseptic.

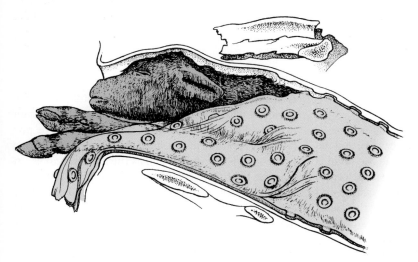

Figure 4.13 Signs of placenta separation before birth of the calf.

The vulval lips are examined and parted gently to enable the vestibule to be seen. If fetal parts or fetal membranes are protruding, complete inspection of this area may not be easy. Any fetal membranes should be identified. The chorioallantois normally breaks quite early in the calving process. It is a pale blue membrane with fine blood vessels and is attached by cotyledons to the uterine wall. The amnion, which may still be intact as the 'water bag' is gray, transparent, and virtually avascular. Care should be taken not to rupture the amnion at this stage of the examination. Premature rupture of the amnion *may* lead to an increased rate of stillbirth, loss of natural lubrication, and inefficiency of uterine contractions. The moistness and color of the vaginal mucosa is noted as is evidence of pressure necrosis, bruising, previous scarring, or any abnormal discharge or odor. Fresh blood may arise from the fetal placenta or from damage to the soft tissues of the birth canal and unless profuse is probably not significant. The lubricated hand held with the fingers and thumb arranged in a cone shape is introduced into the vagina.

OBSTETRICIAN'S CHECK LIST

Inspect vulva

Vaginal discharge?
↓
Presence of unpleasant odor?
↓
Presence of fetal membranes?
↓
Which membranes are present?
↓
State of fetal membranes
↓
Are they fresh or decayed?
↓
Presence of fetal parts?
↓
Identification of fetal parts

The degree of dilation, elasticity of the walls, and the degree of existing lubrication is noted. As the hand is advanced it passes over the external urethral orifice with its diverticulum, which will admit a finger tip and lies on the vaginal floor where it passes over the pubis. The presence of any tears, abnormal structures, or fibrosis is noted and may suggest either damage at an earlier calving or lay interference. The hand is advanced towards the cervix, which is mostly situated just anterior to the pelvic brim. If the cervix is closed the protruding but softening external os (sometimes containing a mucus plug) can be identified but when fully dilated the cervix cannot be distinguished as the vaginal wall continues as the uterine wall. If the cervix is partially closed it should be palpated for evidence of scar tissue and the obstetrician's hand is opened from within the cervix to see if it can be dilated further.

It is quite easy to fail to recognize the closed cervix in cases where the fetal forelimbs have entered the bony pelvic canal. The limbs may be thought to be within the vagina still enclosed in the fetal membranes when in fact the cervix, which may be ventrally displaced (Fig. 4.14), is tightly closed and the calf is still fully within the uterus. This error should be avoided if careful and systematic examination of the anterior vagina is routinely performed.

If the cervix cannot be detected but the passage of the hand is obstructed by a spiraling vaginal wall uterine torsion (see above) may be present. The uterine wall is beyond the cervix and is recognized by the presence of elevated caruncles mostly still attached to the placental cotyledons. Less commonly access to the uterus may be obstructed by downward deviation of the uterus (see above).

The size of the bony pelvis should next be determined. The dorsoventral diameter extends from the sacrum above to the pubis below while the lateral diameter extends between the inner surfaces of the wings of the ilia. The size of these diameters can be estimated in handbreadths as the obstetrician's hand moves from side to side and up and down enclosed in the vagina.

The presence of a fetus within the birth canal may make some of the above observations difficult or impossible since the fetus may occupy most of the space available leaving little room for the obstetrician's hand.

Examination of the fetus

As it approaches the vulva, the bovine fetus is normally enclosed within the amnion. The distended amnion helps to dilate the birth canal and should not be purposefully ruptured at this stage. Accidental rupture may occur (and is not disastrous) as the obstetrician examines the birth canal. The amniotic fluid, if healthy, is thick, slippery, and pale yellow in color. The fetus is examined with the hand to determine its presentation, position, and posture. In hypoxic fetuses the amniotic fluid may be stained green by fetal meconium and if the fetus is dead the fluid may have a fetid smell.

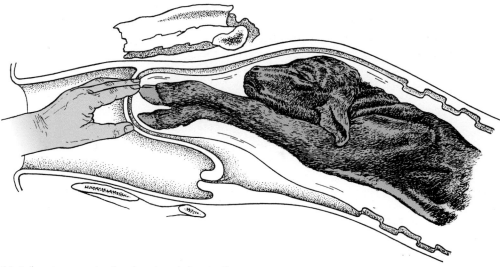

Figure 4.14 Failure to recognize the closed cervix (see text).

Examination of the fetus must be done methodically and with care. In normal presentation a fetal foot is often the first structure encountered and it must be identified as either a fore- or hindfoot. The limb is examined from the hoof upwards attempting to identify each joint and the direction in which it flexes. If the calf is large the degree of joint flexion possible may be very limited. The limbs are identified as indicated below:

- *Forelimb*: fetlock and carpus flex in the same direction followed by elbow in the opposite direction. The shoulder flexes in the opposite direction to the elbow and the obstetrician's hand passes upwards onto the neck and head and downwards onto the thoracic wall (Fig. 4.15 top).
- *Hindlimb*: fetlock and hock flex in the opposite direction. The stifle flexes in the opposite direction to the hock. The obstetrician's hand passes up from the stifle region onto the hip, hindquarters and adjacent tail (Fig. 4.15 bottom).

Note: It is extremely important to identify the lower portions of the limbs with great care because an initial error can be compounded higher up the limb with elbow and hock and also stifle and shoulder being confused. If two limbs are present, careful palpation and relating them to other parts of the fetal body should enable the obstetrician to ascertain whether they belong to the same or two different calves. The obstetrician should try to build up a mental picture of the disposition of the fetus. The arms tire easily while this inspection is being done and taking a short rest outside the birth canal will enable muscles to relax and fingers to become more sensitive again. However, insertion and removal of the hands and arms increases the risk of damage to the birth canal and, despite the above advice, should be kept to a minimum.

It should now be possible to describe the presentation, position, and posture of the fetus. The calf should be in an anterior longitudinal presentation, dorsal position, and in a posture in which the extended head and neck are resting on the extended forelimbs.

Evidence of fetal life

- Positive response to pedal withdrawal and palpebral reflexes.
- Response to pressure on the eyeball or pinching the nose or ear.
- Sucking reflex if fingers are placed in the calf's mouth.
- Contraction of the anal sphincter when a finger is inserted.
- Spontaneous movement of the fetus, but excessive movements of the extremities or the tongue may indicate a developing hypoxia. Discoloration of the amniotic fluid with green meconium is a further sign of fetal compromise. Fetal breathing or bellowing

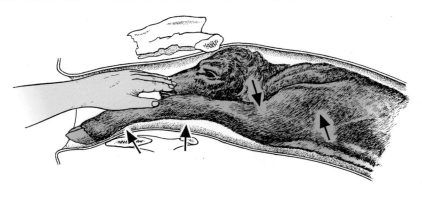

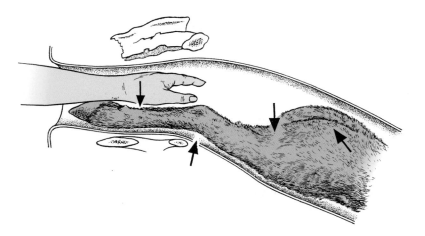

within the uterus may indicate impending placental collapse and imminent fetal death. Delivery in such cases should be immediate but passage through the birth canal without the support of placental circulation is a life-threatening experience for such fetuses and there may be insufficient time for a cesarean section. Apparent spontaneous but not genuine fetal movement can be caused by straining activity in the cow.

Note: a negative response to appraisal of reflexes does not necessarily confirm fetal death, especially in cases where the fetus is so tightly impacted in the birth canal that it is unable to move in response to stimuli. Less commonly, a non-responsive fetus may simply be in a somnolent phase.

- If the fetal head is protruding from the vulva the ocular mucous membranes may be inspected. They should be pink in a healthy, well-oxygenated calf. Cyanosis indicates at least a degree of hypoxia. Extreme pallor of the membranes may suggest that the fetus is severely anoxic.

- Detection of fetal pulse in the metacarpus or metatarsus is occasionally possible but is also made difficult by maternal straining.

If sophisticated equipment is available the following may be tried but straining movements of the cow make recording difficult:

- Detection of heart beat by Doppler or B-mode ultrasonography or by detection of the fetal electrocardiograph. A long Doppler rectal probe can be inserted alongside a small fetus to rest against the chest wall giving clear signal of the heart rate.
- Po_2 and Pco_2 in the fetal blood can be measured if a blood-gas machine is available. A blood sample is taken from the metacarpal or metatarsal vein of the calf if the vessels are accessible. An immediate estimation of Po_2 and the fetal pulse rate can be obtained by means of pulse oximetry techniques. The attachment of a pulse oximeter to the ear or tongue of the calf during delivery is not always easy.

Evidence of fetal death

- Absence of positive signs of life (subject to the caveat concerning impacted fetuses).
- Blood staining of the amniotic fluid occurs 12 hours after fetal death and the development of corneal opacity commences; 72 hours after death collapse of the eyeball may begin – a useful observation if the fetal head is visible or palpable.
- Sterile autolysis of the fetus commences immediately after fetal death and if infection gains access via the cervix, putrefactive decay occurs with fetal emphysema and possibly the complication of septicemia and toxemia in the cow.
- Degeneration and separation of the placenta with loss of fetal fluids.

Obstetricians are strongly advised not to predict the successful birth of a living fetus at an early stage of the examination or before attempted delivery.

Rectal examination is seldom a useful routine procedure in evaluating cases of bovine dystocia except to detect displacement of the maternal broad ligament in cases of uterine torsion or if the cervix is undilated.

DIAGNOSIS OF THE CAUSE OF DYSTOCIA AND THE PLAN FOR ITS TREATMENT

As a result of the above vaginal examination, the disposition of the calf should be known and there should be an indication of the cause of dystocia and state of the fetus.

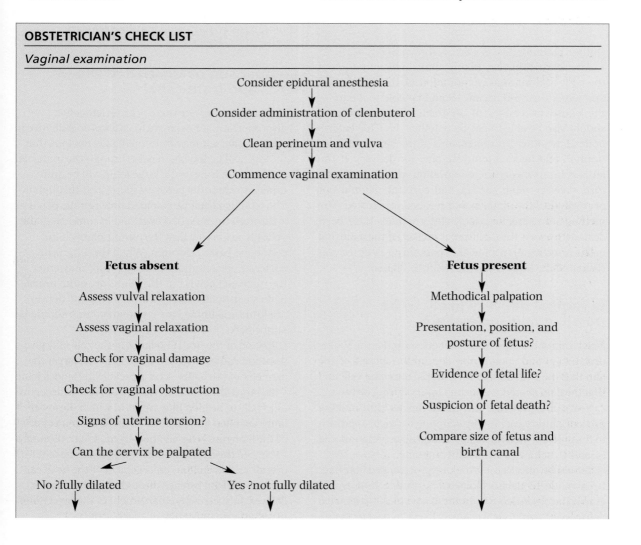

OBSTETRICIAN'S CHECK LIST

Vaginal examination

Consider epidural anesthesia

Consider administration of clenbuterol

Clean perineum and vulva

Commence vaginal examination

Fetus absent

Assess vulval relaxation

Assess vaginal relaxation

Check for vaginal damage

Check for vaginal obstruction

Signs of uterine torsion?

Can the cervix be palpated

No ?fully dilated   Yes ?not fully dilated

Fetus present

Methodical palpation

Presentation, position, and posture of fetus?

Evidence of fetal life?

Suspicion of fetal death?

Compare size of fetus and birth canal

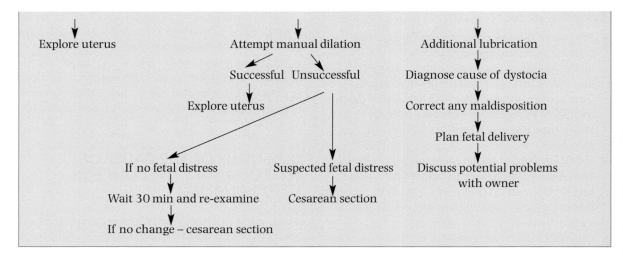

MANIPULATIVE DELIVERY

Outline plans for delivery are as shown in Fig. 4.16.

After careful history taking, clinical examination of the cow, and manual examination of the birth canal and fetus, the obstetrician should be able to diagnose the cause or causes of dystocia. The obstetrician should also be able to decide whether the fetus is alive or dead, whether the dimensions of the birth canal are normal, and make a tentative plan for delivery. If the fetus is in an incorrect presentation, position, or posture, delivery often cannot and certainly should not proceed until the abnormality has been corrected. The methods of correcting such abnormalities have been dealt with above. Fetal delivery is unlikely if the maternal pelvis is too small to allow it to pass through or the soft tissues of the birth canal are not fully dilated.

Is vaginal delivery likely to be possible and successful?

This is one of the most important questions for the bovine obstetrician and upon it may depend the success of the aim that the fetus should be delivered alive and well and that the dam should not sustain injury during delivery.

Years of experience may make the decision-making process a little easier but by adopting a logical approach to the problem even an inexperienced obstetrician should be able to achieve a successful outcome.

To simplify the decision-making process, attempts have been made to devise foolproof formulae that would enable the obstetrician to decide in advance of attempted delivery if vaginal delivery was likely to be successful.

Such formulae have not been found to be reliable and in most cases trial traction may be necessary.

Comparison of the size of the fetus and birth canal

- In some cases where there is gross fetopelvic disproportion, for example in cases of misalliance in young heifers, it may be immediately obvious that the calf will be too big to pass through the maternal pelvis. In such cases the large fetus will be quite unable to enter the pelvis let alone pass through it. The fetal head can be palpated through the pelvis as if through the bars of a cage and in some cases the pelvis is so narrow that the obstetrician's hand cannot be passed through. When the fetus is in posterior presentation the lower limbs may enter the maternal pelvis but the thighs are quite unable to do so. In such cases attempts at vaginal delivery are futile and immediate cesarean section should be performed.
- Palpation of the head and limbs of the calf may give some indication of its size. In general, the larger the diameter of the limbs – and especially the fetlock joints – the larger the calf. This observation can be deceptive, especially in Belgian Blue cattle, in which the lower limbs are often quite slender whereas the upper parts of the limbs are large and heavily muscled. Although the size of the fetal head can be an indication of its overall size, edematous enlargement of the head can occur if the fetal passage through the birth canal is delayed. In such cases enlargement of the head is not necessarily an indication of a large calf.

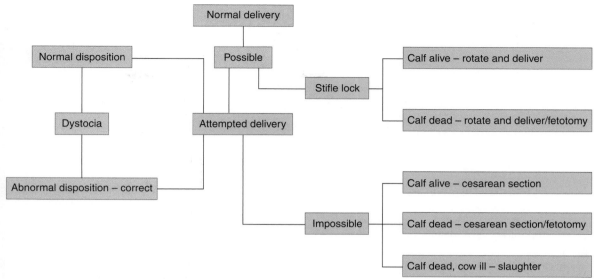

Figure 4.16 Outline plan for manipulative delivery (modified from Schuijt & Ball 1980).

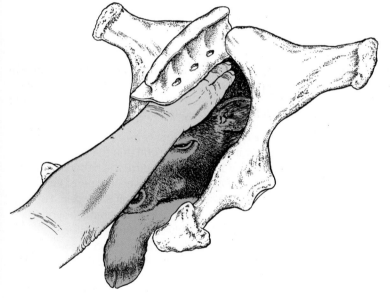

Figure 4.17 Comparison of the size of the fetus and the birth canal.

- The posture of the calf may also give an indication of its size. If the forelimbs are crossed-over within the birth canal it may indicate tight intrapelvic pressure forcing the elbows medially. This is not an entirely reliable observation because crossing of the forelimbs may also occur in very small calves.
- Detailed comparison of the size of the fetus and the birth canal is normally carried out as part of the vaginal examination. The lubricated hand is advanced to the presenting parts of the fetus within the pelvis

and is then moved in a circular fashion around the fetus, estimating the amount of space between fetus and pelvis (Fig. 4.17). The widest parts of the calf are normally the shoulders and pelvis. The narrowest parts of the maternal bony pelvis are normally the sacropubic diameter in the dorsoventral plane and the interilial diameter laterally. If the fetal head is tightly wedged into the pelvis it is unlikely that the fetal shoulders will be able to pass through. If the obstetrician's hand can be passed with ease around

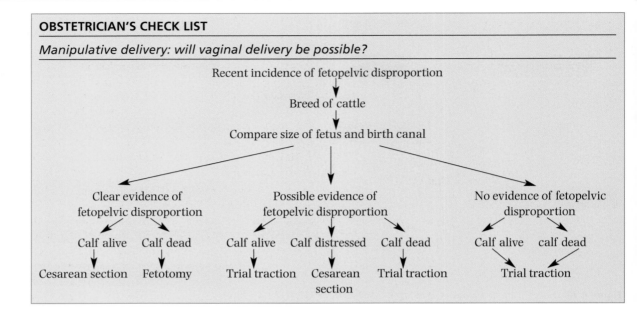

OBSTETRICIAN'S CHECK LIST

Manipulative delivery: will vaginal delivery be possible?

the fetal shoulders within the maternal pelvis then fetal delivery per vaginam should normally be possible.

- When the calf is in posterior presentation the obstetrician's hand is moved up the hindlimbs of the calf in an attempt to palpate the hindquarters and to see whether the hand can be passed between them and the maternal pelvis. If the hand can pass readily between the maternal pelvis and the hindquarters of the calf, including the thighs, hips, and tail head then vaginal delivery is likely to be possible. If the lower limbs only have entered the maternal pelvis and are occupying most of the available space it is unlikely that the wider thighs, hips and tail head will be able to enter or pass through the maternal pelvis.

- Trial traction: unless it is very clear that fetopelvic disproportion is present, an attempt at assisted delivery by 'traction', i.e. pulling, should be made. Traction should always be used with care and with limited force. *It must be remembered that the viability of the calf is often higher after cesarean section than it is after forced extraction.* Thus if it seems likely that great efforts will be needed to deliver the calf per vaginam, the chances of calf survival will be reduced. In such circumstances, cesarean section – if performed promptly – may give the calf a better chance of survival. If delivery is proving difficult, progress does not seem to be made, or it is felt there

is risk of damage to the fetus or its mother then traction must be abandoned for an operative delivery – usually cesarean section.

Trial traction

The following procedure is used:

1. The obstetrician should ensure adequate assistance is available and that the assistants are aware of how the procedure will be carried out.
2. The availability of all equipment required for assisting the delivery of the calf is checked. 100 mg doxapram hydrochloride is prepared in a syringe with a needle attached ready to administer immediately to the calf should spontaneous respiration not occur (see Resuscitation of the calf section, p. 75).
3. Strict hygiene and generous lubrication are used at all times.
4. The obstetrician checks again that the presentation, position, and posture of the fetus are normal.
5. Ropes or chains are applied to the fetus.
6. Traction is applied manually or with a calving aid or obstetric pulley.

Fetus in anterior presentation

Ropes are normally applied to both the fetal head and the forelimbs. If the head is fully within the pelvis or vagina

OBSTETRICIAN'S CHECK LIST

Preparing for trial traction

Minimum assistance required

Manual delivery – 2   Calving aid delivery – 1
   assistants   assistant

Assemble and check all equipment

Explain procedure to assistant(s)

Check restraint of patient

Ensure cow can arch her back

Ensure cow can lie down

Strict attention to hygiene

Ensure adequate lubrication

Check fetal presentation, position, and posture

and is unlikely to slip back then ropes need only be applied to the forelimbs. If there is any doubt it is safer to apply ropes to both the head and the legs. Chains may be used on the legs but are unsuitable for the head. If ropes are to be placed on both the head and legs of the calf, the head rope should always be placed in position first. If the leg ropes are attached first there may be insufficient room for the head rope to be placed in position with ease.

Application of the head rope A large loop is made in the end of the rope. The loop should always be larger than might seem necessary because it may be easily tightened when attached to the head but cannot be opened using one hand within the cow. The loop is carried into the vagina and placed carefully behind both ears of the calf. Before it is tightened, the lower end of the loop is placed within the mouth of the calf. Before tightening, a check is made to ensure the rope is still behind the ears of the calf – it can easily slip forward off the poll when the lower part is being placed in the mouth (Fig. 4.18A). Once the obstetrician is sure of the secure attachment of the head rope it is pulled tight and the end is handed to an assistant, who maintains gentle pressure on it while the leg ropes are attached to prevent it becoming loose.

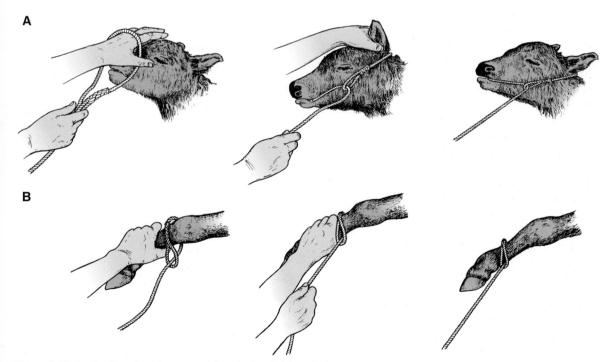

A

B

Figure 4.18 Application of calving ropes. (A) to the head, (B) to the leg.

Note: There are alternative methods of attaching the head rope but it should *never* be looped around the lower jaw – traction applied to the jaw can cause serious damage.

Application of the leg ropes A loop that is large enough to be slipped with ease over the calf's foot and slid up above the fetlock joint is made at the end of the calving rope. The loop is held in position with one hand and is then pulled tight with the other hand (Fig. 4.18B). Great care must be taken to ensure that the leg ropes are secured above the fetlock. If they are applied below the fetlock, damage to the joint or to the hooves can occur. Once the ropes are in position, gentle traction should be applied to them to prevent them coming loose and slipping down the limb.

Manual traction The ropes are attached to short lengths of broom handle using a clove hitch (Fig. 4.19). If chains are used, the handles are attached to their ends or along their lengths. The point of attachment in both cases is initially 25–30 cm from the calf. If two assistants are available, a leg rope is handed to each while the obstetrician or another assistant holds the head rope. Pulling is controlled by the obstetrician. The direction of pull is important – as the calf enters the pelvis the pull should be directed slightly dorsally; as the head passes through the pelvis it should be directed horizontally backwards; and once the head

has passed through the pelvis the direction of pull should be downward towards the cow's hocks. This subtle alteration of the direction of pull will allow advantage to be taken of the greatest diameters of the pelvis and also allow the calf to maintain a profile that will reduce its diameter.

It is essential that the cow is allowed to arch her back and hence tilt her own pelvis during both natural and assisted deliveries. Pulling the calf backwards instead of downwards and backwards will prevent her from doing this and from presenting the greatest dorsoventral pelvic diameter for the calf to pass through.

During delivery one foreleg should be pulled slightly in advance of the other. This will help reduce the width of the fetal shoulders as they pass through the pelvis.

Make a note of the time before commencing to pull the calf – it is essential to limit the duration of traction to a maximum of 10 minutes if little progress is being made.

Pulling should be timed to coincide with straining by the cow, thus increasing the efficiency of her efforts. Occasionally – and if epidural anesthesia has been used – no maternal straining occurs and the fetus must be delivered entirely by the obstetrician and assistants. As pulling commences, traction is applied to each rope in turn – right leg, left leg, and head.

Progress is watched carefully as delivery proceeds. If the calf moves easily backwards it is likely that

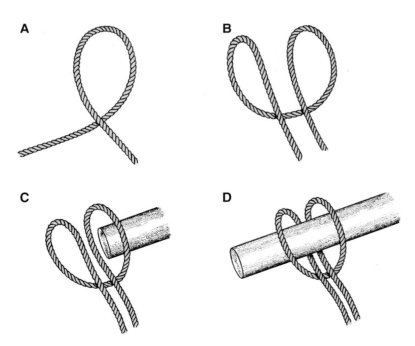

Figure 4.19 Manual traction – the ropes are attached to short lengths of broom handle using a clove hitch.

delivery will be comparatively easy. The greatest resistance to delivery occurs as the fetal shoulders and rib cage enter the maternal pelvis. Externally this coincides with the passage of the head through the vagina and vulva and it may appear to be the head that is causing difficulty.

The obstetrician should assist passage of the head through the caudal vagina and the vulva. The dorsal vaginal wall is quite fragile at this point and the poll of the fetal head can easily stretch and rupture the tissues, allowing prolapse of submucosal fat to occur. Damage can be prevented by pressing the fetal head downwards and using the back of the hand to elevate the dorsal vaginal wall (Fig. 4.20).

When the head and shoulders have passed through the vulva, traction should be applied simultaneously to the head and legs. At this stage delivery should be completed as soon as possible because the umbilical cord may be becoming compressed with a threat to fetal survival. The fetus can only survive for about 6 minutes without access to fresh supplies of oxygen. If the calf is large and it is thought that stifle lock may occur, the calf may be rotated through 45° after the head and shoulders have been delivered (see below).

Arrest of the fetus during delivery – stifle lock ('hip lock') During delivery, the calf – especially a large calf of the continental breeds – may appear to become stuck as the thorax of the calf passes through the vulva (Fig. 4.21). The cause of the problem is believed to be the impaction of the fetal stifles against the brim of the maternal pelvis. The calf may start to breathe because the umbilical cord is compressed but the efficiency of breathing is compromised by compression of the fetal abdomen and delivery should be

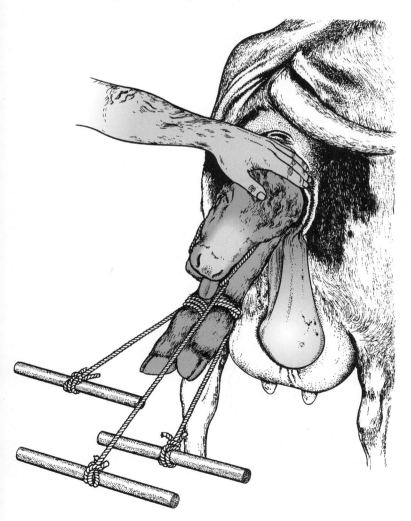

Figure 4.20 Assisting delivery of the head by pressing it downwards and elevating the dorsal vaginal wall.

Figure 4.21 Stifle lock can arrest the calf during delivery (see text).

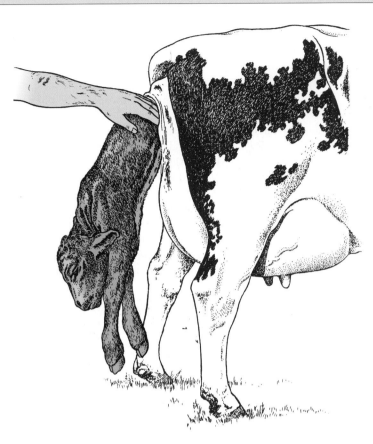

completed as soon as possible. In almost every case it is possible to overcome the problem of stifle lock if it occurs during assisted delivery. The problem is much more serious if it occurs during unattended delivery. In such cases the fetus becomes progressively more impacted into the maternal pelvis and spontaneous delivery becomes impossible (Fig. 4.22).

If the fetus becomes impacted with stifle lock during delivery it should be repelled slightly into the uterus and rotated through 45° about its long axis and traction applied again. If this fails, the obstetrician's arm should encircle the fetus, which is moved in a wide circle around the vulva while traction is maintained by the two assistants. By this method first one stifle and then the other is lifted into the pelvis and delivery is possible.

In very rare cases the fetus may remain impacted and its life becomes progressively at risk. In these circumstances it may help to cast the cow, roll her on her back, and try traction again – the forces of gravity helping the calf to occupy the widest dorsal part of the maternal pelvis and allowing the stifles to enter the pelvis.

If attempts at delivery of the fetus in stifle lock fail – and once the fetal thorax has been delivered it cannot be replaced in the uterus – the calf will inevitably die and may then be delivered by fetotomy (see Chapter 12).

Once the fetal pelvis has passed through the birth canal delivery is completed quickly, the calf is released from its calving ropes and it is examined for signs of life and resuscitated if necessary (see Resuscitation of the calf, p. 75). The calving ropes should be retrieved quickly to avoid them becoming lost in the bedding.

If the fetus fails to move through the birth canal at all during attempted delivery traction should be stopped. Further lubrication is placed around the fetus and it is carefully re-examined to ensure that a maldisposition has not been overlooked and that the extremities to which traction has been applied do belong to the same calf. If an error has been made it must be corrected and a further attempt at delivery by traction made. If the fetus is thought to be small enough to be delivered with ease but will not move, the possibility of a fetal monster – such as a conjoined twin – should be considered. In most cases

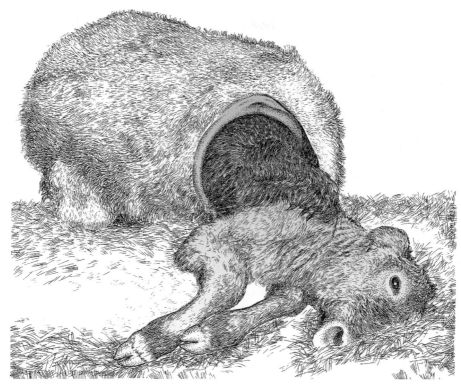

Figure 4.22 Impaction of the calf resulting from stifle lock in an unattended calving. Fetotomy is necessary.

it will be impossible to reach the hind end of the presenting fetus to confirm that this is the case.

If delivery by traction is not successful within 10 minutes it should be abandoned and the calf delivered by cesarean section if it is alive or by fetotomy or cesarean section if it is dead.

OBSTETRICIAN'S CHECK LIST

Delivery of calf in anterior presentation: manual delivery

Apply calving rope to head
↓
Apply calving ropes to forelegs
↓
Attach calving ropes to handles
↓
Pass one leg rope to each assistant
↓
Head rope – to assistant or obstetrician
↓
Apply traction as cow strains
↓
Note time traction first applied
↓
Advance one foreleg in front of the other
↓
Adjust direction of pull with stage of delivery
↓
Ease poll of calf through vulva
↓
Rotate calf through 45° if stifle lock occurs
↓
Complete delivery of calf

If no progress in 10 minutes
↓
Check presentation, position and posture
↓
Consider further brief trial traction/
cesarean section

Application of traction by calving aid or pulleys

Although the use of mechanical calving aids is banned in some countries they are nonetheless extremely useful and safe in professional hands. In cases where only one assistant is available, judicious use of the calving aid may be the means by which the calf can be safely delivered.

Whenever calving aids are used the obstetrician must always be aware of the potential force of their pull. The aid can exert a pulling force of 400 kg, compared with a force of 150 kg exerted by two persons pulling and the normal expulsive force of the calving cow, estimated at 75 kg. Excessive traction can cause severe damage to the calf. Fracture of one or both metacarpals may occur and overextension of the hindlimb as it is pulled through the maternal pelvis may cause femoral nerve damage with subsequent quadriceps atrophy (Fig. 4.23).

Calving aids are usually designed to pull alternately on the two forelegs of the calf and, if required, to exert a constant pull upon the head. In most cases the aid has its own short calving ropes for attachment to the fetal legs as in manual traction. The ropes are attached to the calving aid by knots, which fix into the hooks

on the aid (Fig. 4.24). A normal calving rope is attached to the head of the calf with the other end being either attached to a special hook on the aid or – if it is decided to apply manual traction to the head – to a short length of broom handle.

The position of the calf is checked and lubrication applied as in manual delivery. The HK calving aid (Fig. 4.24) is placed behind the cow with its horizontal bar resting against the perineal area just below the vulva. In the case of the Vink calving aid (Fig. 4.25) the instrument rests against the perineum receiving further support from the maternal pelvis. The ropes on the calf are attached and tightened by moving the ratchet lever backwards and forwards. The shaft of the aid is directed backwards and downwards as pulling is commenced and is held in place by the obstetrician's foot. The head of the calf is eased through the vulva as in manual delivery. The obstetrician may experience slightly greater resistance to delivery as the fetal shoulders and thorax and then its hindquarters pass through the maternal pelvis.

If the calf is large the handle of the aid may be too short for the ratchet to pull the entire fetus from the birth canal and the fetus may lodge, as in a stifle lock obstruction. Further traction can be applied manually, although this may be a little difficult as the short ropes of the aid are not designed for the application of manual traction. In these circumstances the obstetrician and assistants should grasp the calf's legs and pull it manually until it is delivered. Extension handles are available with some calving aids, which enable larger longer calves to be delivered without interruption.

If there is a suspected problem with stifle lock the calf should be repelled and rotated through 45° as in manual delivery (see p. 70).

It is advisable that only the force exerted by the obstetrician using one hand on the ratchet lever of the calving aid should be used. If the fetus fails to move, its posture should be checked after further lubrication, as in manual delivery, and a further attempt at traction using the aid made. If no progress is made within 10 minutes, delivery by traction should be abandoned and the calf delivered by cesarean section or fetotomy.

If an obstetric pulley is used it is usually attached to both limbs of the calf and traction is applied to both simultaneously. The mechanical advantage of the system must be constantly borne in mind and the force exerted on the calf, which may be in excess of 400 kg, must be remembered.

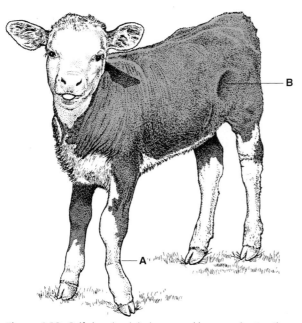

Figure 4.23 Calf showing injuries caused by excessive traction. (A) Fractured metacarpus, (B) quadriceps atrophy caused by femoral nerve paralysis.

Under no circumstances whatever can the use of additional and excessive force by the use of vehicles, etc. ever be condoned.

OBSTETRICIAN'S CHECK LIST

Delivery of calf in anterior presentation: calving aid delivery

Apply calving rope to head
↓
Apply special calving aid ropes to forelegs
↓
Attach ropes to calving aid
↓
Obstetrician applies traction as cow strains
↓

↓
Adjust direction of pull with stage of delivery
↓
Ease poll of calf through vulva
↓
Release calf and rotate through 45° if stifle lock occurs
↓
Attach ropes to calving aid
↓
Complete delivery

If no progress in 10 minutes
↓
Check presentation, position, and posture
↓
Further brief trial traction/cesarean section

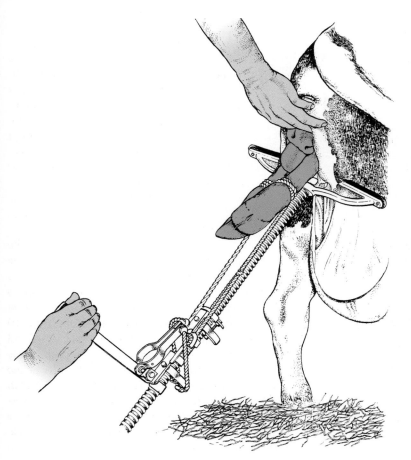

Figure 4.24 Delivery of the calf using an HK calving aid.

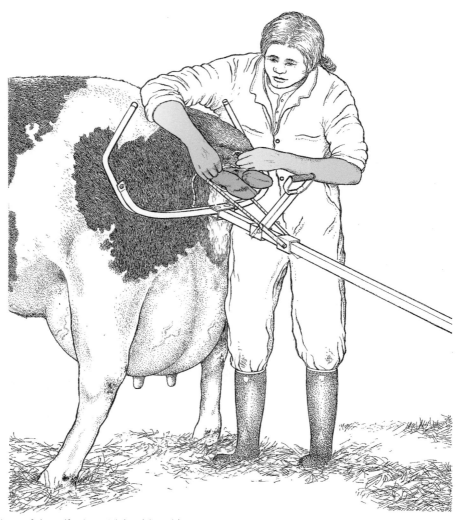

Figure 4.25 Delivery of the calf using a Vink calving aid.

Fetus in posterior presentation

Pulling should never be started with the calf in posterior presentation unless the obstetrician is sure that sufficient help is available. Delivery of the calf in posterior presentation is more hazardous than when the calf is in anterior presentation. The umbilical cord may break early in delivery and unless delivery is completed quickly the calf may become hypoxic and inhale amniotic fluid and drown.

Manual traction Ropes or chains are applied to both hindlimbs just above the fetlock joint. Lubrication is applied generously within the birth canal and around the fetus especially around the hindquarters and over the tail head. The tail should be pulled down to lie between the calf's legs. If it is allowed to curl forward by or over the tail head it will increase the presenting diameter of the calf, increase the resistance to delivery, and the risk of damage to the dorsal wall of the vagina. The legs are examined to ensure they are both hindlimbs and belong to the same calf.

As traction commences, one hindleg is pulled slightly in advance of the other to reduce the diameter of the hindquarters as they enter the maternal pelvis. Traction is applied by the two assistants with pulling coinciding with maternal straining. The direction of pull is slightly upwards as the calf enters the pelvis, backwards as it starts to go through the pelvis, and then downwards and backwards.

As the tail head of the calf approaches the caudal vagina and vulva it should be covered by the obstetrician's hand, which lifts the dorsal vaginal wall and shields it from the sharp bony prominence of the tail head, which might otherwise cause laceration.

Once the hips have passed through the pelvis, traction is applied equally to both hindlimbs and the speed of delivery is increased. This should ensure that – at a time when the umbilical cord is likely to be compressed or to rupture – the calf is able to reach and breathe atmospheric air as quickly as possible. Some resistance may be encountered as the fetal thorax passes through the maternal pelvis.

If the fetus fails to move at all during attempted delivery traction should be halted and the fetus examined to ensure that the posture of the calf is as expected and the limbs belong to the same calf.

If no progress is made within 10 minutes, delivery by traction should be abandoned and the calf should be delivered by cesarean section or by fetotomy.

OBSTETRICIAN'S CHECK LIST

Delivery of calf in posterior presentation: manual delivery

Check sufficient help is available
↓
Apply calving ropes to hindlegs
↓
Pass one calving rope to each assistant
↓
Apply traction as cow strains
↓
Note time traction first applied
↓
Advance one hindleg in front of the other
↓
Adjust direction of pull with stage of delivery
↓
Ease tail head through the vulva
↓
Rotate calf through 45° if delivery is delayed
↓
Complete delivery of calf

Application of traction by calving aid or pulley

The same general principles for use apply as in the delivery of the calf in anterior presentation (see p. 72). The special knotted calving ropes are attached to the aid

and, after further lubrication of the birth canal and fetus, delivery is attempted. As with manual delivery the obstetrician should place a hand over the tail head as it approaches and passes through the vulva. As in the case of anterior presentation the dangers of excessive traction must be remembered. Separation of one or both femoral head epiphyses may be sustained if the calf in posterior presentation is subjected to excessive pulling force. If delivery by traction is unsuccessful within 10 minutes it should be abandoned and the calf delivered by cesarean section or fetotomy.

OBSTETRICIAN'S CHECK LIST

Delivery of calf in posterior presentation: calving aid delivery

---

Check sufficient help is available
↓
Apply special calving rope to each hindleg
↓
Apply traction as the cow strains
↓
Adjust direction of pull with stage of delivery
↓
Ease tail head through vulva
↓
Rotate calf through 45° if delivery is delayed
↓
Complete delivery of calf

RESUSCITATION OF THE CALF

The following procedure should be followed:

1. *Clearing the airway*: in many cases spontaneous breathing occurs as soon as the calf is born. Inevitably some fluid will be present in the lungs and mucus that might have been inhaled during birth should be encouraged to drain out in the early postparturient phase to help establish a clear airway. The calf can be held up by its back legs and swung backwards and forwards, although this may be difficult with a heavy calf. Alternatively, the calf may be briefly suspended by its legs from a convenient beam or hung over a door (Fig. 4.26). The chest is slapped gently to dislodge mucus. If suction is available it should be used to ensure removal of mucus from the mouth, pharynx, larynx, and nasal passages.

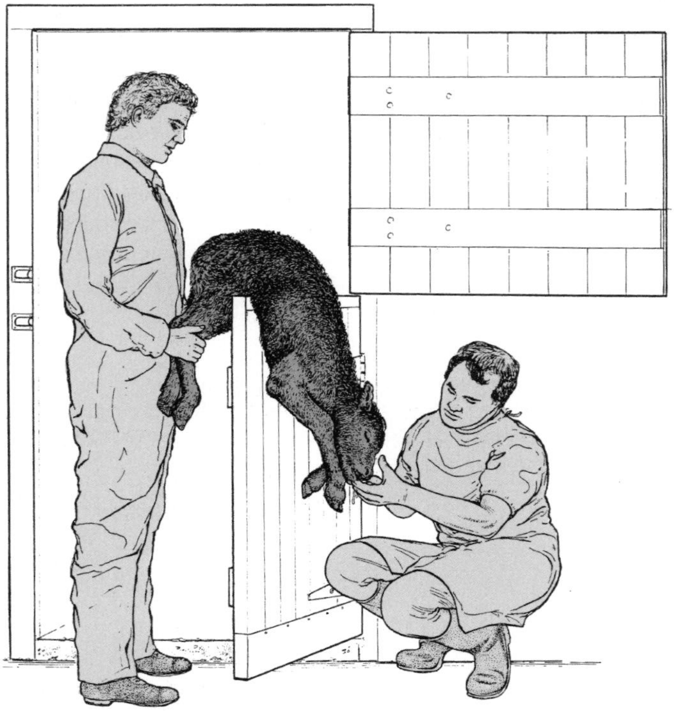

Figure 4.26 Resuscitation of the calf (see text).

2. *Fetal heart beat*: check for the visible or palpable apex beat of the heart. Check for vital signs including palpebral reflex and spontaneous movement. If there are no vital signs, an attempt to establish a heart beat is unlikely to be successful. However, external cardiac massage or an intracardiac injection of adrenaline (epinephrine) may be tried. Auscultate the chest for any evidence of cardiac activity. Look for signs of earlier fetal death such as corneal opacity.

3. *Establishment of respiration when the heart is beating*: if spontaneous respiration is not present it can be stimulated by pinching the fetal nose or feet, pricking the nasal filtrum, tickling the nasal mucosa with straw, or by splashing cold water on the head. If these methods are ineffectual, respiration may be further stimulated by quickly giving the calf 40–100 mg doxapram hydrochloride by intravenous injection or sublingual application. The distended jugular vein is usually clearly visible in the neonatal calf. The calf should normally take its first breath within 30 seconds of delivery. After the first breath there may be a period of apnea and, providing the mucous membrane color is good and the heart beat strong, this is not necessarily a cause for concern. In the healthy calf, further gasping movements are made before shallow respiratory movements are made.

Oxygen therapy: can be supplied by face mask or endotracheal tube. It may be possible to aid fetal intubation by holding the larynx between the finger and thumb of one hand and passing the tube over the tongue to be inserted into the stabilized larynx. Once in position, the endotracheal tube is inflated and gentle positive pressure applied to inflate the lungs. Maximum survival time without oxygen entering the lungs is 4–6 minutes and hence the advantage of having resuscitation equipment available *before* fetal delivery is commenced.

Inflation of the fetal lungs using an esophageal tube: in the absence of an endotracheal tube, or if attempts to intubate the calf fail, this technique can be tried. Two people are required to use the technique effectively. A small (foal size) stomach tube is passed into the calf's esophagus. Applying positive pressure through this will dilate the calf's abomasum but not inflate its lungs. The esophagus is obstructed distal to the end of the tube by compressing it between the finger and thumb. The calf's mouth is held tightly closed and its nostrils are covered. Air or oxygen is passed or blown into the stomach tube. The gas – unable to pass into the abomasum or escape through the mouth or nostrils – can only pass into the trachea and lungs. The lungs are inflated in this way until normal breathing is established. Inflation of the lungs can also be aided using a Cox calf resuscitator. This has a face mask through which air is supplied using a cylinder-shaped resuscitator pump. The esophagus is closed as described above to ensure that the 800 mL of air supplied by the pump passes into the lungs. It is suggested that after 10 pumps the calf is turned onto its other side to ensure both lungs become inflated.

4. *Artificial respiration*: may be used if cardiac function is present but there is no respiration even after administration of doxapram hydrochloride and encouraging the calf to gasp (see 3. above). After clearing the airways (see 1. above) the calf is laid on its side with head and neck extended. The upper chest wall is raised and lowered, holding it by the humerus and the last rib. Excessive pressure should not be applied externally to the ribs because of the possibility of fracture or damage to underlying organs such as lungs and liver. If spontaneous breathing still fails to occur an attempt may be made, if equipment is available, to intubate the calf and provide positive-pressure ventilation. Mouth-to-mouth respiration should be avoided – it is ineffective and carries zoonotic risks.

5. *Breathing difficulties*: hyperpnea or dyspnea may indicate dysmaturity of the fetal lungs or possibly a severe, life-threatening cardiac anomaly. Cardiac murmurs in the bovine neonate are not necessarily pathological and occasionally an asymptomatic atrial septal defect with attendant murmur is present for the first few days of life. The most common important cardiac anomaly is the ventricular septal defect; persistent patent ductus arteriosus is less commonly encountered. A careful clinical examination should be carried out and if fetal pulmonary atelectasis is suspected dexamethasone and antibiotic treatment may be given. For further discussion on the treatment of neonatal dyspnea (after cesarean section) see Chapter 11. Dyspnea may also be an indication of severe blood loss from the umbilical vessels or internal damage to the chest or abdomen sustained during delivery.

6. *Signs of fetal acidosis*: signs of immediate postpartum acidosis in the calf include:
   i   superficial mainly abdominal breathing
   ii low fetal heart rate
   iii prolonged jugular filling time
   iv poor body muscle tone
   v   absence of a pedel reflex.

7. *Estimation of the degree of acidosis*: the degree of fetal acidosis can be determined immediately if a blood-gas machine is available. In the field, the time to attain sternal recumbency (T-SR) has been found to be a useful indicator of the degree of acidosis affecting the calf (Schuijt & Taverne 1994). These authors found that T-SR was 4.0 ± 2.2 minutes after unassisted delivery, 5.4 ± 3.3 minutes after assisted delivery, and 4.5 ± 3.1 minutes after cesarean section. When severe traction was used, T-SR rose to 9.0 ± 3.3 minutes. A T-SR of >15 minutes was an ominous sign of severe acidosis with poor short- and longer-term survival rates. These findings also suggest that delivery by traction may cause the calf greater stress in some cases than delivery by cesarean section.

8. *Treatment of acidosis*: if there is no sign of spontaneous improvement, an attempt may be made to correct the acidosis by giving 250–500 mL of 4.2% sodium bicarbonate solution by *slow* intravenous injection.

   Untreated acidosis can lead to poor colostral uptake and a shortening of the period during which the calf is normally able to absorb antibodies. Other problems, such as abomasal atony, general dullness, and reluctance to move or suck from the cow, may be seen.

OBSTETRICIAN'S CHECK LIST

Postnatal management of the calf

A: visible signs of life

Spontaneous breathing – monitor and watch for signs of acidosis

↓

Heart beating but no respiration

↓

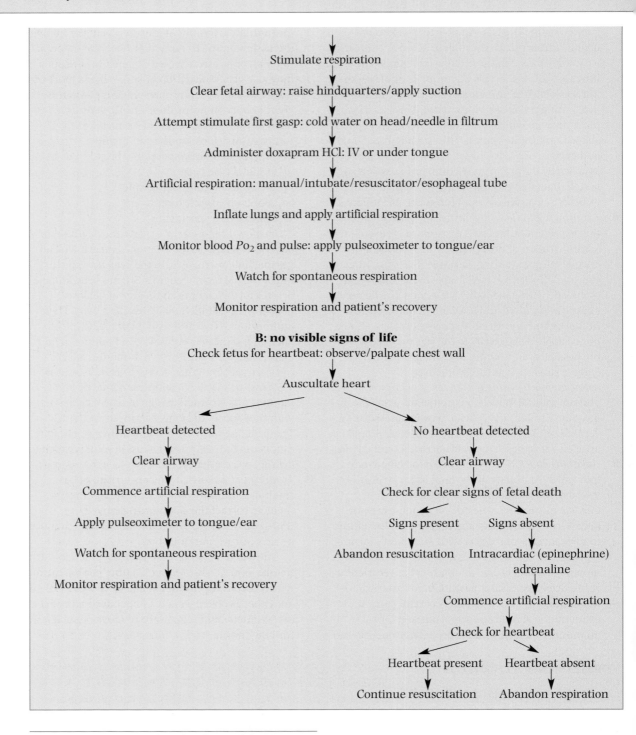

POSTNATAL CHECK OF THE COW

After delivery of the calf the uterus must always be checked for evidence of another fetus. This process is repeated after each calf until the obstetrician is sure that the uterus is empty. The birth canal is checked for signs of damage and hemorrhage. Uterine involution usually commences immediately after the birth of the calf. If uterine tone feels low (the uterine walls are flabby) 20 IU of oxytocin should be given by

---

OBSTETRICIAN'S CHECK LIST

Postnatal check of cow

Explore uterus for further fetus(es)
↓
Assess and deliver further fetus(es)
↓
Ensure uterus is empty
↓
Check for vaginal and uterine damage
↓
Repair any accessible damage
↓
Assess myometrial tone
↓
Administer oxytocin if tone poor
↓
Consider antibiotic cover
↓
Consider need for analgesia
↓
Consider need for additional drug therapy
↓
Administer calcium if required
↓
Further treatment for mastitis if present
↓
Advice regarding postnatal management
↓
Arrange prebreeding check at 21 days

---

intramuscular injection. The udder is checked again for signs of mastitis.

FURTHER CARE OF THE COW AND CALF

It is important that effective bonding between the calf and its mother develops. This is more likely to happen if the cow and calf are left quietly alone but care must be taken to ensure that the calf is not damaged if the cow or heifer is aggressive towards it.

The calf should be encouraged to suck colostrum within 6 hours of birth. The navel should be dipped in iodine or sprayed with antibiotic aerosol as soon after birth as possible. The navel should be checked at intervals after delivery to ensure that delayed hemorrhage from the umbilical vessels is not occurring. There should be negligible blood loss from the navel of the normal calf. Vessels from which blood loss is occurring should be ligated. In neglected cases where severe blood loss has occurred, a blood transfusion may be required.

The cow should be monitored carefully after calving for evidence of any of the postparturient problems that are discussed in Chapter 13.

THE OVERDUE BIRTH – PROLONGED GESTATION

Many cases presented with a history of suspected prolonged gestation are found to have a normal pregnancy. In some cases the owner may have miscalculated their prospective calving date. In other cases the cow may have returned to estrus after her initial service. A further service was given but not recorded and the cow becomes pregnant again but not to her initial service. The breeding history and service records of animals in this category should be checked and the possibility of an unrecorded service reviewed.

All cases of suspected prolonged gestation should be examined carefully. A general clinical examination precedes the gynecological examination. Rectal examination including ultrasonography should reveal whether the cow is still pregnant and if so whether her pregnancy is normal or abnormal. The possible findings are as follows:

- *Normal pregnancy*: there may be clear evidence that the age of the existing pregnancy is not that suggested by the cow's records. Examination of the uterus, palpation of the fetus (if possible), the presence of fremitus in the middle uterine arteries, and the size of the cotyledons should enable the approximate stage of pregnancy to be determined. The cow's records are altered and she is returned to the herd. A further examination should be planned a month later to check that the pregnancy is progressing normally.
- *Abnormal pregnancy with a dead fetus*: there are two possible problems in such cases: The fetus had died and is either mummified or macerated. The clinical signs of these conditions in cattle and their diagnosis and treatment are discussed in detail in Chapter 2.
- *Abnormal pregnancy with a living fetus*: this is the least likely diagnosis but remains a possibility. In such cases parturition has failed to occur at the normal time. A single cow or a number of animals in the herd may be affected. In most cases the fetus has a defect affecting the hypothalamic – anterior-pituitary – adrenal axis; other anatomical defects may also be present. The normal endocrine changes in the fetus that precede its birth fail to occur. Pregnancy continues almost

indefinitely beyond the normal time of parturition. Fetal growth is restricted only by placental capacity.

Three genetic abnormalities causing prolonged gestation in cattle have been identified. Fetal pituitary abnormalities are found in each case:

1. Fetal giantism with pituitary hypoplasia occurs in Holstein–Friesian and Ayrshire cattle. Pregnancy may be prolonged by up to 150 days. The fetus may weigh up to 80 kg and show signs of postmaturity such as abnormally long hair and hoof growth. Dystocia is a serious problem if parturition should occur naturally or is induced.
2. Prolonged gestation associated with severe craniofacial defects has been reported in Ayrshire, Jersey, and Guernsey cattle. Unlike cases of fetal giantism, the fetus ceases to grow from 7 months gestation onwards.
3. In the third condition, seen in Hereford cattle, multiple skeletal defects, including arthrogryposis, accompany pituitary hyopoplasia.

Prolonged gestation has also been caused by exposure to mucosal disease virus and by toxic alkaloids found in plants such as the skunk cabbage (*Veratrum californicum*). Blue tongue and akabane viruses cause similar problems.

Fetal abnormalities – especially craniofacial defects – may be palpable per rectum in cases of prolonged gestation and can be confirmed by ultrasonographic scan. Prolonged gestation may be terminated by induction of birth. An intramuscular injection of cloprostenol (500 μg) and dexamethasone (20 mg) is given. Parturition normally commences 24–72 hours later. Dystocia due to fetopelvic disproportion or maldisposition may occur. Parturition should be monitored and assistance with birth given if necessary.

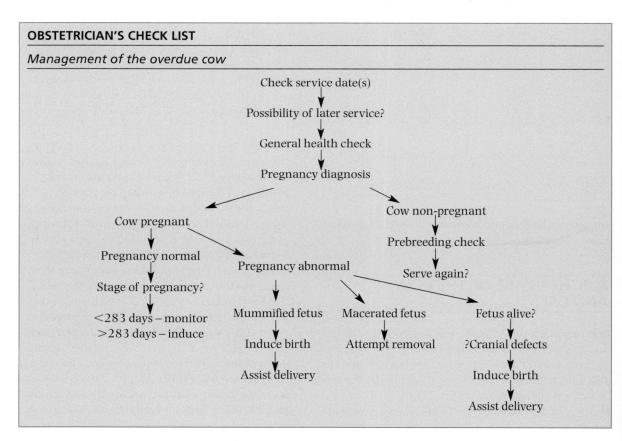

OBSTETRICIAN'S CHECK LIST

Management of the overdue cow

Check service date(s)

Possibility of later service?

General health check

Pregnancy diagnosis

Cow pregnant — Cow non-pregnant

Pregnancy normal — Pregnancy abnormal — Prebreeding check

Stage of pregnancy? — Serve again?

<283 days – monitor / >283 days – induce

Mummified fetus — Macerated fetus — Fetus alive?

Induce birth — Attempt removal — ?Cranial defects

Assist delivery — Induce birth

Assist delivery

REFERENCES

Schuijt G, Ball L 1980 In: Morrow DA (ed) Current therapy in theriogenology. WB Saunders, London, p. 247–257

Schuijt G, Taverne MAM 1994 The interval between birth and sternal recumbency as an objective measure of the viability of new born calves. Veterinary Record **135**:111–115

Chapter 5

DYSTOCIA IN THE MARE

Parturition in the mare is normally a rapid and quite violent process. Once the birth process is under way, placental separation or functional deterioration is likely to occur much more quickly than in other species. Fetal death or damage – including development of the neonatal maladjustment syndrome – due to hypoxia may occur. *Any reported case of equine dystocia must be treated as an emergency and attended immediately.* Fetal maldisposition is an important cause of equine dystocia predisposed to and complicated by the long head, neck, and limbs of the foal. If recognized early in the birth process it can often be corrected without difficulty, sometimes by an experienced stud groom. Where such experienced help is not available the obstetrician must be called without delay.

If not identified quickly the maldisposed fetus may become impacted in the maternal pelvis by strong abdominal straining and uterine contractions. Correction of the abnormality – often now complicated by fetal death – is much more difficult in such circumstances.

Supervision of equine birth must be quiet and unobtrusive because any disturbance may delay initiation of parturition. In many studs use is made of remote control video cameras, one-way windows, and observation points allowing good observation of the parturient mare without disturbance. Assistance may be given quickly if there is the slightest suspicion of any abnormality likely to compromise birth.

ANTENATAL CARE

Pregnancy diagnosis by rectal ultrasonography of the uterus is performed in many mares at 14–18 days after covering and before the mare is likely to return to estrus. Twin pregnancy can often be detected at this stage by the identification of two separate vesicles each containing a conceptus. A further ultrasonographic examination should be performed at 28–35 days to minimize the risk of missing twin conceptions and to check that the fetus is alive. Triplet pregnancies can occur in the mare and a thorough examination of the uterine body and horns is advised to avoid missing them. Most equine twin pregnancies end in abortion, often at about 7 months of gestation. Premature lactation may be seen in such animals. Restlessness, sweating, and mild colic may precede the passage of the twin foals. One is often mummified and the other may be living but non-viable. Rare cases of twin pregnancy persist to term when two small foals may be born and dystocia through simultaneous presentation, fetal maldisposition, or uterine inertia may be a complication. For these reasons, early diagnosis of equine twins is desirable. If equine twins are diagnosed one conceptus can be destroyed by crushing per rectum. Alternatively, the whole pregnancy may be terminated by an intramuscular injection of prostaglandin F2α (500 μg cloprostenol or 5 mg dinoprost). This should be carried out before day 35 of pregnancy, when the endometrial cups form and prostaglandin F2α is not effective. After termination the mare may be served again.

A further confirmation of pregnancy may be carried out at 6–10 weeks of gestation to ensure that unexpected fetal loss has not occurred since the original positive pregnancy diagnosis was made. In many mares no further veterinary attention is given unless it is needed at the birth of the foal.

Novice breeders should be advised about the care of their mare during pregnancy. Normal feeding should continue with grazing in the summer and concentrates and hay in the winter. Mares in poor condition on a low-protein diet and with a heavy parasite burden may fail to maintain their pregnancy. Moderate exercise throughout gestation is beneficial but strenuous riding should be avoided in the last trimester of pregnancy. Novice breeders should also be given details of normal birth and the signs of dystocia, and told to seek help immediately if the mare shows any signs of abnormality.

Mares with a history of previous abortion should be subjected to special care during a subsequent pregnancy. Thoroughbred mares will have been screened for evidence of infections such as equine viral arteritis, contagious equine metritis, *Klebsiella*, and *Pseudomonas* before covering. Vaccination against equine herpesvirus-1 is used on some studs. The uterine health of problem mares is carefully checked before service at an appropriate time by a stallion whose venereal health has also been checked.

Once pregnancy is confirmed, problem mares should be checked at intervals throughout pregnancy. Monthly or more frequent examinations are carried out depending on the history of the mare. A general health check and the following procedures are carried out on each occasion:

- *Rectal examination*: to ensure uterine enlargement and fetal growth are normal. The ovaries are also palpated as they move forward out of reach as pregnancy progresses. As birth approaches the presentation, position, and posture of the fetus are checked. The fetus is usually in anterior presentation, ventral position with the head and forelegs extended towards the pelvic inlet as birth approaches.
- *Ultrasonographic examination*: of the uterus, the placenta, the fetus, and its fetal fluids. Fetal growth and movement are monitored. The fetal heart rate should be reasonably steady and faster than that of the mare. The chorion should be closely applied to the endometrium. Areas of separation or thickening of the chorion may indicate that placental function is suboptimal and the risk of pregnancy loss is increased. Fetal fluids should be non-echogenic and free from any solid material.
- *Vaginal examination*: is carried out with strict attention to hygiene. The cervix is observed through a vaginal speculum and is checked for closure and the absence of an abnormal discharge. Any purulent material should be cultured and antibiotic therapy may be required.
- *Plasma progesterone*: may be monitored each time the mare is examined. A decrease in plasma progesterone, especially at a stage of pregnancy at which previous abortion has occurred, may indicate that the pregnancy is at risk. In such cases natural progestin production by the placenta may be supplemented by the administration of the synthetic progestagen altronogest; 2.2 mg altronogest/50 kg body weight are given orally each day. The efficacy of this treatment has not been scientifically evaluated but obstetricians may be under great pressure from owners to use it. If used, the drug should be withdrawn slowly before parturition is due.

INCIDENCE OF DYSTOCIA

The incidence of dystocia in mares has been much less well documented than in cattle. However, a very comprehensive survey involving over 600 cases of equine dystocia was carried out by Vanderplassche (1993) at Ghent Veterinary School in Belgium.

Dystocia occurs in about 4% of Thoroughbred mares, with a higher incidence (in the above survey) in Belgian Draft horses, in which double-muscling of the fetus may cause problems with fetopelvic disproportion. Dystocia may be also more common in Shetland ponies. The incidence of elbow flexion as a cause of dystocia in this breed is quite high. Fetopelvic disproportion is occasionally seen in this and other small breeds. The Shetland foal has a relatively large head and this may prevent the forelegs from becoming fully extended as they enter the birth canal. This may predispose to dystocia due to incomplete extension of the elbow joints. Dealing with dystocia in such small breeds can be difficult because of the lack of space in the birth canal.

The fetus is in anterior presentation in nearly 99% of normal equine births, in posterior presentation in only 0.9%, and in transverse presentation in 0.1%. Although the foal is in a ventral position during late gestation, it normally assumes a dorsal position during delivery. The foal may occasionally fail to move completely into the dorsal position and may be presented in a lateral position. All the maldispositions described in the calf also occur in the foal.

The incidence of dystocia is higher in mares foaling for the first time but may increase again as the mare becomes older. In general it may be advisable not to breed from mares below the age of 4 years or over the age of 20.

CAUSES OF DYSTOCIA

Published details of the survey by Vanderplassche (1993) are insufficient to provide an exact breakdown of the component causes. The survey related to mares seen in a referral clinic and thus reflects the more serious

Table 5.1 Causes of dystocia in the mare		
	No. of cases	**%**
Foal in anterior presentation	408	68
Lateral deviation of the head	237	40
Other postural abnormalities,	171	28
malpositions, and fetal monsters		
Foal in posterior presentation	95	16
Breech presentation	47	8
Hock flexion	24	4
Other abnormality	24	4
Foal in transverse presentation	98	16
Complete bicornual pregnancy	47	8
Partial bicornual pregnancy	51	8
Total	601	100

causes of dystocia referred for specialist assistance. Some causes of dystocia such as uterine inertia, which may mostly be dealt with in practice, are not listed. Table 5.1 shows the broad categories into which the causes of dystocia fell.

SPECIFIC CAUSES OF EQUINE DYSTOCIA

Details of the more important causes of dystocia are described below.

FAILURE OF THE EXPULSIVE FORCES

Uterine inertia

Primary uterine inertia

This is mostly the result of voluntary suppression of parturition caused by disturbance of the mare as foaling approaches. In nervous mares even the slightest sound or movement may be sufficient to inhibit birth and hence the need for totally unobtrusive observation in this species. The mare is restless and uneasy and birth appears imminent but foaling does not commence. The cervix is usually partially open and can be manually dilated without difficulty. The chorioallantois is normally intact.

Treatment   If the chorioallantois is intact and there is no evidence of fetal distress the mare may be left completely alone for up to 20 minutes. In some cases, parturition will recommence spontaneously in the now undisturbed patient. In other cases the mare is so

disturbed that she continues to inhibit parturition. In such cases birth should be induced with an intravenous injection of oxytocin. Although this can be incorporated in a drip and be given over a period of 1 hour an intravenous bolus injection appears equally satisfactory and is more easily managed. A dose of 2.5–15 IU oxytocin is used, depending on the size of the mare. The mare should go into labor within 15 minutes of injection and may show signs of sweating and mild colicky pain. For further details concerning induction of birth in the mare see Chapter 15.

The induced birth should be carefully supervised and fetal delivery assisted by moderate traction if necessary.

Secondary uterine inertia

Secondary uterine inertia follows another primary cause of dystocia such as fetal maldisposition. In such cases the primary dystocia is corrected and fetal delivery assisted by traction.

Following delivery in both categories of uterine inertia, uterine involution after the birth of the foal should be encouraged by administration of 10–30 IU oxytocin given by intramuscular injection.

Failure of the abdominal expulsive forces

This usually results from damage to the integrity of the abdominal musculature, which compromises its ability to assist in straining to expel the fetus. Ventral hernia may occur in older multiparous mares as a result of senile changes and increasing fetal weight in late pregnancy. It may also arise as a result of injury. The ability of affected mares to foal unaided is compromised and assistance (by traction applied to the foal) when parturition commences may be necessary. In severe cases of ventral hernia downward deviation of the uterus may occur. The foal's exit from the displaced uterus is obstructed and assisted delivery is necessary to bring the foal up into, and then through, the maternal pelvis (for details of fetal delivery, see Downward deviation of the uterus, p. 86).

Rupture of the prepubic tendon in mares

Rupture of the prepubic tendon should always be suspected if severe painful edema is seen on the ventral surface of the abdomen of the mare in late gestation. The edema forms a plaque-like layer up to 15 cm deep in some mares (see Fig. 2.4). The edema pits on pressure and digital pressure causes evidence of pain. The condition may be more common in heavy breeds of horse. *Note*: non-painful edema is frequently seen in mares in late gestation. It is thought that the presence of the growing fetus causes partial obstruction of maternal lymphatic and venous drainage. This latter type of edema usually disappears completely without treatment within 48 hours of foaling.

Treatment   The development of painful edema may initially indicate threatened rather than actual rupture of the tendon. An ultrasonographic scan of the tendon may help assess the degree of damage. In any case, the ventral abdominal floor should be supported by strong canvas strapping fixed round the abdomen. The abdominal floor and the damaged or threatened tendon are thus supported indirectly by the vertebral column. Surgical repair of the tendon and its insertion into the pubis – where the rupture usually occurs – is not normally feasible. The mare is kept under observation and assistance given with foaling if required.

Rupture of the tendon may cause displacement of one of the mare's teats but lactation and access by the foal are not normally affected. In many cases the foal is reared normally but after weaning the mare should be retired from further breeding.

OBSTRUCTION OF THE BIRTH CANAL

Bony tissue obstruction

Pelvic injury compromising the patency of the pelvic canal is uncommon in horses. If such injury had been sustained the mare should not be bred. If she is found to be in foal after injury, arrangements should be made for an elective cesarean section. If the problem is undiscovered until dystocia occurs, attempts should be made to guide the fetus past any obstruction. If this is not possible then immediate cesarean section might allow delivery of a living foal. Fetotomy can be used to divide and deliver a dead foal.

Soft tissue obstruction

As in other species, soft tissue obstruction of the birth canal may affect any part from the vulva to the uterus.

Many Thoroughbred mares have had the dorsal two-thirds of their vulval orifice stitched by Caslick's operation as an aid to conception. The stitched tissues should be opened with scissors up to a week before foaling to prevent tearing at birth. On some studs, an experienced stud groom opens the stitched vulval lips during the first stage of labor. The vulval lips are normally sutured again shortly after birth of the foal and passage of the placenta if it is intended to breed from the mare again.

Vaginal obstruction

This is relatively uncommon in mares. In older mares a squamous cell carcinoma may involve the caudal vagina and vulva. Melanomas may be found in the vagina of gray mares and may also occasionally interfere with fetal delivery. In neither case should such mares be bred from again but, providing the tumor is not too large, it may be possible to guide the lubricated foal past the obstruction during delivery. If problems are encountered or anticipated, cesarean section may be required.

Varicose veins occur in the vaginal wall of some older mares and may project into the lumen. Physical obstruction to the passage of the foal is seldom a problem. Hemorrhage can occur spontaneously during pregnancy or at parturition. Such hemorrhage is rarely life-threatening and is dealt with by standard hemostatic measures. These include packing the vagina with damp toweling or coagulation of the vessels using a gauze pad soaked in 10% formol saline. If these methods fail, the vessels should be ligated under epidural or general anesthesia. Hemorrhage from the uterine arteries is described in Chapter 13.

The cervix

Obstruction of the cervix of the mare is rarely a cause of dystocia unless the cervix has suffered damage and scar tissue formation at an earlier birth. The normal equine cervix can be dilated manually with relative ease at any stage of pregnancy or parturition. Scar damage from a previous foaling should have been noted during inspection of the cervix at the previous postnatal check. Severe damage may compromise conception and may necessitate cesarean section if dystocia occurs and manual dilation proves impossible.

Torsion of the uterus

Uterine torsion can occur during pregnancy or as a cause of dystocia at parturition. The condition is relatively uncommon, with approximately 50% of cases occurring after 7 months of pregnancy and 50% at term. The two forms of uterine torsion will be considered separately.

1. Torsion of the uterus during pregnancy

Clinical signs   Uterine torsion should always be considered when signs of colic occur in mares during late gestation. Mild colic can occur in any pregnant mare and may be associated with fetal movements and pressure on pelvic nerves and blood vessels. Such colics are non-progressive and usually resolve rapidly without treatment. Occasionally, analgesia may be required. Any more serious or persistent colic should be fully investigated. In summary, a full history is taken and the mare subjected to a complete clinical examination in case a serious gastrointestinal problem has developed incidentally in the pregnant mare. A rectal examination is performed to examine the accessible parts of the abdomen for signs of abnormality involving the gastrointestinal tract. A stomach tube is passed to check for evidence of gastric reflux and the abdomen is auscultated to assess bowel activity. An abdominal paracentesis is performed to obtain a sample of peritoneal fluid. The latter technique is often unproductive in late pregnancy because paracentesis at this time usually results in the collection of allantoic rather than peritoneal fluid.

Specific findings with uterine torsion during pregnancy include:

- mild to quite severe unremitting colic
- slight elevation of the pulse; packed cell volume is usually normal
- normal bowel activity and sounds
- scant but normal peritoneal fluid
- rectal examination: reveals displacement of the uterus and its broad ligaments. The pregnant uterus lies laterally and is displaced from its normal midline position
- vaginal examination: usually no abnormality. Most cases during pregnancy are precervical and have little effect upon the vagina.

During rectal examination the uterus may be felt to deviate sharply laterally and downwards instead of being readily palpable in the midline. The fetus may not be palpable and the uterus is immobile. The broad ligaments are displaced and may be tense, especially on the side of the animal towards which the uterus is rotated. Thus if the uterus is rotated to the right the right broad ligament may be palpated per rectum as a tense band running from the right sublumbar region down to and under the uterus. The left broad ligament runs from the dorsal aspect of the displaced uterus to the left sublumbar area. Right and left uterine displacement occur with equal frequency.

Treatment The state of the uterine wall must be taken into account: it may have been compromised if the torsion has been present for some time. Fetal compromise may have also occurred if the placenta has been damaged. Fetal death may occur in cases of prolonged torsion. Economic considerations are also important, as is the quality of the surgical facilities available. Three methods of treatment may be considered:

1. *Replacement of the uterus by manual manipulation*: an attempt is made to grasp the uterine wall per rectum, rock the uterus from side to side, and then swing it back into the correct position. Great care must be taken to avoid damaging the rectal and vaginal walls and this method is only likely to be successful if the uterine torsion is recent and the fetus small. If successful, the uterus resumes its midline position and the signs of colic rapidly resolve.
2. *Rolling the mare under general anesthesia*: this can be attempted if the previous method fails, but should not be used in late gestation. The mare is placed on the side to which the torsion is directed and then sharply rolled over in the direction of the twist. It may be necessary to repeat the procedure and external pressure on the uterus and fetus may be supplied using a board – on which an assistant stands – as in the cow. The procedure is not without risk but may be considered if laparotomy is not possible for economic or other reasons.
3. *Replacement of the uterus via laparotomy*: this can be attempted in the standing or recumbent mare.

    Standing flank laparotomy in the sedated mare and under local infiltration anesthesia is performed on the side towards which the torsion is directed. A small incision is made in the center of the sublumbar fossa initially to allow the obstetrician's hand to grasp the uterus. The uterus is rocked backwards and forwards away from and towards the operator and then turned back into its correct position. Occasionally, bilateral incisions may be required.

    Ventral midline laparotomy is performed under general anesthesia and allows better access to the abdomen and uterus. Good surgical facilities are mandatory. The direction of the torsion is checked and an attempt made to rock or replace the uterus into its correct position. If satisfactorily replaced, the uterus and its broad ligaments should be in their correct position and under normal tension.

    The abdomen may be more readily checked for gastrointestinal abnormalities during a ventral midline laparotomy. If the uterine wall is compromised it may be possible to repair damage and if there is clear evidence of fetal death then cesarean section can be employed to remove it. Severe damage or disruption of the blood supply to the uterine wall carries a grave prognosis.

Preoperative antibiotic and non-steroidal anti-inflammatory therapy are recommended.

Management of the mare and fetus after correction of uterine torsion   The prognosis following treatment – especially rolling or surgery – must be guarded. There is a risk of placental separation with fetal death, uterine rupture, peritonitis, or other postprocedure complications. In one survey, 70% of foals known to be alive at surgery were born alive at term.

Following correction of uterine torsion, the foal should be monitored carefully after treatment. A transabdominal ultrasonographic scan should be performed daily to monitor the fetal heart beat and the clarity of the amniotic fluid. The scan should be carried out daily for the first week and weekly after that until term. Fetal survival will depend on whether there has been any compromise of placental function. It has been suggested that a compromised placenta produces insufficient progestins to maintain pregnancy; 2.2 mg/50 kg body weight daily of the synthetic progestagen altrenogest can be given orally to the mare in such cases in an attempt to support maintenance of pregnancy. The drug is withdrawn slowly and with reducing dose towards the end of pregnancy. The efficacy of the drug therapy has not been scientifically proven.

2. Torsion of the uterus as a cause of dystocia at term

Clinical signs   Suspicions of uterine torsion may arise if there are signs of colic and delay in the early stages of birth. In parturient mares the point of torsion is normally anterior to the cervix. Vaginal examination may reveal some constriction of the birth canal and displacement of the broad ligaments may be confirmed on rectal examination. The fetus may be displaced anteriorly and not as easily palpated as in other forms of dystocia. In some cases the uterine torsion is associated with an abnormal disposition of the foal, which may be found in a lateral or ventral position.

Treatment   If good surgical facilities are available an immediate cesarean section is advisable to deal with this abnormality. If immediate surgery is not contemplated and access can be gained to the fetus an attempt should be made to correct the torsion by rotating the fetus and surrounding uterus back into its normal position. The obstetrician's hand is fully inserted into the birth canal and the fetus is grasped by the neck or shoulder. The fetus and uterus are rocked from side to side and then sharply turned in the opposite direction

to the torsion. Several attempts may be necessary to correct the problem. Once the torsion has been dealt with the fetus should be delivered manually. Great care must be taken as the viability of the uterine and possibly vaginal walls may have been compromised or more severely damaged by interference with the blood supply during the period of torsion. Gentle massage of accessible tissues may encourage relaxation and facilitate delivery.

If rotation of the uterus per vaginam is not successful a ventral midline approach to the uterus should be made at surgery. At laparotomy the uterus is inspected and rotated into its correct position. It may be advisable to deliver the foal by cesarean section to avoid further complications. Standard postoperative care and management are required.

Rolling the mare at term is accompanied by grave risks of uterine rupture and should not be attempted.

Downward deviation of the uterus

This may be a problem in mares that have suffered a ventral hernia. If the pregnant uterus passes into the sac of the hernia the fetus may hang almost vertically down from the pelvis. Exit from the uterus may be occluded and fetal delivery is compromised. The start of parturition should be closely monitored and manual assistance given with delivery of the foal. The severity of the hernia may be reduced and fetal delivery assisted by support for the ventral abdominal wall. A canvas sling passing around the abdomen and supported by the mare's spine may be found useful as in cases of rupture of the prepubic tendon (see p. 83). Fetal delivery is more easily completed in the recumbent mare. The abdominal floor may be raised in the quiet standing mare by using a sack under the abdomen held and lifted by two assistants one on either side of the patient. In a nervous mare, sedation or casting may be necessary to cause her to lie down. Traction is applied to the foal to bring it up into and through the maternal pelvis.

FETOPELVIC DISPROPORTION

This is seldom a problem in mares although it has been reported in Belgian Draft mares where double-muscling, which greatly increases fetal size, occurs. It is occasionally seen in other breeds including ponies. Prolonged gestation in mares, in total contrast to the position in cattle, does *not* result in fetal oversize. In fact, quite the reverse. Foals are quite frequently carried for 4 weeks or more past the expected delivery date (330 days post-service) and it is possible that their foals may be smaller rather than larger than normal. Fetal maturity and size are usually related to placental competence and prolonged gestation may be an indication that the placenta is not functioning as well as normal. Fetal life in such circumstances is seldom at risk. The rarity of fetopelvic disproportion in mares means that vaginal delivery should be possible in cases where fetal disposition and the birth canal are normal. In those rare cases where it is believed (and confirmed by trial traction) that the fetus will not pass through the pelvis it may be delivered by cesarean section or fetotomy. The fetus may be larger than normal in cases of transverse presentation with the foal having developed as a 'bicornual' pregnancy (see p. 88).

Fetal monsters

Fetal monsters are less common in horses than in cattle but their presence should be suspected if the delivery of what appears to be a normal fetus does not proceed as expected. At all cases of dystocia those parts of the foal that are palpable should be examined for evidence of abnormality.

Cases of hydrocephalus with gross enlargement of the cranium have been reported. The deformed head may be too large to pass through the pelvis.

Ankylosis of one or more limb joints may interfere with delivery. In some foals a persistent lateral deviation of the neck ('*wry neck*') may make delivery difficult as the neck tends to spring back into its abnormal position when the head is released. Such foals may show slow improvement after birth although help with sucking the mare may be required. The occurrence of other monsters such as schistosomus reflexus in horses is very rare.

Treatment of cases of dystocia caused by fetal monsters   This depends on the extent and nature of the abnormality. In a case of hydrocephalus in which the foal is dead, the abnormal cranium may sometimes be removed using the embryotome. In cases of wry neck, which cannot be manually corrected, the embryotome may also be used to remove the head and allow delivery of the dead fetus. If the fetus is known to be alive and manual correction of the maldisposition has proved impossible, cesarean section might be indicated. Partial fetotomy is extremely useful to assist delivery of a dead foal in cases of ankylosis of limb joints.

FETAL MALDISPOSITION

This category comprises the major causes of equine dystocia. The long neck and limbs of the foal predispose it to maldisposition and the violent expulsive efforts of the parturient mare rapidly and irreversibly compound the problem. The length of the extremities may make correction of maldispositions more difficult in the mare than in the cow. The risk of uterine rupture by the long extremities or during attempts to correct their position is also high.

Many of the maldispositions that affect the foal are also seen in the calf. They are considered in great detail in Chapter 4. Their treatment is summarized in this section and the reader is advised to consult Chapter 4 if more detail is required. Those maldispositions more commonly seen in the horse, such as the 'dog sitting' position of the fetus, will be considered here in detail.

Treatment   The principles of treatment of fetal maldisposition are broadly the same in mares as in cows. The nature of the fetal maldisposition is diagnosed by inspection of visible fetal parts and methodical palpation of the fetus per vaginam. Before delivery can be achieved the fetus must be restored, where possible, into the correct presentation, position, and posture for birth. The fetus must be repelled back into the uterus to allow the obstetrician space to correct abnormalities of head or limb posture. Generous application of obstetric lubricant will aid manipulation of the fetus, including repulsion. In quiet mares fetal repulsion may be achieved by firmly pushing the fetal head, chest, or hindquarters away from the pelvic inlet. If maternal straining makes this maneuver difficult, an epidural anesthetic may be administered; 10–15 mL of 2% lidocaine (lignocaine) may be given into sacrococcygeal space or the first intercoccygeal space. Pulling the mare's tongue out of the side of her mouth sometimes helps to reduce straining and may be used before an epidural anesthetic is given. Relaxation of the uterine muscles may also assist in the correction of maldispositions and can be achieved by the use of 200–300 μg clenbuterol given by intravenous or intramuscular injection. Correction of maldispositions may be more readily performed in the standing mare. The recumbent mare should be encouraged to rise if manipulation of the fetus is proving difficult.

Deviated extremities are identified and if possible returned to their correct anatomical position.

Damage to the uterine wall may be minimized by the obstetrician cupping the sharp points of the deviated extremity in the hand as it is returned to its normal position. Once the maldisposition has been corrected the mare should be assisted to deliver the foal as quickly as possible.

If manual correction is impossible, the alternatives are to proceed to cesarean section or fetotomy. If facilities for cesarean section are not available or if the foal is dead, fetotomy (often partial) may provide the only course of action. The foal will not usually survive for more than an hour in second-stage labor and thus in many cases of dystocia it may already be dead. If there are any doubts concerning the living state of the foal when fetotomy is to be performed it can be destroyed by intrathoracic injection of 40–50 mL pentobarbitone sodium.

FETAL MALPRESENTATION AND MALPOSITION

Malpresentation

Posterior presentation

This condition occurs in only about 1% of normal equine births but accounted for 16% of dystocia cases seen in the Ghent survey (Vanderplassche 1993). Posterior presentation of the foal apparently predisposes to difficulty at birth. Fifty per cent of the foals in posterior presentation were also in lateral position as they entered the birth canal. This caused the fetus to be impacted against the pelvic brim or wing of ilium.

Before the fetus is delivered it should be repelled and, when necessary, rotated back into a dorsal position. As in other species, delivery of the fetus in posterior presentation is generally more hazardous than when the fetus is in anterior presentation. If the fetus becomes hypoxic it may attempt to breath and inhale amniotic fluid. This problem is exacerbated by premature rupture or by compression of the umbilical cord, which is likely to occur during delivery in this presentation. Once delivery in posterior presentation is started it should be completed as quickly as possible. For this reason the obstetrician must ensure that adequate assistance is available before attempting to deliver the fetus.

Transverse presentation

This rare presentation – occurring in only 0.1% of natural births – is always associated with dystocia;

16% of cases of dystocia in the Ghent survey were associated with the fetus in this presentation. Cesarean section is required to deliver the fetus in most cases.

Etiology   In normal equine pregnancy the fetus commences its development in one uterine horn. After 6 months gestation it also occupies part of the uterine body. The placenta also extends into the nonpregnant uterine horn.

In transverse presentation, fetal occupancy of the uterus is abnormal and is almost always associated with a *bicornual pregnancy*. Fetal development commences in one uterine horn and as the fetus grows it enters the other uterine horn rather than the body of the uterus. The placenta develops fully in both horns and, as a result, some fetuses become larger than normal. Fetal movement is somewhat restricted and a degree of joint ankylosis may occur. A further complication is that the unoccupied uterine body does not grow and expand as much as it does in a normal pregnancy. The exit from the uterus at the cervical end of the uterine body may therefore be smaller than normal and the fetus poorly accessible to the obstetrician. Natural birth is quite impossible.

Clinical signs   Although the birth process starts it makes no progress because the uterine contractions of first-stage labor do not move the fetus towards the pelvis but impact it further into the two uterine horns. Vaginal examination may reveal a poorly developed uterine body, the fetus far forward in the uterus and only just palpable through its fetal membranes by the obstetrician's finger tips. In most transverse pregnancies the fetus is in a ventral position and the feet are directed towards the maternal pelvis. Other parts of the fetus are not palpable (Fig. 5.1).

A *ventrotransverse presentation* not associated with bicornual pregnancy has also been described in the mare. In this abnormality the fetus is thought to have developed chiefly in the uterine body. At birth all four fetal legs enter the birth canal and the fetus becomes impacted with both head and hindquarters away from the pelvic inlet.

Occasionally, a *dorsotransverse presentation* is encountered, in which case the obstetrician may be able to palpate the spinal column of the fetus and possibly its neck or croup (Fig. 5.2).

Treatment   If the fetus is alive, immediate cesarean section is advisable, and even if the fetus is dead this may be the best course of action. Fetotomy may be possible but the fetus is normally so far forward from the

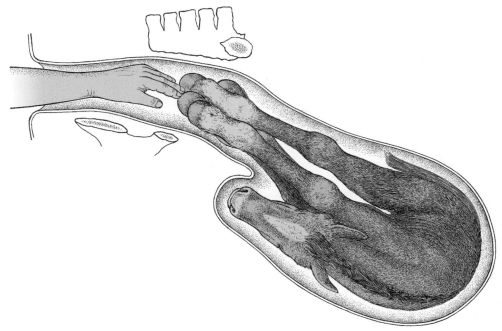

Figure 5.1 Bicornual pregnancy in the mare. The foal is in a ventrotransverse presentation. The uterine body is poorly developed and vaginal delivery is impossible.

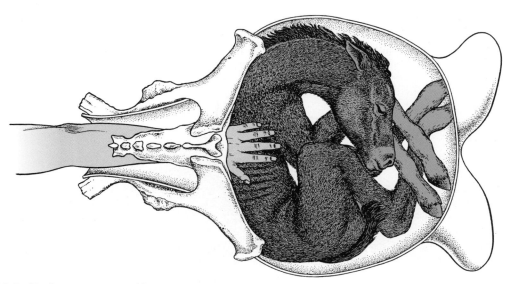

Figure 5.2 Foal in dorsotransverse position.

cervix that access is extremely difficult. Very occasionally it may be possible to reach one end of the fetal body, bring it to the pelvic inlet and deliver the fetus per vaginam.

Vertical presentation

A form of dystocia seen very occasionally in the horse (and extremely rarely in the cow) is sometimes described as being a 'vertical presentation'. This is the '*dog sitting position*' in which the fetal head, neck, and forelimbs are in the vagina accompanied by the distal extremities of both hind limbs.

Clinical signs   Initially, birth may appear normal with the fetal forelegs and head appearing at the vulva. Unproductive straining follows and no progress is made. Vaginal examination reveals that the forelegs are less advanced in the birth canal than normal (this may also be seen in cases of elbow flexion, see p. 93). In some cases the head and part of the thorax pass through the vulva. The fetus cannot be moved caudally even when modest traction is applied, even though it appears that delivery is underway and should now be easy and uncomplicated.

This lack of progress – being abnormal and unexpected – should indicate an unusual situation requiring further careful vaginal examination. Such examination is not easy because the presence of the fetus in the birth canal makes access difficult. The lubricated hand is advanced into the vagina beside or beneath the fetus and towards the pelvic brim. In cases of the dog sitting position the hindfeet are found resting on the pelvic floor (Fig. 5.3) The position of the hindlimbs – with hips flexed and hocks extended – prevents any further advance of the fetus into the birth canal.

Treatment   If the problem is diagnosed at an early stage it may be possible for the hindfeet to be cupped in the obstetrician's hands and lifted off the pelvic floor and placed back in the uterus. The hindlimbs are placed as far forward from the pelvic inlet as space will allow. Traction is applied to the head and forelegs of the fetus and it is delivered. There is still a risk that the hindfeet may damage the uterine floor.

If the hindfeet cannot be reached or dislodged it has been suggested that the anterior end of the fetus could be repelled into the uterus. Traction is applied to the hindlimbs to convert the presentation into a posterior presentation in a ventral position. The fetus is rotated into a dorsal position and delivered by traction. Although possible, this complex manipulation is likely to be difficult.

Cesarean section would be difficult unless the fetus could be repelled into the uterus enabling it to be removed at laparotomy. Correction of the maldisposition by laparotomy and hysterotomy may be an alternative to full cesarean section. A small opening in the uterus is made. The obstetrician reaches forward in the uterus to identify the displaced limbs, which are lifted from the pelvic floor and carefully extended back into the uterus. The fetus is delivered by traction and the small opening in the uterus and the laparotomy wound are closed.

If manipulative delivery is impossible, fetotomy may present the only method of resolving the problem if the fetus is dead. Using the embryotome with the wire looped over the fetal head and neck the fetus should be

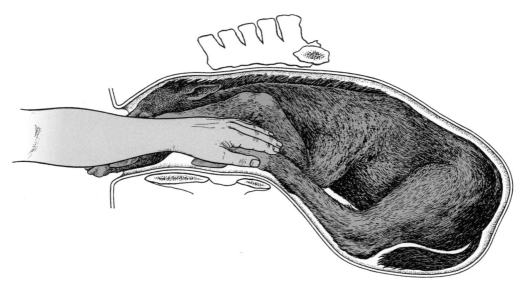

Figure 5.3 Fetal malposture – foal in the 'dog sitting' position.

sectioned in the lumbar region. The front end of the fetus is delivered by traction. Fetal viscera should be removed manually. The caudal part of the spinal column is repelled converting the fetal remnants into a posterior presentation. Traction applied to the hindlegs should allow delivery to be achieved preceded if possible by rotation to place the fetus into the dorsal position.

Malposition

The foal is normally born in the dorsal position but during gestation it lies in the uterus in a ventral position. The fetus starts to rotate into the dorsal position during the first stage of labor. The hindquarters and legs of the foal usually rotate from ventral to dorsal position during the second stage of labor as the foal is born. Failure of this rotation to occur will lead to a malposition, which may be left or right lateral or ventral – in the latter case the foal being 'upside down' in the birth canal. The dorsal surface of the foal's body is rather more pointed than that of the calf and its shape is accommodated by the contour of the inner dorsal surface of the maternal pelvis. Any malposition may interfere with the delivery of the foal. Malposition may occur in the foal in either anterior or posterior presentation.

The malposition is diagnosed by examination of the foal's position in relation to that of its mother. It must be corrected by obstetric rotation whereby the foal is turned on its long axis into the dorsal position. This is achieved repelling the fetus and then applying lateral direct pressure to the shoulder region of the fetus assisted if appropriate by a rocking movement. The maneuver is greatly assisted by generous application of obstetric lubricant to the fetus and the birth canal.

Strong uterine contractions and straining may impact the malpositioned fetus and make repulsion and rotation difficult. In this case, a degree of rotation can often be achieved during delivery by applying traction combined with rotation. Downward pressure is exerted on one fetal limb and upward pressure on the other as traction is applied.

Malposture

This extremely important category of equine dystocia is caused by displacement of the fetal head and/or forelegs with the fetus in anterior presentation. Hock and hip flexion may complicate delivery of the fetus in posterior presentation. Natural movements by the foal during birth help it to assume the correct posture for delivery. If the foal is dead, unwell, or deformed, these natural movements do not occur and the risk of dystocia is increased. In most cases, non-productive straining is seen, sometimes combined with an abnormal appearance of fetal parts at the vulva. For example, the head and a single forelimb or two forelimbs without the head.

Lateral deviation of the head

This abnormality was the single most common cause of dystocia in the Ghent survey, being responsible for 40% of all the equine dystocia cases. The deviation may arise sporadically or may be caused by the condition of wry neck, in which the fetal neck is 'permanently' deviated laterally.

Clinical signs   The fetal forelegs are found within the vagina or protrude through the vulval lips. Intense maternal straining fails to move the fetus. Vaginal examination confirms the absence of the fetal head in the pelvis but the base of the neck is palpable and deviates sharply to the right or left (Fig. 5.4).

Treatment   The long neck and head of the foal may mean that the fetal muzzle may be lying near its hindquarters. Space is required to accommodate correction of the abnormality and the fetus must be repelled as far back into the uterus as possible. This may be assisted by standing the mare on a sloping surface with her hindquarters raised and the use of epidural anesthesia. Generous lubrication is mandatory.

The base of the neck is located and followed forwards until the head is located. The head is brought towards the pelvis, initially by pulling the skin of the neck, an ear or inserting the finger into an eye socket or the mouth until the head is brought closer to the obstetrician. If possible, the obstetrician encloses the fetal muzzle to protect the uterus and the head is guided round and up into the pelvis.

The head of the foal is much longer than that of the calf and bringing it round into the pelvis is proportionately more difficult (Fig. 5.5).

Once the head has been located, ventral flexion of the fetal neck will provide more space to correct the displacement of the head.

If correction of the abnormality is impossible, cesarean section or fetotomy may be required.

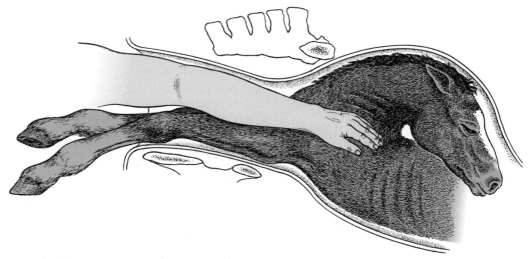

Figure 5.4 Fetal malposture – lateral deviation of the head.

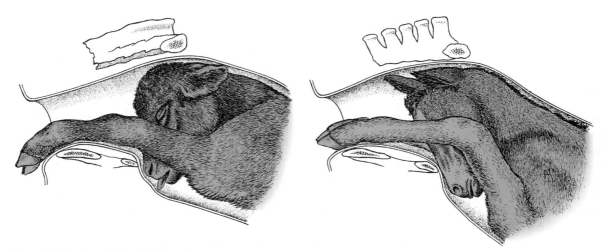

Figure 5.5 The head of the foal (right) is much longer than the head of the calf (left) and manipulation into the correct posture is more difficult.

Downward deviation of the head

Clinical signs   Varying degrees of this abnormality are seen. The long nose of the foal can quite easily catch on the maternal pelvic brim causing the fetus to be presented in the vertex posture. In severe cases the head may be pushed down between the forelegs in the breast–head posture.

Treatment   Slight downward displacements such as in the vertex posture may be corrected by repelling the fetus and lifting the fetal muzzle up onto the pelvic floor. The long fetal head may require the poll of the head to be further repelled to allow space for the muzzle to be lifted into the pelvis. In cases of severe downward deviation it may be necessary to repel a forelimb into the uterus to permit access to the head and to allow it to be retrieved and brought up into the pelvis. The foreleg is brought back up into the pelvis and delivery by traction follows. If manual correction proves impossible, delivery must be by cesarean section or fetotomy.

Dystocia in the mare caused by the foot–nape malposture in the foal

This rare dystocia is not believed to occur in cattle and is caused partly by displacement of the fetal head and partly by displacement of the forelegs.

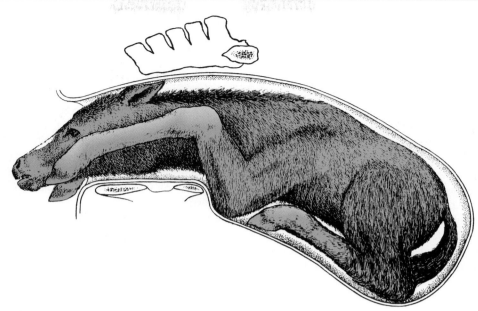

Figure 5.6 Foal malposture – incomplete extension of the elbow.

Clinical signs   Attention is drawn to the case by severe non-productive straining by the mare. Vaginal examination reveals the fetal head in a normal extended position in the vagina. The fetal forefeet are found resting on the dorsal surface of the fetal head or neck. The legs may cross over each other and the tips of the hooves may be directed towards the roof of the vagina. If the dystocia is not rapidly corrected there is a grave risk that the hooves may penetrate the vaginal roof possibly producing a rectovaginal fistula.

Treatment   The foal is repelled and the upper limb is lifted from its position across the fetal neck and placed alongside the head. The second limb is dealt with in a similar manner. The fetal head is lifted upwards and the legs placed just underneath the head. Both legs are extended and the fetus is delivered by traction.

Retention of a forelimb

This may involve carpal flexion, incomplete extension of the elbow, or shoulder flexion involving one or both forelimbs.

1. Carpal flexion

Clinical signs   In many cases when only one limb is affected, the fetal nose and the distal extremity of one foreleg are visible at the vulva but, despite straining, the mare makes no progress. Vaginal examination will normally reveal the other limb either at the pelvic inlet or in the vagina. The anterior surface of the flexed carpus

is palpable and the long slender limbs of the foal may allow the flexed carpus to enter the vagina and come almost up to the vulva.

Treatment   The fetus must be repelled as far as possible. The flexed carpus is repelled, pushed upwards and forwards into the uterus to bring the fetal foot within reach of the obstetrician. The foot is cupped in the hand and brought up into the pelvis. If both legs are in carpal flexion, both must be retrieved and brought into the pelvis. In some cases a calving rope may be used to help correct the abnormality (see Carpal flexion in Chapter 4, p. 53). If the foal is dead and the deviated limb impacted, it can be sectioned just below the carpus with the embryotome to allow fetal delivery.

2. Incomplete extension of the elbow

This condition may be more common if the fetal head is larger than normal and appears to be seen more frequently in Shetland ponies than in other breeds.

Clinical signs   The fetal nose and the tips of the feet may appear together at the vulval lips. The feet are not in advance of the nose as they are in normal birth. The fetus appears to be completely impacted and does not move even when the mare strains vigorously. Vaginal examination – if space permits – reveals that the fetal elbows are flexed and the olecranon process of each is impacted against the anterior edge of the maternal pelvic brim (Fig. 5.6).

Treatment   The problem is normally easy to correct. The fetus is repelled and, after lubrication, one limb is pulled into an extended position. The second limb is extended in a similar fashion and the foal delivered by traction.

3. Shoulder flexion

Bilateral shoulder flexion in the foal is rare and more commonly one limb only is involved.

Clinical signs   The fetal head and one limb protrude from the vulva. The second forelimb is absent but the shoulder joint on that side is palpable. The proximal portions of the retained forelimb can be felt in a flexed position lying alongside the fetal thorax.

Treatment   The fetus is repelled and an attempt made to retrieve the retained limb. The limb is grasped around the humerus and the shoulder joint is extended. The obstetrician's hand is transferred to the radius as soon as possible and the carpus is brought up to the pelvic inlet. The carpal flexion is corrected by the method described above.

If the foal is dead and it is impossible to retrieve the deviated limb it can be removed by fetotomy. The fetotomy wire attached to an introducer is dropped between the upper forelimb of the foal and its thoracic wall. The wire is threaded through the embryotome and the muscular attachments of the limb are readily sawn through allowing removal of the limb and fetal delivery.

Retention of a hindlimb

Hock flexion and hip flexion involving one or both hindlimbs can occur in the fetus in posterior presentation.

1. Hock flexion

Clinical signs   The tip of the fetal tail may be seen at the vulva and the flexed hocks are palpable at the pelvic inlet. If one limb only is involved the other leg can be extended and protruding through the vulva.

Treatment   The long legs of the foal make this a potentially difficult and hazardous procedure. Great care must be taken to avoid damage to the uterine floor by the sharp hoof of the foal during the process of correction. The fetus is repelled into the uterus as far forward as possible. Using plenty of lubrication, the hock is pushed upwards and forwards. The obstetrician's hand slides down the metatarsus to seek the fetal foot. The foot is cupped in the hand and is lifted into the pelvic canal, thus allowing the limb to be extended and delivery to proceed. For further details of alternative manipulation used in the calf and applicable to the foal, see Chapter 4, p. 94.

If the foal is dead and the malposture cannot be corrected manually, the lower part of the limb may be removed by fetotomy.

2. Hip flexion (breech presentation)

Clinical signs   Only the tail of the foal may be visible at the vulva and sometimes – if the tail lies alongside the fetal body – nothing is visible, despite intense non-productive straining. Vaginal examination reveals the hindquarters of the foal either engaged in the maternal pelvis or lying in front of or below the pelvis. Occasionally, only one limb is flexed and the other is extended into the birth canal.

Treatment   The fetus is repelled from the pelvic inlet and an attempt made to locate one of the hocks. This is gently raised up to the pelvic inlet. Once there it is dealt with as a case of hock flexion (see above). If the second limb is involved it is dealt with in a similar manner. A calving rope may be used to assist in retrieving the hock (see Chapter 4).

If manipulative delivery is impossible, cesarean section or fetotomy may be used.

Delivery of an equine breech presentation in an uncorrected malposture   If the fetus is small and the mare's pelvis capacious, it *may* be possible to deliver the foal without attempting to retrieve the retained hindlimbs. Ropes are passed (using the introducer of an embryotome) between the thigh and the body wall of the fetus on both sides. Traction is applied and the fetus is guided rump first into the pelvis. Further traction is applied and the foal delivered. *This is a potentially hazardous procedure with severe consequences if the fetus become impacted in the maternal pelvis during delivery.* Severe damage to the cervix will probably be sustained by the mare, making her unfit for future breeding. The technique is not recommended unless all other methods fail or are unavailable.

DYSTOCIA DUE TO MULTIPLE BIRTH

Every effort is made – at least in Thoroughbred and other controlled breeding establishments – to avoid twin pregnancy. In many cases the twin pregnancy – through placental insufficiency – will end in abortion at about 7 months gestation. Occasionally the pregnancy goes on to term, when two small foals are born. Dystocia can occur if:

- either fetus is malpresented
- simultaneous presentation of the fetuses occurs

- uterine inertia, which is rare in mares, occurs as a result of overstretching of the uterus.

Clinical signs and treatment   The presence of twin foals may have been discovered after formation of the endometrial cups at 35 days and a decision made to allow the pregnancy to continue to term. Such a foaling should be carefully supervised and assisted as required. Early vaginal examination should be performed and action taken to deliver the foals manually if uterine inertia is present. If two fetuses are presented simultaneously at the pelvic inlet or within the vagina, one is repelled and the other delivered by traction. Maldispositions are dealt with in the manner described for singleton foals suffering this abnormality.

DYSTOCIA CAUSED BY FETAL DEATH

Fetal death during pregnancy in the mare is normally followed by abortion. If the foal dies at term dystocia may arise through: (1) failure of the foal to adopt the normal birth posture; (2) loss of fetal fluids, which impedes normal delivery through lack of natural lubrication. Failure of the cervix to dilate (as may occur in similar circumstances in cattle) is seldom a problem in mares, in which the cervix can normally be manually dilated without difficulty.

Treatment   This is attempted by manually dilating the cervix, introducing generous amounts of lubricant into the uterus, correcting any maldisposition, and attempting to deliver the foal by traction. Before treatment in cases in which the fetus is thought to have been dead for some time, a full evaluation of the mare should be performed. Antibiotic and non-steroidal anti-inflammatory therapy is advisable before delivery is commenced. If the mare looks unwell and shows signs of abdominal pain, a peritoneal tap is useful to check for the presence of early peritonitis, which would worsen the prognosis of the case. Ultrasonographic guidance may assist in obtaining peritoneal rather than allantoic fluid.

For further discussion on additional methods of dealing with the emphysematous fetus, see Chapter 4, p. 56.

SIGNS OF DYSTOCIA IN THE MARE

Thoroughbred mares are very closely supervised as birth approaches. Many pony mares foal in the open without supervision. Prediction of the time of birth in the horse is notoriously difficult. Gestation length is very variable and even the same mare may show considerable variation in the length of her gestation during different pregnancies. Mares prefer to give birth in conditions of quiet and solitude. Observation by stable staff for approaching foaling may itself disturb the mare and delay birth for many hours or even days. Such observation must be very discreet but must nonetheless be thorough because, if dystocia is thought to be present, it must be dealt with as a matter of urgency.

Specific signs of dystocia include:

- Prolonged first-stage labor: the mare is restless for much longer than normal.
- Straining without any progress being made.
- The presence at the vulva of an abnormal combination of extremities – two forefeet alone may indicate that the head is deviated laterally. The fetal head and one forelimb may indicate that one limb is abnormally disposed in shoulder or carpal flexion. A more subtle abnormality – but a serious one – is that observed in cases of elbow flexion. In this abnormality the fetal forefeet are level with the nose instead of being in front of it (Fig. 5.6).
- Any abnormal vaginal discharge or odor, which might indicate signs of fetal death.

APPROACH TO A CASE OF DYSTOCIA IN THE MARE

Speed of attendance

The importance of rapid attendance to foaling cases has already been mentioned but is so important that it is repeated here. While waiting for the arrival of the obstetrician the owner could be advised to keep the mare standing and walking to minimize nonproductive straining. Clean, warm water and help should be arranged. Separation of the chorion from the endometrium occurs in some cases of dystocia and also after induced birth. The red-colored velvety chorion may appear unruptured at the vulva, with fetal parts palpable through it and the amnion. This is sometimes termed a 'red bag foaling'. Experienced owners and grooms should be advised to open the chorion quickly, but carefully, with scissors while awaiting the obstetrician.

OBSTETRICIAN'S CHECK LIST

Call received

Brief history taken
↓
Advice to owner *re* immediate treatment
↓
Keep mare walking/reduce straining
↓
Open vulva if sutured
↓
Open chorion if 'red bag foaling'
↓
Obstetrician – check equipment
↓
Attend mare urgently

On Thoroughbred stud farms an experienced head groom is sometimes instructed to perform a vaginal examination of the mare as she enters second-stage labor. If both forefeet and the head of the fetus are present the mare is left to foal without assistance, although her progress is monitored carefully. If the fetal presentation is not normal, the head groom may make minor adjustments to the fetal posture and, if necessary, the obstetrician is called immediately.

Preparations for foaling

In case problems occur the owner should be encouraged to have the mare in an accessible, roomy box. Light, electricity, and a good supply of warm water should be readily available. Foaling outside is possible if the weather is good but observation in such circumstances can be difficult and the lack of facilities, should help be required, is a disadvantage. The mare should wear a head collar at all times so that she can be caught with ease in any circumstances.

Even normally quiet mares can become agitated and violent as birth approaches. They may lie down or get up very quickly and lash out with their hindlegs or strike out with their forelegs during foaling, and such behavior may become more violent if dystocia occurs.

A foaling mare should be approached with great caution and the obstetrician should always be alert and ready to take evasive action if violent behavior – often unpredicted – occurs.

A tail bandage should be fitted and changed daily and it is advisable, for safety reasons, to remove the mare's shoes. If the mare has had her vulval lips sutured by Caslick's operation before breeding the sutured area should be snipped open with a pair of scissors.

Position of the mare, assistance, and restraint

A reliable assistant holding the mare's head is essential. If she is already lying down and her hindquarters are accessible she may be approached quietly and a preliminary vaginal examination may be carried out without the mare rising. If she is nervous or standing it is advisable to have a second assistant holding her tail and steadying her hindquarters. Two persons may be required to apply traction to the foal. If only one assistant is available to hold the mare's head the use of a calf puller to apply careful traction during fetal delivery can be helpful. A calf puller should be used only in exceptional circumstances, and then only by the obstetrician. This is not likely to be necessary in Thoroughbred establishments. If the mare is lying in a corner where her hindquarters are not accessible to the obstetrician she must be encouraged to rise and moved round so that such access is possible.

Sedation

This is advisable in nervous mares but the level of sedation must be such that the ability to stand can be maintained. Detomidine hydrochloride provides effective sedation at a dose of 10–20 µg/kg given by intravenous or intramuscular injection.

Epidural anesthesia

This is not necessary for routine equine obstetric work. If straining makes examination or manipulation difficult, or if fetotomy is required, epidural anesthesia will be beneficial; 10–15 mL of 2% lidocaine (lignocaine) hydrochloride is injected via the sacrococcygeal space or the first intercoccygeal space using strict aseptic technique. It is sometimes less easy to locate the injection site in mares than in cows. Careful palpation for the depression between adjoining dorsal spines of vertebrae and locating the point of maximum flexibility of the tail base is often helpful.

Protective clothing

Unless the mare is very quiet it is not advisable for the obstetrician to wear a long parturition garment. The rustling of the garment may frighten the mare and its length may inhibit the obstetrician taking rapid evasive action if the mare becomes suddenly violent. Normal washable clothing and waterproof overtrousers will be useful.

Equipment

- Three nylon ropes (such as calving ropes), preferably of different colors and with cylindrical wooden handles with which to apply traction.
- A mechanical puller, such as the HK calving aid, is useful in professional hands (only) if little skilled help is available.
- A fetotomy kit if available.
- A supply of obstetric lubricant, oxytocin, tetanus antitoxin, local anesthetic, clenbuterol, antibiotics, a sedative (such as detomidine hydrochloride). Doxapram hydrochloride and oxygen may be required for the foal.

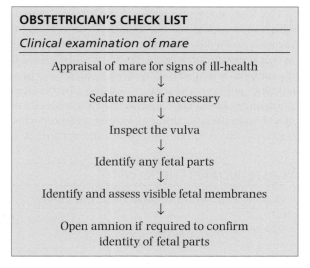

OBSTETRICIAN'S CHECK LIST

Arrival at stables

Further history taken briefly
↓
Expected foaling date?
↓
Management during pregnancy?
↓
Problems during pregnancy?
↓
Duration of labor?
↓
What has been observed so far?
↓
Discuss restraint of mare
↓
Assess available assistance
↓
Seek further assistance if required and available
↓
Approach mare with caution

General examination of the mare

A brief appraisal of the mare is required and more detailed examination is made if she appears unwell. Heavy sweating at foaling is quite normal, as are signs of colicky discomfort and groaning. The problems of

acute hypocalcemia and acute mastitis (quite common in the cow) are very seldom seen in the parturient mare.

The presence of visible fetal parts and placental tissue is observed. The outer surface of the chorion is a deep red color and has a velvety appearance. Occasionally, especially in induced birth, the chorion does not rupture as the foal enters the pelvic inlet. In such rare cases ('red bag delivery' or 'red bag foaling') the chorion appears as a conical red projection emerging from the vulval lips. If it does not rupture spontaneously it should be opened carefully using a pair of scissors.

In most cases, any fetal parts are covered by the amnion, which is more fibrous and less transparent than in the cow. If the amnion is very opaque it may be difficult to identify any fetal parts visually. Palpation of the fetal parts usually allows them to be readily identified. If there is still doubt concerning the identity of fetal parts, the amnion can be opened by tearing or the careful use of scissors.

OBSTETRICIAN'S CHECK LIST

Clinical examination of mare

Appraisal of mare for signs of ill-health
↓
Sedate mare if necessary
↓
Inspect the vulva
↓
Identify any fetal parts
↓
Identify and assess visible fetal membranes
↓
Open amnion if required to confirm identity of fetal parts

Vaginal examination

The genital tract of the mare is susceptible to infection and the obstetrician must pay very strict attention to hygiene. The whole perineal region is washed thoroughly and the obstetrician's lubricated hand is passed through the vulva into the vagina. Once the obstetrician's hand is within the vagina the mare does not normally kick out behind herself.

If the vulva is not easily dilated the obstetrician should check again that the upper parts of the vulval lips are not constricted by an earlier Caslick's operation. If such constrictions remain they should be removed by carefully cutting between the vulval lips up to the dorsal commissure to restore the full vulval orifice.

The vagina and its contents are explored systematically, as in other species. The mare has a large external urethral orifice (with no diverticulum) lying on the pelvic floor. In some mares foaling for the first time a hymenal remnant may be present just in front of the external urethral orifice. In most cases it causes no problem but it can occasionally obstruct the vagina. It may be possible to push it to one side or gently tear through its thin non-vascular structure with the fingers. Occasionally, it may be necessary to carefully incise the hymen with a scalpel.

The cervix of the mare is usually level with the brim of the pelvis. The external os protrudes caudally into the vagina and distinct dorsal and ventral frenulae are palpable when the cervix is closed. The equine cervix is much softer and less fibrous than that of the cow and can in most cases be readily dilated with expanding digital pressure. If fully dilated the cervix blends with the vaginal wall and cannot be recognized.

The fetus is usually enclosed within the amnion, which in horses seems particularly closely applied to the fetus and tightly stretched by the head and forelegs as they enter the birth canal. The fetus, still enclosed in the amnion, is palpated with care to establish its presentation, position, and posture and also whether there is evidence of fetal life. This examination is performed exactly as in the calf. Although fetopelvic disproportion is a rare cause of equine dystocia, an attempt is made to compare the size of the fetus with the soft and bony tissue dimensions of the birth canal. The hand is passed back past the long head of the fetus and along the neck to the shoulders. If the lubricated hand can be moved comfortably between the fetus and the maternal pelvis vaginal delivery is likely to be possible. Trial traction is certainly justified. The presence of more than one fetus is also very uncommon but care must be taken to ensure that any fetal parts palpable belong to the same foal.

If the presentation, position, or posture of the foal is abnormal the amnion must be opened to enable the obstetrician to examine the fetus more directly, confirm the maldisposition, and attempt corrective action. Firm finger pressure is required to penetrate the equine amnion and, occasionally, it may have to be opened carefully with scissors.

If there is evidence of fetal maldisposition, this must be corrected before delivery can take place, Repulsion of the fetus is necessary in most cases and is achieved by applying pressure to the fetal head. In cases of elbow flexion, repulsion is followed by extension of the limbs to enable the elbows to enter the birth canal. In more severe malpostures, considerable fetal repulsion is necessary to provide room to manipulate the misplaced extremities into their correct position. Encouraging the recumbent mare to stand may facilitate the correction of fetal maldispositions. Great care must be taken to protect the uterine and vaginal walls from damage during fetal manipulation.

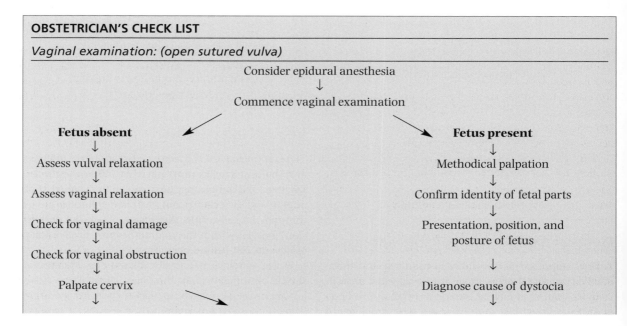

OBSTETRICIAN'S CHECK LIST

Vaginal examination: (open sutured vulva)

Consider epidural anesthesia
↓
Commence vaginal examination

Fetus absent
↓
Assess vulval relaxation
↓
Assess vaginal relaxation
↓
Check for vaginal damage
↓
Check for vaginal obstruction
↓
Palpate cervix
↓

Fetus present
↓
Methodical palpation
↓
Confirm identity of fetal parts
↓
Presentation, position, and posture of fetus
↓
Diagnose cause of dystocia
↓

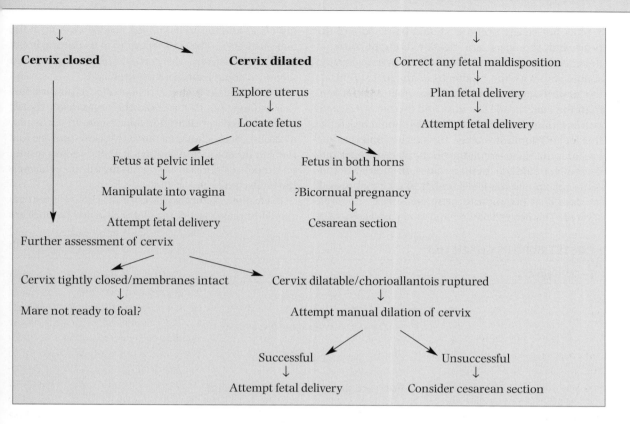

MANIPULATIVE DELIVERY

The obstetrician should check that the foal is in the correct presentation and that there appears to be space between the foal and the pelvis. Generous amounts of obstetric lubricant should be introduced into the birth canal. Ideally, help should be given to the mare when she is lying down. If she is standing she may be left for a short time until she lies down, but prolonged delay is not justified in case the foal is already becoming hypoxic. Sometimes fetal maldispositions can be corrected more easily in the standing mare.

If the mare foals – or is assisted to foal – in the standing position the foal's umbilical cord may rupture prematurely. In such circumstances, flow of blood from the placenta back into the fetal circulation may be impaired and there may be resultant tissue hypoxia.

Sometimes, the mare does not lie down to foal – either when being assisted or when foaling naturally. Premature rupture of the umbilical cord can occur in such circumstances and does not always have serious consequences.

If the foal is of normal size, has entered the birth canal and the mare is straining, delivery may be achieved by two persons each grasping a fetal leg just above the fetlock. As the mare strains, each leg is pulled in turn under the obstetrician's instructions. The direction of pull is initially backwards and then downwards towards the mare's hocks. If a little more traction is required, ropes may be applied to the foal's legs just above the fetlock joints. They may be tied onto cylindrical wooden handles and traction applied to alternate forelegs with the aid of ropes and handles (see also Figs 4.18 and 4.19).

In cases where the foal's head has not engaged in the pelvis, an additional rope should be applied to the head – using the same technique as in the calf – before the leg ropes are placed in position. Traction is applied in sequence to each foreleg and then the head, with the greatest effort coinciding with the mare's straining.

If only one person is available to help with delivery, the HK calf puller – or similar instrument – may be used in exceptional circumstances to apply traction. This is used in the same way as it is used in the cow and can be equally effective. It should be used only by the obstetrician and with the same limitations on the degree of traction exerted as in the cow (see Chapter 4, p. 72).

Slow but steady progress should be made and the head and shoulders are steadily brought through the vulva. Once the thorax has been delivered, traction should stop with the hindlimbs of the foal still inside the mare's vagina. Amniotic remnants are removed from the foal's head. The nose and muzzle are cleared and breathing is monitored. The foal should be left like this for 5–10 minutes while the uterus contracts and squeezes the blood circulating in the placenta back into the foal's circulation. In many cases, the mare will suddenly get up and the foal's umbilical cord ruptures. If the cord does not rupture spontaneously it should be severed. The obstetrician's hand is placed against the umbilicus and the cord is pulled steadily away from the foal's abdomen. The cord separates at its natural break point. Alternatively, the cord should be ligated and sectioned about 5 cm from the umbilicus.

If traction fails to move the foal after 5 minutes, further pulling should cease and the obstetrician should check the foal's presentation once again. In particular, a careful check should be made to ensure that the foal is not in the dog sitting position, with its hindfeet resting on the pelvic floor preventing further advance through the birth canal.

If a further attempt at delivery by traction fails the case should be reassessed. If the foal is alive and facilities are

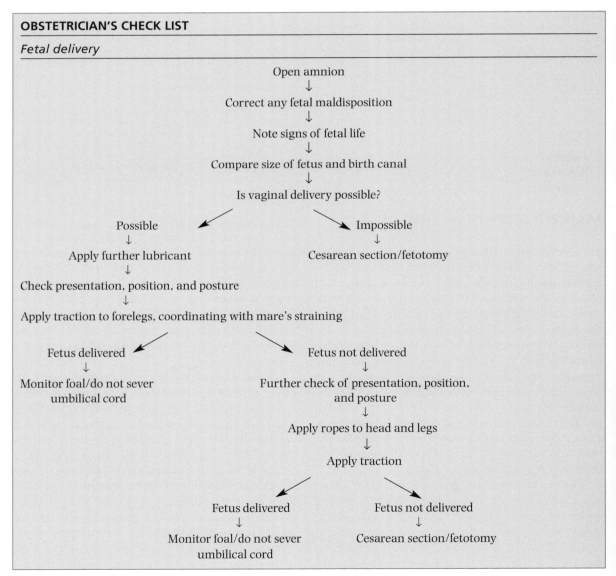

OBSTETRICIAN'S CHECK LIST

Fetal delivery

Open amnion
↓
Correct any fetal maldisposition
↓
Note signs of fetal life
↓
Compare size of fetus and birth canal
↓
Is vaginal delivery possible?

Possible ← → Impossible
↓ ↓
Apply further lubricant   Cesarean section/fetotomy
↓
Check presentation, position, and posture
↓
Apply traction to forelegs, coordinating with mare's straining

Fetus delivered ← → Fetus not delivered
↓ ↓
Monitor foal/do not sever   Further check of presentation, position,
umbilical cord   and posture
↓
Apply ropes to head and legs
↓
Apply traction

Fetus delivered ← → Fetus not delivered
↓ ↓
Monitor foal/do not sever   Cesarean section/fetotomy
umbilical cord

available, delivery by cesarean section may be used. If the foal is dead but readily accessible, fetotomy may be used.

RESUSCITATION OF THE FOAL

If the foal fails to breath at birth, the thorax is palpated for evidence of an apex heart beat. If the heart is beating respiration may be stimulated by administration of 40–100 mg of doxapram hydrochloride given intravenously or sublingually. The pharynx and larynx should also be cleared by suction and oxygen given by face mask. Should breathing fail to commence, artificial respiration should be given. A Cox foal resuscitator can also be used at this point. This has a resuscitator pump through which additional oxygen can be supplied via a face mask.

In this serious situation, concern about premature rupture of the cord is less important than starting the foal breathing. Positioning the foal safely for artificial respiration may entail rupturing and temporarily applying artery forceps to the cord. The foal is laid on its side with head and neck extended. The upper chest wall is raised and lowered holding the uppermost humerus and the last rib. If spontaneous respiration still fails to occur, an attempt should be made to intubate the foal (if suitable equipment is available) and provide positive-pressure ventilation. For further details of fetal resuscitation see Chapter 4, p. 75.

FURTHER CARE OF THE MARE AND FOAL

The foal's navel should be dipped in a weak iodine solution or 2% chlorhexidine solution; alternatively, it may be sprayed with an antibiotic aerosol. The mare's teats are checked for patency. Mare and foal are best left alone to enable bonding to take place. Discreet observation should continue in case the mare becomes mildly colicky and uncomfortable as she attempts to expel her placenta. There is also a small risk that she may accidentally tread on the foal. The foal may need assistance to stand if it has not spontaneously gained its feet within 2 hours of birth.

The foal may need help finding the teats and learning to suck, especially if, as quite often occurs, the mare's udder is uncomfortable as milk builds up in the udder. Meconium production and passage should be observed carefully. Meconium is usually passed within 12 hours of birth and retention is associated with colic. Resolution of the problem usually follows careful administration of an enema.

Urine production and passage should also be monitored. Urachal patency with leakage of urine through the umbilical stump may occur. In colt foals, discomfort may arise through inability to pass urine through the

---

OBSTETRICIAN'S CHECK LIST

Postnatal care of the foal

A: Visible signs of life

Do not sever umbilical cord intentionally
↓
Clear fetal airway
↓
Attempt to stimulate first gasp: cold water on head/needle in filtrum
↓
Administer doxapram HCl IV or under tongue
↓
Artificial respiration: manual/foal resuscitator
↓
Inflate lungs and apply further artificial respiration
↓
Monitor pulse and blood P_{O_2}
↓
Apply pulsoximeter to ear or tongue
↓

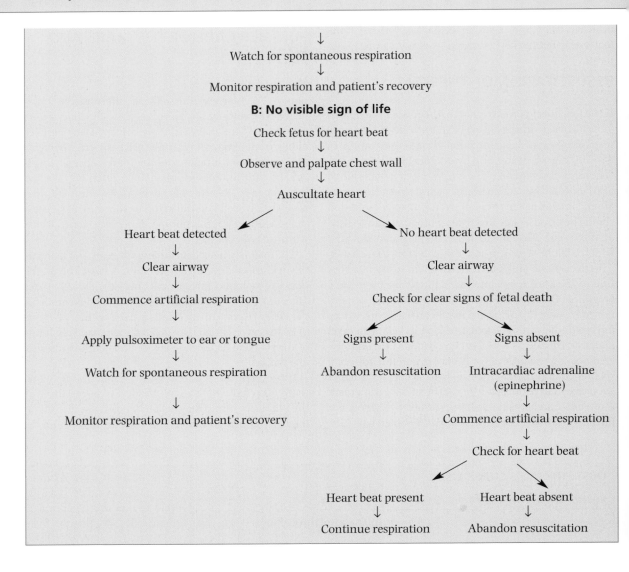

penis. The clinical signs may closely resemble those of meconium retention. The history of observed meconium passage and a digital rectal examination reveal no abnormality. Very occasionally, the penis is apparently stuck within the prepuce by smegma-like material that prevents its extrusion. Penile extrusion is essential to allow comfortable passage of urine in colt foals. If untreated the condition might progress to a ruptured bladder. The problem is readily resolved by washing the prepuce and penis with a mild soapy solution and introducing obstetric lubricant into the prepuce. The penis is then gently but firmly drawn out from the prepuce using the fingers – a procedure normally followed by immediate urination and relief of colicky

signs. The general health of the foal must be closely observed because neonatal septicemia and the neonatal maladjustment syndrome may develop at an early stage.

The mare should stand within 15 minutes of foaling and if she has not done so spontaneously should be encouraged to rise. Occasionally, a foaling mare will become cast by getting herself in an awkward position in the stable from which she cannot easily rise. She may have her head so close to a wall or corner that she cannot extend her forelegs in the normal way before rising. In many cases she does not seem able to move herself into a suitable position. She may appear distressed and ill but in many cases is simply cast. In such cases the head should be pulled round away from the obstruction and the mare stimulated by knee pressure from the obstetrician over her ribs. Most mares will rise easily and with apparent relief.

The mare normally passes her placenta within 3 hours of the foal's birth. The presence of the placenta, especially if parts hang down onto the mare's hocks may cause irritation and restlessness. The placenta is normally passed with its gray–blue allantoic surface outermost. The placenta has the gross appearance of a pair of bloomers with one large leg – from the pregnant horn – and a smaller leg from the non-pregnant horn. After the placenta is passed it should be removed from the foaling box immediately. The problem of retained placenta is dealt with in Chapter 13. In mares that have had a previous Caslick's operation, the vulval lips are cleaned, freshened and resutured in preparation for the next breeding season.

OBSTETRICIAN'S CHECK LIST

Postnatal care of the mare

Check uterus for a further foal
↓
Check birth canal for damage
↓
Check uterine involution
↓
Administer oxytocin if poor uterine involution
↓
Advise owner about placental retention
↓
Arrange to replace Caslick sutures

PROLONGED GESTATION – THE OVERDUE MARE

Pregnancy lasting over 330 days is not uncommon in mares. Fortunately it is not normally followed by the birth of a very large foal and dystocia caused by feto-pelvic disproportion. The cause of prolonged gestation in mares is usually that the fetal placenta is either small or its function compromised. Local areas of chorionic necrosis or detachment may be present, restricting the area of efficient placenta available to the foal. Gestation may be prolonged by several weeks, and occasionally up to 2 months. Fetal maturity in the mare cannot be predicted by gestational length. The window of viability in foals is narrow and premature induction of birth can result in the loss of the foal. Birth should not be induced in mares with prolonged gestation until the obstetrician is sure that the fetus is mature.

Cases of suspected prolonged gestation should always be examined without delay. The mare's service date is checked and the possibility of later services investigated. The mare should be given a full clinical examination to check her general health. Signs of approaching parturition, including relaxation of the pelvic ligaments, vulval lengthening, and mammary development may be present. These signs are not always reliable indicators of approaching birth. Pregnancy diagnosis should be performed to check that she is pregnant. Rectal examination enables the uterus and fetus to be palpated and the approximate stage of pregnancy determined. The viability of the fetus can also be determined. The cervix should be inspected or palpated to ensure that it is closed and that there is no abnormal discharge coming from the uterus. Ultrasonographic scan per rectum and transabdominally will enable the viability and pulse rate of the fetus to be observed. The placenta should be examined carefully to see if areas of placental separation from the endometrium or placental thickening are present. The fetal fluids are also viewed ultrasonographically to ensure that they are non-echogenic.

If milk is present in the udder a sample can be taken for calcium, sodium, and potassium assay. Milk calcium levels of over 40 mg/dL are indicative of fetal maturity; levels below 12 mg/dL are indicative of fetal dysmaturity. Assessment of fetal maturity and the induction of birth is discussed in greater detail in Chapter 15.

If birth does not appear imminent and the fetus is considered dysmature, the mare should be examined at intervals of 14 days to monitor the progress of her pregnancy. The owner should be advised to keep a close eye on her for signs of foaling.

OBSTETRICIAN'S CHECK LIST

Management of the overdue mare

Check service date(s)
↓
Check details of antenatal care
↓
Full clinical examination
↓

$\downarrow$

Vaginal examination – check cervix

$\downarrow$

Rectal examination – check uterus and fetus

$\downarrow$

Ultrasound scan of fetus, fluids, and placenta

$\downarrow$

Milk in the udder? – assay calcium, sodium, and potassium

$\downarrow$

Advise *re* monitoring mare

$\downarrow$

Arrange follow-up visit

REFERENCE

Vanderplassche M (1993) Dystocia. In: McKinnon AO, Voss JL (eds) Equine reproduction. Lea & Febiger, Philadelphia, p 578–587

Chapter 6

DYSTOCIA IN THE EWE

Lambing time and the periods that precede and follow it are the times of greatest veterinary activity within most sheep flocks. Obstetric work forms a substantial part of a flock's veterinary care. It is essential that the obstetrician has a good understanding of both normal and abnormal parturition in sheep. Treatment of simple dystocia cases is often undertaken by the shepherd, with more serious cases being brought to the veterinary surgery for professional care.

INCIDENCE

A number of surveys have suggested that the incidence of dystocia in ewes is approximately 3%, although the level of assistance at lambing given in closely supervised flocks may be much higher. The incidence of dystocia may be higher in ewe lambs carrying a single fetus and also in the heavier lowland breeds. The tendency to use large breeds for commercial crossing has, in some surveys, resulted in a higher incidence of dystocia due to fetopelvic disproportion. Little dystocia is seen in highland breeds or among feral sheep. Problems that may have a hereditary predisposition to dystocia, such as a small pelvic size, tend to be naturally eliminated in such groups. Over 90% of lambs are delivered in anterior presentation but the incidence of dystocia is proportionally and significantly higher in lambs in posterior presentation. In one survey, over 80% of lambs in posterior presentations had one or both fetal hindlimbs flexed.

CAUSES OF DYSTOCIA

Analysis of a number of surveys suggests that the incidence of the various causes of ovine dystocia presented for veterinary attention is as shown in Table 6.1.

Table 6.1 Causes of dystocia in the ewe

Cause	%
Fetal maldisposition	50
Obstruction of the birth canal	35
Fetopelvic disproportion	5
Fetal monsters/abnormalities	3
Others	7

Data from: Blackmore DK 1960 Some observations on dystocia in the ewe. Veterinary Record 72:631–636, Hughes-Ellis T 1958 Observations on some aspects of dystocia in the ewe. Veterinary Record 70:952–959, Jackson PGG 2003 Unpublished data, Thomas JO 1990 Survey of the causes of dystocia in sheep. Veterinary Record 127:574–575.

All surveys have shown that fetal maldisposition (especially lateral deviation of the head) and obstruction of the birth canal (especially failure of the cervix to dilate – ringwomb – are the most common causes of dystocia in sheep. These and other causes of dystocia are discussed in greater detail below.

SPECIFIC CAUSES OF DYSTOCIA IN THE EWE

Details of the more important causes of dystocia in the ewe follow below.

FAILURE OF THE EXPULSIVE FORCES

Uterine inertia

This is relatively uncommon in sheep.

Primary uterine inertia

Birth may be inhibited or delayed through fear, such as may occur through worrying of sheep by dogs. Primary uterine inertia is occasionally seen in young, inexperienced ewe lambs who, through apparent anxiety, do not actually get on with lambing. Assisted delivery and supervision of the establishment of mothering may be all that is required. Although hypocalcemia can occur both before and after lambing, it is rarely associated with uterine inertia in sheep. Primary uterine inertia may occasionally occur in severe cases of pregnancy toxemia.

Secondary uterine inertia

This may develop as a result of another cause of dystocia, such as an uncorrected fetal maldisposition. Its presence may be noted during the correction of the primary cause of dystocia. Sometimes after a first maldisposed fetus has been delivered the tone of the uterine wall is found on palpation to be very low. Specific treatment of such secondary inertia is seldom required because further fetuses are normally manually delivered. However, postdelivery administration of oxytocin will encourage uterine contraction, encourage passage of the placenta, and help prevent uterine prolapse.

Failure of abdominal expulsive forces

This may occur as a result of disease or previous injury. In cases of severe debility through poor feeding, or in advanced cases of pregnancy toxemia, the ewe may be too weak or ill to lamb spontaneously. The cervix may open at term, there is some evidence of uterine contraction, but fetal delivery does not take place. Manual delivery is normally possible and the ewe is supported by intensive nursing and medical care.

Abdominal wall ruptures or hernias are occasionally seen in ewes. Ventral rupture may occur as a result of rough handling during pregnancy. A tear occurs in the ventral abdominal wall musculature allowing the gravid uterus to pass through the abdominal wall and lie subcutaneously. The risk of complete breakdown of the abdominal wall is small but the ability of the animal to strain is compromised. Assistance with fetal delivery in affected ewes should be anticipated and planned. The udder may be displaced in such cases, making access to one of the teats by the lamb difficult.

Less common are umbilical and perineal hernias in ewes. Perineal hernias are either unilateral or bilateral and are recognized by the presence of reducible swellings in the perineal region. These are seldom life threatening unless the urinary bladder becomes trapped, but they can compromise the ability of the ewe to strain. Assisted delivery of the lambs may be required.

OBSTRUCTION OF THE BIRTH CANAL

As in other species, this may be caused by either bony or soft tissue obstruction.

Bony obstruction

This is uncommon, although the pelvis may be small in some ewe lambs (see Fetopelvic disproportion, p. 111). In some sheep, including Scottish Blackface ewes, the dorsal surface of the pubic symphysis is both sharp and prominent. In some cases this may partially obstruct the passage of the fetus. It may also cause damage to the vaginal or uterine floor as the obstetrician is manipulating the fetus prior to delivery. Great care should be taken to avoid accidentally exerting downward pressure on this sharp prominence if soft tissue damage is to be avoided.

Soft tissue obstruction

This may involve any section of the birth canal from the vulva to the cervix.

Vulval obstruction

This can result from injury at a previous lambing or occasionally through lack of normal prelambing relaxation. In most cases, gentle stretching of the vulva with the well-lubricated fingers will result in sufficient relaxation to permit passage of the obstetrician's hands and fetal delivery.

Vaginal obstruction

This is uncommon, especially in parturient ewes. It may result from either failure of normal tissue relaxation or from previous injury, including scars from the insertion of sutures to retain a vaginal prolapse. In many cases gentle stretching will overcome the problem but where this fails cesarean section may be required.

Obstruction of the birth canal by vaginal prolapse   Vaginal prolapse is a common complication of late pregnancy in sheep. In the majority of cases the prolapse does not prevent spontaneous delivery of the fetus, especially if the prolapse has been secured with a

T-shaped plastic retainer. If sutures have been used they must be removed before birth to prevent tearing of the vulval lips. Occasionally, and especially if the prolapse has been damaged, the vagina is severely edematous and swollen, with resultant occlusion of its lumen. In most cases, and using generous amounts of lubricant, the obstetrician is able to guide the fetus through the prolapsed organ without causing further damage. Very occasionally, if severe laceration has occurred, delivery by cesarean section might be necessary.

The cervix

Obstruction of the cervix (often termed *ringwomb*) is a major cause of ovine dystocia. The cervix fails to dilate sufficiently to allow fetal delivery per vaginam, or it may show only partial dilation. The exact etiology of the condition is not known but studies have suggested a number of predisposing factors. These include a failure of the normal complex process of cervical relaxation, induration of the cervix through previous injury, uterine inertia, and fetal maldisposition – especially breech presentation. Abnormally high levels of estrogen in the diet have also been blamed for 'outbreaks' of cases of ringwomb. In some cases this is associated with the presence of estrogenic *Fusarium* spp. molds in the food or bedding. The incidence of ringwomb on farms varies considerably. Numerous cases may occur in one season but the following year, although management is ostensibly the same, the incidence may be much lower.

It has also been suggested that in neglected cases of dystocia the cervix may open normally and then close again before fetal delivery, thus producing what might be described as secondary obstruction of the cervix. In some cases it may be possible to gently dilate the closed cervix manually, and this should always be attempted first. If manual dilation fails, cesarean section is usually required. A number of drugs, including estradiol, vitamin D, calcium borogluconate, prostaglandin E, and a range of 'uterine relaxants' have been used in an attempt to open the cervix. Evaluation of such treatments is difficult and none has been found to be entirely reliable. If the cervix is genuinely obstructed, fetal life will be at risk and delivery by cesarean section should not be delayed. Further details about the evaluation and treatment of the closed cervix are given below (p. 115).

Torsion of the uterus

Uterine torsion is rare in sheep and results in partial or complete obstruction of the caudal part of the uterine body, preventing passage of the lamb. Uterine torsion usually occurs (as in cattle) at the beginning of first-stage labor. It is usually detected when a vaginal examination is carried out to determine why an expected birth has not proceeded at the anticipated rate. An internal examination reveals that the vagina is obstructed caudal to the cervix. Displaced folds of vaginal mucosa converge conically as the hand is advanced. If the degree of torsion is less than 180° it may be possible to pass the hand beyond the obstruction and past the dilated cervix to palpate the lamb. Complete obstruction may occur if the degree of torsion is greater than 180°. Torsion may be clockwise or anticlockwise.

If the obstetrician's hand can reach the lamb, correction of the torsion may be achieved by rotating the lamb and surrounding uterus back into its correct position. Rotation in such cases is greatly facilitated by raising the hind end of the ewe to allow gravitational forces to move the uterine contents away from the pelvic inlet. If the vagina is completely obstructed, rolling the ewe may be attempted as in the cow but in most cases cesarean section is performed.

Downward deviation of the uterus

This may be seen in cases of ventral hernia or rupture of the prepubic tendon. These abnormalities occur mainly in older ewes heavily pregnant but often in poor bodily condition. Muscular damage – spontaneous or as the result of trauma – allows the gravid uterus to fall into the hernia sac and to come to lie under the ventral abdominal skin. Death through hemorrhage and shock may occur acutely in some cases immediately after trauma. In other cases, pregnancy continues to term. Spontaneous birth may not be possible in such cases for two reasons: The abdominal straining required for fetal expulsion is absent or very inefficient and the exit from the uterus may be obstructed by the uterine deviation. The commencement of birth in such cases can easily be overlooked and supervision should be especially vigilant as assistance will almost certainly be required. Vaginal examination will reveal that the uterine body deviates sharply downwards just beyond the pelvic brim. The weight of the gravid uterus may cause the cervical region of the uterus to be pulled tightly downwards, occluding its lumen. The obstetrician's lubricated hand can normally be introduced beyond the obstruction with comparative ease and the fetus(es) delivered manually. Delivery is easier if the ewe is lying down or if an assistant gently raises her ventral abdominal wall.

FETAL MALDISPOSITION

This is the most common cause of ovine dystocia. Abnormalities of posture are particularly common and an analysis of a number of surveys of dystocia suggests the following broad distribution of this type of abnormality shown in Table 6.2.

In many cases of fetal maldisposition in ewes, abnormalities of presentation, position and posture may be seen at the same time, often involving more than one fetus in the litter. In most cases, repulsion of the maldisposed fetus is required before postural defects can be corrected. The presence of other fetuses within the uterus may limit the amount of repulsion possible.

Malpresentation

Over 95% of lambs are born in anterior presentation. *Posterior presentation* does not always result in dystocia. Delay in the delivery of lambs in this malpresentation may result in their asphyxiation through inhalation of fetal fluids. Assisted delivery by traction is advisable. Malposture due to hock or hip flexion frequently complicates this posterior presentation. Such malpostures must be corrected before delivery is attempted.

Transverse presentation is seen chiefly in cases where more than one fetus is present in the uterus. The fetus lies across the pelvic inlet unable to be delivered without assistance and obstructing the delivery of other fetuses in the litter. In some cases the back of the fetus is presented at the pelvic inlet (dorsotransverse presentation). In other cases the limbs and possibly the fetal

head are presented (ventrotransverse presentation). Transverse presentation is treated by repelling the fetus and applying further repulsion to one end of the fetus and easing the other end towards the pelvic inlet. (Ideally the hind end of the lamb should be pulled towards the pelvic inlet as only two extremities have to be guided into position.) The transverse presentation is converted into a longitudinal presentation, the fetus and birth canal are lubricated and delivery is completed by gentle traction.

Malposition

Lambs in ventral or lateral position are quite frequently seen. Malposition is often complicated by malposture and simultaneous presentation. Where possible cases of fetal malposition should be converted into the normal dorsal position before delivery is attempted. This is achieved by repulsion of the fetus and lubrication of the fetus and birth canal. The fetus is then rotated around its long axis into the dorsal position and delivery is completed by careful traction.

Malposture

Fetal malposture is the most common cause of dystocia in the ewe. Nearly 70% of the causes of dystocia listed in Table 6.2 are in this category. Multiple birth is very common in sheep and in cases of dystocia more than one member of the litter may have an abnormal posture.

Lateral deviation of the head

This is the most common single cause of dystocia in ewes. The degree of displacement of the head varies greatly. It may be slightly displaced from being able to enter the maternal pelvis normally or the head and neck may lie back against the lamb's body. If the case has been untreated for some time fetal fluids will probably be lost and the uterine wall may be tightly applied to the fetus. Correction of the maldisposition may be difficult in such cases and great care must be taken to avoid damaging the uterine wall. Lubrication is introduced into the uterus and the fetus is repelled by exerting pressure on the base of its neck. The deviated head is cupped in the obstetrician's hand and brought round and up into the pelvis (see Fig. 7.1). In some horned breeds the fetus has prominent horn buds and these and the fetal mouth should be covered by the obstetrician's hand to prevent uterine damage.

Table 6.2 Fetal maldisposition in sheep	
Type	**% of maldispositions**
Lateral deviation of the head and neck	41
Shoulder flexion	6
Carpal flexion	10
Bilateral hip flexion (breech)	8
Hock flexion	4
Simultaneous presentation	17
Transverse presentation	14

In some cases access to the deviated head may be difficult because of the presence of the fetal forelegs in the pelvis. To gain access to the head one fetal foreleg can be flexed and repelled back into the uterus. Once the deviated head has been correctly positioned the flexed foreleg can be retrieved and the lamb delivered by traction.

Retention of a forelimb

This is quite frequently seen and results from either shoulder or carpal flexion; 16% of the cases listed in Table 6.2 were in this category. One or both limbs may be involved (Fig. 6.1). If both limbs are retained the fetal head may pass through the vulva without the legs. In this position the head may become enlarged and edematous and fetal life may be compromised unless prompt delivery is achieved. In a very small fetus it may be possible to deliver the lamb with one shoulder flexed without correcting the malposture. It is better obstetric practice, however, to correct all maldispositions before attempted delivery. The fetus is repelled, lubrication is applied and the retained forelimbs are identified. Shoulder flexion is first converted into a carpal flexion posture. The fetal foot is cupped in the hand and brought up into the pelvis. The second leg (if affected) is retrieved and its malposture is corrected in a similar manner.

Occasionally the fetal head obstructs the passage of the obstetrician's hand into the uterus to retrieve the retained forelimbs. In such cases the head should be repelled slightly to allow access to the forelimbs. Before repulsion a cord snare or the loop of a lambing instrument (Fig. 6.2) should be placed to secure the head for later retrieval. Once the malposture is corrected the lamb is delivered by gentle traction.

Retention of a hindlimb

Although posterior presentation is relatively uncommon in sheep assistance with delivery is often required. Cases of unilateral or bilateral hip or hock flexion are encountered and require assistance. In bilateral hip flexion (breech presentation) the fetal tail may be seen protruding from the vulva. Breech presentation may also be complicated by, and predispose to, failure of the cervix to dilate. If the lamb is very small, spontaneous or assisted delivery of the uncorrected breech presentation may occur. Whenever possible the malpresentation should be corrected into a posterior presentation with extended hindlimbs before delivery.

In cases of *hock flexion* (Fig. 6.3) the fetal hocks are presented at the pelvic inlet obstructing the passage of the lamb into the pelvis. To allow delivery, the fetus is first

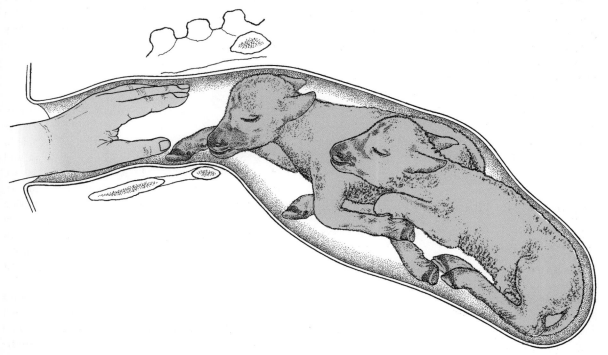

Figure 6.1 Fetal maldisposition – lamb with carpal flexion. The second lamb has a similar malposture.

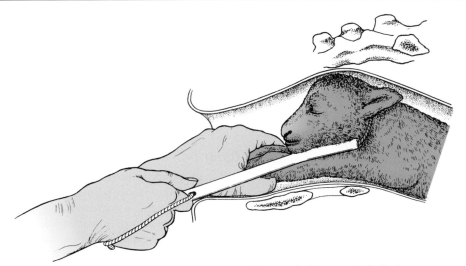

Figure 6.2 A lambing snare can be used to apply traction to the fetal head when space is limited.

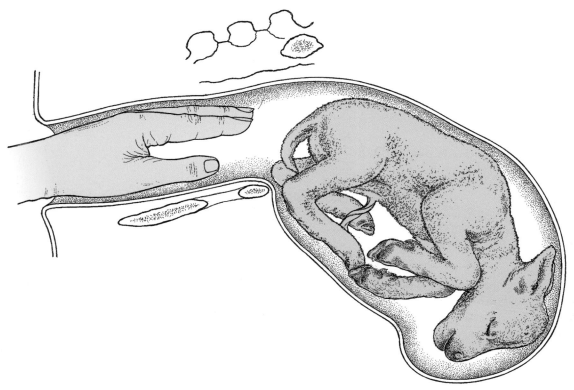

Figure 6.3 Fetal maldisposition – lamb with bilateral hock flexion.

repelled by exerting pressure (after the application of lubrication) on the hindquarters. The obstetrician's hand follows each limb in turn down to the fetal foot. The foot is enclosed in the hand, the hock is further flexed, and the foot is lifted over the pubis into the maternal pelvis. The procedure is repeated for the second limb if this is also in malposture.

If the fetus is presented in *hip flexion* the fetus is first repelled and lifted slightly within the uterus by applying pressure to its hindquarters. The obstetrician's hand follows one hindlimb down until the hock is reached. The hock is gently flexed and brought towards the pelvic inlet and is now in a hock flexion position. The foot is cupped in the obstetrician's hand and is brought back and extended into the pelvis. The second leg is retrieved in a similar fashion and the lubricated lamb is delivered by traction. If the lamb has very long legs there is a risk that, during conversion of the hip flexion to hock flexion, the fetal foot might damage the uterus. In such cases the obstetrician should attempt to reach the fetal foot and cup it in the hand and flex the hock. The foot should be retained in the hand as further correction of the dystocia is carried out by lifting the foot and extending it into the maternal pelvis.

Simultaneous presentation

The presence of multiple fetuses is very common in sheep and should be anticipated at all times. Although many litters with multiple fetuses are delivered spontaneously; 17% of the cases of dystocia in Table 6.2 were caused by simultaneous presentation. In most cases two fetuses are involved in dystocia cases in this category. If individual lambs are very small three lambs or very occasionally more may be involved.

Dystocia from simultaneous presentation may arise in a number of ways:

- *Uterine inertia*: caused by overstretching of the myometrium, especially in debilitated animals.
- *Simultaneous presentation of two or more fetuses*: the lambs may be in the same presentation or, more frequently, one is in anterior presentation and the other in posterior presentation.
- *Maldisposition*: of the first, second, or subsequent fetuses.

Initial vaginal examination of such cases can be confusing. A number of extremities are found within the pelvis or at the pelvic inlet. There is little space available for the obstetrician's hand. Examination is aided if the ewe is standing so that her uterine contents fall away slightly from the pelvic inlet. The hindquarters of the ewe may be raised slightly but this should be for a short period only. With the aid of generous lubrication the presenting parts are examined methodically to identify individual lambs and their presentation, position, and posture. A mental picture is built up of the lambs and how delivery will be attempted. If two lambs are presented with one in posterior presentation the latter should be delivered first. Only two extremities have to be guided into the pelvis compared with three in the case of the lamb in anterior presentation. For further discussion, see the section Approach to a case of dystocia in the ewe, p. 112.

FETOPELVIC DISPROPORTION

This problem is more common when litter size is small but the size of the individual lamb is large. Many ewe lambs produce only a single lamb in their first litter. Such animals are themselves not fully grown and their pelvic size may also be quite small. This type of dystocia may be further predisposed by the increasing use of heavier breeds of ram, e.g. the Texel to produce a large, rapidly growing commercial lamb. The lamb – especially a male lamb – may be simply too big to pass with ease through the maternal pelvis. Assisted delivery with generous lubrication may be required and in some cases, if the disproportion is severe, cesarean section will be necessary.

FETAL MONSTERS

These are occasionally seen and if large in size or diameter may cause dystocia. Most of the monsters described in cattle also occur in sheep. In addition, lambs with one or more accessory limbs are sometimes seen. Dystocia associated with edematous lambs has been reported in Beulah speckle-faced sheep. In all cases an attempt at vaginal delivery is made. If this proves impossible the abnormal fetus is delivered by cesarean section or fetotomy.

DYSTOCIA CAUSED BY FETAL DEATH

Death of one lamb or all the lambs in the litter in late pregnancy or at term may arise from a number of causes. Lack of space in the uterus may compromise placental function as fetal demands increase. Infections such as *Chlamydia psittaci* may cause abortion and also the death of one or all of the lambs in late pregnancy. Exposure to toxic agents, severe metabolic disease, and stress can also result in fetal death. In some cases fetal death results in failure of initiation of birth. Cervical opening in such cases may be incomplete and ascending infection gains access to the uterus. No signs of first- or second-stage labor may be seen and the ewe is examined only when an abnormal vaginal discharge or decaying placenta is seen at the vulva.

A number of the infectious agents that cause fetal death are zoonotic and animals in which fetal death is suspected should be examined with gloved hands and strict attention to hygiene. If the ewe is in very poor condition or moribund, attempted treatment may compromise her welfare and euthanasia may be preferable to treatment. Vaginal examination is carried out with generous lubrication. The fleece of dead lambs, together with the lack of uterine fluid, makes internal examination difficult. Warm water can be introduced into the uterus by stomach tube. Great care must be used as the uterine wall may be in poor condition and easily ruptured. The dead lambs are frequently malpresented having been unable to adopt the correct posture for birth. Access to the uterus may be compromised by incomplete cervical opening. An attempt is made to identify the presentation, position, and posture of the lamb or lambs. It may be possible in some cases to gently dilate the cervix but this is often not possible. After the introduction of additional lubrication an attempt is made to deliver the lambs by careful traction. If a lamb is severely decomposed it can sometimes be delivered by removing small portions of it from the uterus.

If vaginal delivery is impossible, cesarean section, fetotomy, or euthanasia should be considered. The economics of the case must be discussed with the owner. Cesarean section has a poor prognosis in such cases. Access to the uterus by a paramedian incision may be best (see Chapter 11). Fetotomy is only possible if access to the uterus via the cervix is possible. The ewe should be euthanized if other methods of treatment prove impossible, compromise her welfare, or are uneconomic. Good aftercare of the ewe is important in such cases. Antibiotic and non-steroidal anti-inflammatory treatment is given. Fluid therapy is beneficial in cases in which signs of shock are present.

SIGNS OF DYSTOCIA IN THE EWE

Sheep are normally and advisedly closely supervised at lambing time so that any departure from normal can be observed and investigated without delay. Approximate dates of lambing for groups of ewes served during a particular time are normally known and these animals are subject to careful scrutiny as their time for lambing approaches. Some of the signs of dystocia are quite subtle and may easily be missed if supervision is not very good.

In many cases, pregnancy may have been confirmed by ultrasonic scanning and those ewes known to be carrying two or more lambs have been identified. Specific signs of dystocia include:

- The presence of a foul vaginal discharge or decaying placenta at the vulva. This is a serious sign, which may indicate fetal death or attempted abortion and must be investigated without delay.
- An abnormal disposition of the fetus seen at the vulva. For example, a fetal head but no forelegs is seen at or protrudes between the vulval lips. Such an appearance suggests gross fetal maldisposition, e.g. the forelegs being in shoulder flexion.
- A prolonged non-progressive first stage of labor. The ewe may have separated herself from the rest of the flock and may appear uneasy. She may stand for short periods and then lie down. Some straining may occur but the vigorous straining that is characteristic of second-stage labor does not occur. Such signs may suggest that the ewe has ringwomb or is suffering from uterine inertia.
- The ewe strains vigorously for 20–30 minutes or intermittently for 30–60 minutes but no fetus is seen. This suggests the possibility of a fetus in a maldisposition, fetopelvic disproportion, or the simultaneous presentation of two or more fetuses. The second stage of normal birth in sheep may take up to an hour but obvious progress is seen during this time.

As in other species, the dividing line between normal birth and dystocia is not clear cut. Dystocia may be suspected in a ewe that is in fact lambing normally but slowly. As in other species it is better to examine cases that raise even slight suspicions of abnormality to ensure that no true case of dystocia is overlooked.

APPROACH TO A CASE OF DYSTOCIA IN THE EWE

Many cases will be examined in the surgery in a clean room prepared for the purpose. Such a room should be designed in such a way that thorough cleaning and disinfection between cases is possible (for general details, see also Chapter 3).

Equipment

Minimum equipment is required – the obstetrician's hands being the most effective instruments. Parturient sheep are a possible source of zoonotic disease, which may be particularly dangerous to female obstetricians. For this reason the wearing of long-sleeved plastic gloves for lambing work may be advisable. A lambing snare (see Fig. 6.3) is occasionally useful but if this is not available then three lightweight lambing cords may be used. Handles for the cords are seldom necessary and it is unusual for more than one cord to be used at a time. Adequate supplies of obstetric lubricant will be needed, especially if the case has been in labor for a long time. In such cases, natural lubricants are lost and the birth canal and fetus become very dry. A sterile cesarean surgical kit should be available, together with supplies of suture materials, antibiotics, etc.

Additional equipment may be needed if the case is to be attended on the farm. If lighting is known to be poor, a good torch or lantern is a valuable aid. If supplies of hot water are limited, 5 liters taken in a plastic container along with soap and towel from the surgery can make working conditions much better for both obstetrician and patient.

OBSTETRICIAN'S CHECK LIST

Call received

Brief history taken
↓
Check drugs and equipment
↓
See patient as quickly as possible
on the farm or at the surgery

Case history

A brief history of the case is taken. Was the patient unwell in late pregnancy? What was the nature of her illness? Has she experienced previous dystocia? Have any lambs been born already? How many and were they alive or dead? How long has she been attempting to lamb? Has anyone else attempted to treat the case? Have any other ewes in the flock suffered from dystocia recently? In many cases the shepherd will have examined the ewe and will report any abnormalities or damage found or caused accidentally.

General examination of the ewe

It is very important to check the ewe's health status before commencing to deal with her dystocia.

Assessment of her condition score should indicate how well she has been managed during pregnancy, and in particular if her dietary energy levels have been satisfactory. If her dystocia is recognized and presented early she should be in good condition unless her pregnancy has been complicated by pregnancy toxemia. If she has been left untreated for some time, or if treatment was attempted by unskilled hands, she may be in very poor condition. If the uterus has been ruptured and dirty hands used to investigate the dystocia it is possibile that clostridial disease with overwhelming endotoxemia may be developing. In such cases the ewe may show signs of severe depression, toxic mucous membranes, and a degree of dehydration.

Occasionally, her condition may be such that she is unlikely to withstand further treatment and euthanasia is indicated. If she is suffering from severe life-threatening pregnancy toxemia supportive therapy may be necessary before fetal delivery can begin. Mastitis is uncommon in the parturient ewe but the udder should be checked for the presence of milk and the patency of both teats. Milk (initially thick colostrum) is usually present in the udder 12–24 hours before lambing. Absence of milk may suggest that the ewe is not quite ready to lamb, especially if her cervix is found to be closed.

Close inspection of the vulva and vagina may reveal an intact amnion in early cases. In cases of longer duration a detached chorioallantois, ruptured amnion and possibly vulval damage may be seen. Any visible fetal parts should be identified.

OBSTETRICIAN'S CHECK LIST

Evaluation of the ewe

Further history taken
↓
Problems during pregnancy in ewe or flock?
↓
Details of recent management
↓
Pregnancy scanning result?
↓
Previous dystocia (if known)?
↓
Recent dystocia problems in flock?
↓
Help already given by shepherd?

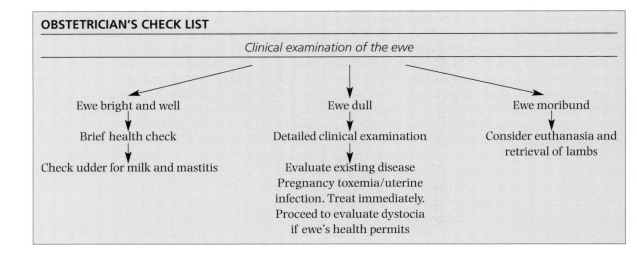

OBSTETRICIAN'S CHECK LIST

Clinical examination of the ewe

Ewe bright and well
↓
Brief health check
↓
Check udder for milk and mastitis

Ewe dull
↓
Detailed clinical examination
↓
Evaluate existing disease
Pregnancy toxemia/uterine
infection. Treat immediately.
Proceed to evaluate dystocia
if ewe's health permits

Ewe moribund
↓
Consider euthanasia and
retrieval of lambs

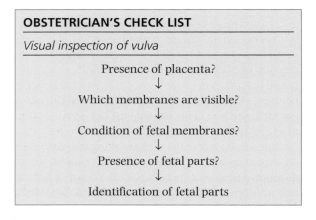

OBSTETRICIAN'S CHECK LIST

Visual inspection of vulva

Presence of placenta?
↓
Which membranes are visible?
↓
Condition of fetal membranes?
↓
Presence of fetal parts?
↓
Identification of fetal parts

Restraint

The ewe may be held in a standing position by an assistant but if she is in a small pen she can be examined and restrained by the obstetrician alone (Fig. 6.4). She should not be held by her fleece, which is easily pulled out in late pregnancy. If the parturient ewe is lying down she may be approached quietly from behind and an internal examination carried without her getting up.

Vaginal examination

Before commencing this examination in a ewe, three important points must always be borne in mind:

1. The obstetrician must constantly be aware of the potentially extreme fragility of the ovine uterus. Internal examinations and manipulations must always be carried out with the utmost care if

accidental iatrogenic rupture of the uterus is to be avoided.

2. It is not necessary or desirable to routinely raise the hind end of the ewe before internal examination or manipulation is carried out. This procedure is stressful and potentially dangerous. It may compromise the ewe's respiration and predispose to uterine rupture. Raising the hind end of the ewe may occasionally be necessary to correct uterine torsion or to deal with a fetal maldisposition that is impacted at the pelvic inlet. In such cases the time the ewe is held in this position should be kept to a minimum.
Most internal manipulations can be carried out with the ewe in the standing position.

3. The genital tract of the ewe is quite susceptible to infection. The highest standards of hygiene and cleanliness must be practiced at all times. It is also extremely important that the veterinary obstetrician sets a very good example, which may be emulated by the shepherd.

If the perineal area is surrounded by dirty fleece, this should be removed using dagging shears before commencing the internal examination. Preferably, all ewes should be dagged before lambing time.

After washing the perineal region thoroughly, the obstetrician's lubricated hand is carefully inserted into the vagina. In most cases this can be done with ease and, unless the cervix is closed or a fetus occupies the caudal birth canal, the hand can readily be passed on through the bony pelvis into the uterus. In small ewes the passage of the hand through the pelvis may only

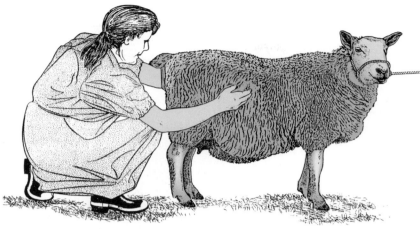

Figure 6.4 Restraint of the ewe for vaginal examination.

just be possible. The presence of the obstetrician's hand in the birth canal usually provokes straining in the ewe. Gentle persistence and moving the hand forward between bouts of maternal straining will allow the birth canal and its contents to be explored and evaluated. The caudal birth canal is carefully palpated for signs of damage, such as tears in the vaginal mucosa.

Evaluation of the cervix

The frequency of ringwomb as a cause of dystocia means that the ewe's cervix should always be carefully evaluated. If the cervix is fully dilated it is not palpable – the vaginal and uterine walls appear to be continuous. Sometimes the cervix is not fully dilated and all degrees of incomplete dilation may be seen. The cervix may be completely closed and careful exploration of the anterior vagina will encounter and identify the external os. If the cervix is completely and tightly closed the ewe may not, in fact, be really ready to lamb. Apparent signs of discomfort may be seen in ewes that have suffered an earlier vaginal prolapse – such animals may appear to be trying to lamb when they are not ready. On palpation the cervix is found to be closed.

If partially dilated, one, two, or three fingers can be inserted into the cervix, which is palpable as a circular ring around the circumference of the vagina/uterine junction. The problem with the partially dilated cervix is deciding whether it is likely to open further and how healthy the lambs are on the other side.

A number of factors involving the cervix, the unborn lamb(s), the duration of parturition, and the readiness of the ewe to lamb must be taken into account in all cases where the cervix does not appear to be fully opened.

Further assessment of the cervix

The cervix should be gently palpated for evidence of previous scar tissue, which may have formed at an earlier lambing and is now preventing the cervix from opening. If firm scar tissue is found, the chances of further cervical dilation are small but even in such cases an attempt at manual dilation should be made.

Manual dilation of the partly closed cervix should always be attempted and in many cases will be successful. The obstetrician's lubricated finger is introduced into the partially opened cervix and is moved around with centrifugal action exerting lateral pressure on the rim of the cervix. Sometimes the cervix will be felt to open like the shutter in a camera in response to pressure and further fingers – initially forming a cone – and eventually the whole hand may be inserted. Further pressure will allow complete dilation of the cervix and access to the lamb(s) in the uterus. Complete manual dilation may require 10 minutes or more to complete. Once the cervix is open it is advisable to deliver the lambs immediately – reports of the cervix closing before the fetuses could be delivered by the ewe make this action advisable. If there has been genuine delay in cervical opening the lambs may be becoming hypoxic and immediate delivery is in any case advisable.

If the partially opened cervix cannot immediately be dilated manually a further period of time may be allowed to see if natural dilation will occur. If the ewe is healthy and the lambs are not believed to be at immediate risk

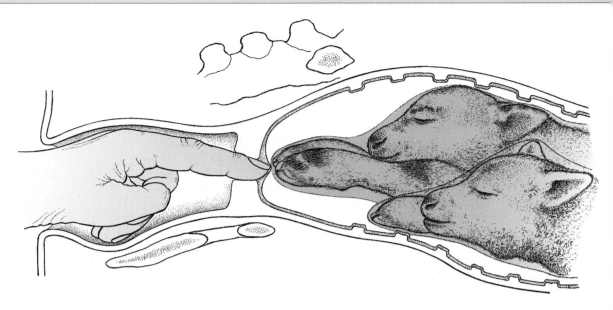

Figure 6.5 Assessment of ewe with 'ringwomb'. The fetal membranes are intact, fetal fluids are present, and the fetus is alive (see also Figure 6.6).

the ewe may be left quietly in comfortable surroundings for a further 30 minutes. Drug therapy may be given at the start of this period.

Drug therapy

As mentioned above, a number of drugs have been claimed to encourage cervical dilation. These include parenteral calcium borogluconate, vetrabutine hydrochloride, vitamin D, estradiol, and the local application to the cervix of prostaglandin E. None has been fully evaluated but on some farms a response to one or more of these treatments has been seen. After 30 minutes the ewe is re-examined and a further attempt is made to dilate the cervix. If this is not possible the lambs should be delivered by cesarean section.

Assessment of the lamb(s) through the partially dilated cervix

In such cases the lamb(s) may be alive and well or dead and decaying. Access to the lambs is restricted but even palpation by the finger may reveal useful information about the lamb and placenta.

- *Is the lamb surrounded by healthy placenta?* Healthy placenta is soft, fluid filled, and does not have an unpleasant smell. Fetal movements may be palpated

(Fig. 6.5). If the lamb is dead the placenta may feel leathery to the touch, has probably lost its fluid contents, and has a foul smell. Separated cotyledons of the chorioallantois may be palpable and occasionally portions of the unhealthy placenta are protruding through the cervix (Fig. 6.6).

- *Is the lamb alive?* The restricted access to the lamb again makes this difficult to ascertain. If the lamb is alive, spontaneous fetal movements may be palpable through the cervix. If the fetal muzzle is touched the fetus may demonstrate a sucking reflex. If access to a fetal foot is possible, pinching the toes will produce the pedal withdrawal reflex in the living lamb.
- *Further evidence of fetal life* This may also be demonstrated by palpating the ewe externally through the flanks and resting the flat of the hands against the body wall. Spontaneous intrauterine movements will indicate fetal life. Hyperactivity within the uterus may indicate threatened fetal hypoxia. Doppler or B-mode ultrasonographic evaluation of the lamb(s) through the ewe's abdominal wall can provide further definite evidence of fetal life by demonstrating fetal movement, including a beating heart.

If the above positive signs of life are absent the lamb is probably dead. If it has been dead for several days it will probably not have instigated the birth process including a possible role in cervical dilation.

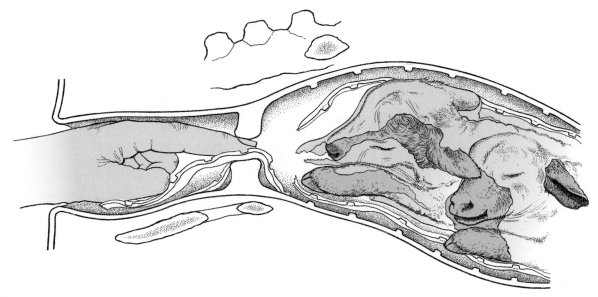

Figure 6.6 Assessment of ewe with 'ringwomb'. The fetal membranes are ruptured, fetal fluids have been lost, and the fetus is dead (see also Figure 6.5).

The readiness of the ewe to lamb must be assessed whenever there are problems of non-dilation or partial dilation of the cervix. If the ewe is not really ready to give birth, the lambs are unlikely to survive. The following questions should be posed and, if possible, answered:

- Do the ewe's service dates suggest that lambing is really imminent and have other animals in her service group lambed already?
- Is milk (colostrum) present in the udder and teats?
- Are the sacrosciatic ligaments, which run between the tuber ischii and the sacrum, fully relaxed?

- Has the vulva lengthened?

If the answer to all the questions is 'yes' then the ewe is *probably* ready to give birth and the lambs should be delivered without delay. If the cervix cannot be further dilated in such cases by hand or with the aid of drugs, cesarean section is indicated. If the lambs are thought to be dead the prognosis for the case is not good, especially if the ewe is depressed and toxemic. For details of the management of the ewe prior to cesarean section if fetal dysmaturity is suspected or is possible, see Chapter 11.

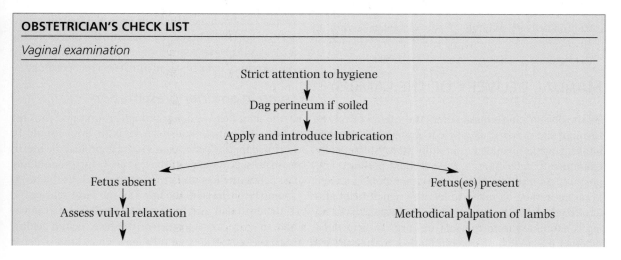

OBSTETRICIAN'S CHECK LIST

Vaginal examination

Strict attention to hygiene
↓
Dag perineum if soiled
↓
Apply and introduce lubrication

Fetus absent
↓
Assess vulval relaxation
↓

Fetus(es) present
↓
Methodical palpation of lambs
↓

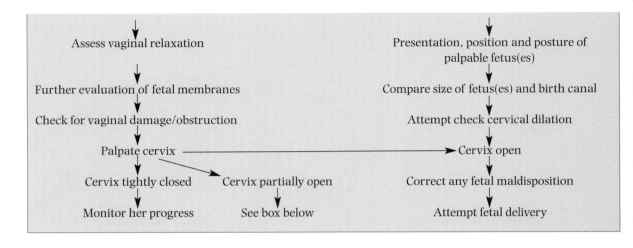

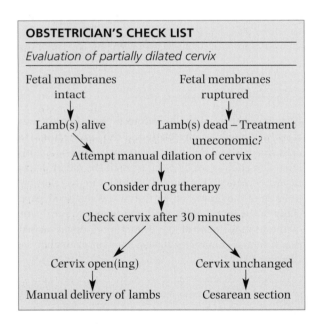

MANUAL DELIVERY OF THE LAMB(S)

As the obstetrician's hand enters the vagina or passes through the cervix it usually encounters one or more lambs. Each lamb must be carefully and systematically examined to determine its presentation, position, and posture. As multiple birth is very common in sheep, great care must be taken to identify which head and fetal legs belong to the same lamb. Each presenting leg is examined from the foot upwards to determine whether it is a forelimb or a hindlimb as in the calf (see

Fig. 4.15). A mental picture of each lamb is built up and a plan made of what is needed to place it into a normal presentation for delivery.

Correction of malpresentations

Most lambs are born naturally in anterior presentation with their head extended and resting on their extended forelimbs. A few lambs are born in posterior presentation with their extended hindlimbs passing through the birth canal first. The malpresented, malpositioned, or malpostured lamb should be moved into a correct anterior or posterior presentation. The obstetrician should always introduce plenty of lubricant into the uterus before attempting to correct any abnormalities. Each displaced extremity is located and brought into its correct position, taking great care to ensure that the fragile uterus is not damaged in the process. It is usually necessary to repel the fetus gently back into the uterus during a break in the ewe's straining efforts to allow room for the extremity to be replaced into its correct position.

Lamb in anterior presentation

If the fetal head is being brought round and into the pelvis, the muzzle and horn buds (if any) should be enclosed in the obstetrician's hand to protect the uterus from possible damage. If the legs are being brought into the pelvis, the feet and prominences such as the hocks should be enclosed in the hand for the same reasons.

If both head and forelegs are displaced it is advisable to correct the posture of the head before dealing with the legs. The head is brought round to the pelvic inlet. Each leg is then retrieved, its posture corrected, and brought into the pelvis. Retrieving the second leg may be difficult as the pelvis is now occupied by both the head and the other forelimb. In such cases the lamb may have to be gently repelled to provide a little more room. If the legs are corrected first there may be insufficient room to bring the head round and up into the pelvis.

Occasionally with this manipulation the head will not remain in the pelvis but falls back as an attempt is made to retrieve the legs. If this happens the head should be held in the pelvis before the legs are retrieved. If the head is close to the vulva the obstetrician may hold it with one hand while the other hand locates and deals with the forelegs in turn. Alternatively, the head can be held by the lambing snare (see Fig. 6.2) or by using a light-weight lambing cord secured around the head and through the mouth as in the calf (see Fig. 4.18).

Lamb in posterior presentation

Correction of malposture in this presentation is normally less complex as only two extremities (instead of three in anterior presentation) must be brought into the pelvis. The obstetrician must take particular care to ensure that the uterus is not damaged by the fetal feet as they are brought into the pelvis, especially following correction of a bilateral hip flexion malposture.

Although very small maldisposed lambs can be delivered without correction of their abnormal posture – this is especially true of the small lamb with unilateral shoulder flexion or in breech presentation – it is not good obstetric practice to to do this.

Delivery of the lamb by traction

Once any malpostures have been corrected, the lamb is ready for delivery.

Fetopelvic disproportion is less common in sheep than in cattle. Before delivery is attempted the size of the lamb should be compared manually with the diameters of the pelvis through which it must pass. If there is any doubt, trial traction should be employed. If this is not successful, cesarean section may be required.

Application of traction

Fetus in anterior presentation   Once the fetus is correctly presented at the pelvic inlet it is ready for delivery. Plenty of obstetric lubricant is placed around the lamb and in the caudal birth canal. Using one hand, the obstetrician eases the head and then each foreleg

in turn back towards the vulva. As soon as the legs are within reach the obstetrician grips them with his or her other hand. Gentle traction is applied in a backwards and downwards direction to the fetal legs while the obstetrician applies traction using the other hand to the head (Fig. 6.7). If the lamb is quite large, traction is initially applied alternately to each forelimb. The head is eased along the birth canal as the legs are moved. If the lamb is small and the delivery is proceeding well, traction can be applied to both forelegs simultaneously. Traction should always coincide with straining efforts by the ewe. The head may be gripped by placing the fingers over the back of the lamb's head and the thumb between the mandibles. If space is restricted, the lamb can be gripped carefully using the eye socket hold. Alternatively, traction may be applied to the head using the lambing snare. Traction should be applied – carefully – only by the obstetrician, without the help of an assistant.

Once the head and thorax of the lamb have been delivered the hindquarters should follow with further moderate traction. Moving the trunk of the lamb from side to side and rotating it slightly on its long axis aid the passage of its hindquarters through the maternal pelvis.

Fetus in posterior presentation   The fetal hindlimbs are brought into the pelvis and, using one hand, the obstetrician gently but firmly pulls both towards the vulva. At this stage one leg is held in each hand – the leg being gripped around or just below the hocks. Traction is applied to each leg alternately until the fetal hips are engaged in the pelvis. Both legs are now pulled in a backwards and downwards direction until the fetus is delivered. When the fetal hindquarters pass through the maternal vulva, the dorsal commissure and caudal vaginal roof should be protected by the obstetrician's hand.

As in other species, posterior presentation increases the risk of fetal asphyxia through early rupture of the umbilical cord and the risk of inhalation of amniotic fluid. Once traction is commenced it should be completed with all possible speed. Adequate lubrication of the birth canal and the fetus are essential and greatly aid the passage of the fetus.

If moderate traction fails to deliver the lamb, its presentation should be checked again carefully, together with its size in relation to that of its mother's pelvis. Further generous lubrication is applied and traction tried again. If the lamb does not move cesarean section will be necessary.

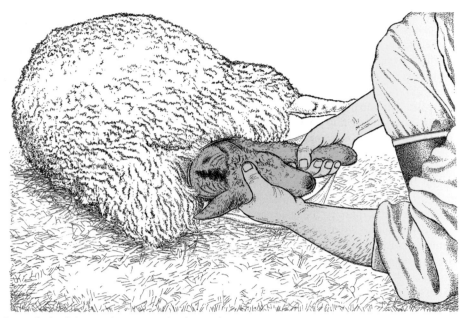

Figure 6.7 Delivery of a lamb in anterior presentation by traction.

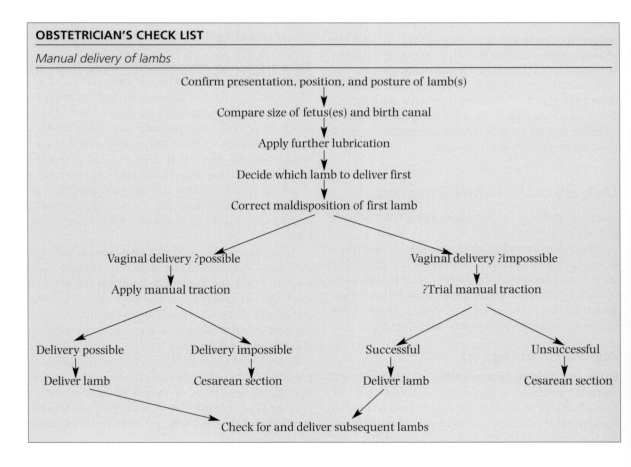

OBSTETRICIAN'S CHECK LIST

Manual delivery of lambs

Confirm presentation, position, and posture of lamb(s)

Compare size of fetus(es) and birth canal

Apply further lubrication

Decide which lamb to deliver first

Correct maldisposition of first lamb

Vaginal delivery ?possible   Vaginal delivery ?impossible

Apply manual traction   ?Trial manual traction

Delivery possible   Delivery impossible   Successful   Unsuccessful

Deliver lamb   Cesarean section   Deliver lamb   Cesarean section

Check for and deliver subsequent lambs

RESUSCITATION AND CARE OF THE LAMBS

As soon as the lamb is delivered it is held up by the back legs and gently shaken to allow fetal fluids and mucus to drain from the mouth, nasal passages, and lungs. Remnants of amnion are removed from the lamb's face. Cardiac function is identified by the presence of an apex beat in the chest. In most cases, breathing will start spontaneously but if not the lamb should be swung carefully but more vigorously backwards and forwards. During such swinging the lamb should be firmly gripped by its back legs just above the hocks because – as it is often covered in natural and artificial lubricant – it may be accidentally dropped.

If breathing has not started, the lamb is laid on its side and artificial respiration is started. This is best achieved by gently lifting the thoracic wall with one hand and the shoulder joint with the other and then releasing the grip. Negative pressure in the chest is achieved by this method and the lungs should be encouraged to inflate allowing air to enter the lungs. Commencement of respiration can be further encouraged by administration of 5–10 mg of doxapram hydrochloride, either intravenously or under the tongue. A small oxygen cylinder with face mask is very useful to enrich any air being breathed in. Alternatively, air may be pumped into the lungs using a Cox lamb resuscitator, which supplies approximately 100 mL of air with each pump through a face mask.

Great care must be taken when compressing the lamb's chest – the ribs are very easily broken and severe damage can unknowingly be done to both the lungs and the liver. Very occasionally the lamb's ribs may be damaged during assisted delivery. If slight rib damage is discovered analgesia should be provided in the form of an injection of flunixin and antibiotic cover prescribed.

Mouth-to-mouth respiration is highly risky for zoonotic reasons and should never be employed in lambs.

As soon as the lamb is breathing, the navel should be sprayed with antibiotic (e.g. oxytetracycline) or dipped in a weak iodine solution. It is then placed near the ewe's head to encourage mothering and the firm establishment of the fetomaternal bond. Subsequent lambs are treated in the same way. Colostrum should be taken in by the lamb within 6 hours of birth and on many farms its intake is ensured by administering 60 mL by small stomach tube to each lamb shortly after birth. A further 60 mL is given later unless it is known that the lambs have sucked. On farms where losses through watery mouth have occurred, lambs may be given a routine dose of an oral antibiotic, such as spectinomycin.

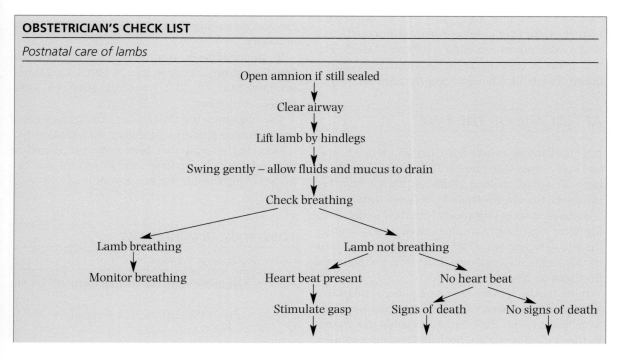

OBSTETRICIAN'S CHECK LIST

Postnatal care of lambs

Open amnion if still sealed

↓

Clear airway

↓

Lift lamb by hindlegs

↓

Swing gently – allow fluids and mucus to drain

↓

Check breathing

Lamb breathing   Lamb not breathing

Monitor breathing   Heart beat present   No heart beat

Stimulate gasp   Signs of death   No signs of death

↓

Administer doxapram   Abandon   Intracardiac
                          resuscitation   adrenaline
                                               (epinephrine)
        ↓   ↓
Artificial respiration   Continue
                                              resuscitation
        ↓
Manual/resuscitator/esophageal tube technique
        ↓
Watch for spontaneous respiration
        ↓
Monitor respiration
        ↓
Place lamb near ewe's head

DELIVERY OF THE REST OF THE LITTER

After the first lamb has been delivered the uterus is again examined for the presence of further offspring. The second lamb is delivered manually and the uterus checked again. This process is repeated until it is ascertained that the uterus is completely empty. The lambs may occupy both horns or one horn may be pregnant and the other non-pregnant. Both horns should be identified – one on either side of the septum – and examined for the presence of further lambs.

The last lamb in the litter can easily be overlooked – especially if the litter size is large. The last lamb often occupies the tip of one uterine horn and the coiled shape of the ovine uterus can make it difficult to reach (Fig. 6.8) unless the obstetrician carefully searches actively to the tip of each horn, however deep that may be.

AFTERCARE OF THE EWE

After the lambs have been born they should be left quiet and undisturbed with the ewe. The ewe licks and stimulates the lambs, making chuckling sounds with her voice, which enable the lambs to recognize their mother.

Some ewes seem very rough with their lambs, pawing them vigorously with their forefeet to encourage them to move and rise. Little damage seems to be done by this action but small weak lambs must be protected from possible injury.

It is advisable to move the ewe and her lambs into a small pen for 24 hours or so to keep the lambs warm and to further establish the family relationship and make it less likely that the ewe and her lambs become separated.

After an assisted lambing, antibiotic cover is usually provided for the ewe. An intramuscular injection of one of the long-acting preparations of penicillin or oxytetracycline is given. If the risk of infection is considered high, antibiotics may be given daily for up to 5 days after the lambing. Antibiotic pessaries may be placed in the uterus. The perineal region of the ewe should be washed with a mild antiseptic solution. Most ewes will have received a booster injection of clostridial vaccine 4–6 weeks before lambing.

Before releasing the ewe her milk supply should be checked – the patency and function of each teat and its associated mammary gland should be checked. Supplementary feeding for the lamb(s) is provided where necessary.

If uterine tone is considered poor after assisted lambing uterine involution may be encouraged by the administration of 20 IU oxytocin given by intramuscular injection.

The ewe is watched closely after lambing for signs of postparturient problems (for details, see Chapter 13).

Once the placenta has been passed it should be removed from the lambing pen to prevent the ewe from choking when trying to consume it.

OBSTETRICIAN'S CHECK LIST

Postnatal care of the ewe

Check the uterus for further lamb(s)
↓
Check the birth canal for damage
↓

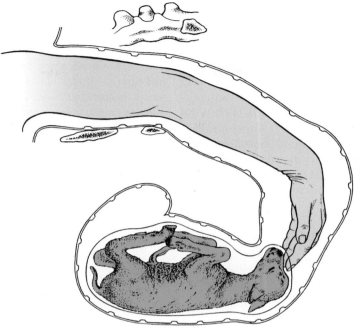

Figure 6.8 The entire uterus must be searched carefully to ensure that the last lamb has not been overlooked.

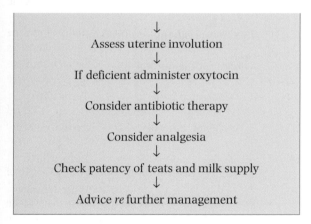

↓

Assess uterine involution

↓

If deficient administer oxytocin

↓

Consider antibiotic therapy

↓

Consider analgesia

↓

Check patency of teats and milk supply

↓

Advice *re* further management

THE OVERDUE BIRTH – PROLONGED GESTATION

Prolonged gestation is not always recognized in the ewe because the exact service date of many ewes is not known. At the end of the lambing season the obstetrician may be asked to examine ewes that were known to be pregnant when scanned but which have not lambed. In most cases, abdominal palpation and ultrasonographic scan will reveal that such animals are no longer pregnant. An earlier unobserved abortion is the most likely cause of this.

Any ewe found to be pregnant after the end of the lambing season should be examined carefully. The possibility of a later service date should be investigated, helped by knowledge of the date that the rams were removed from the flock. If a ewe is found to be pregnant more than 150 days after ram removal the possibility of a true prolonged gestation increases. In some cases the fetus may be mummified. Abdominal palpation may reveal a hard, irregular mass just anterior to the pelvic inlet. Ultrasonographic scan reveals an echogenic mass but no evidence of fetal fluids, the placental cotyledons, or of fetal life. Ewes found to be carrying one or more mummified fetuses are often culled. Their abnormal pregnancy may be terminated by an intramuscular injection of 125 μg of the prostaglandin F2α analog cloprostenol. The mummified fetus is normally expelled from the uterus within 48 hours. Manual removal from the vagina may be necessary.

Ewes in which fetal maceration has occurred are likely to have been detected at an earlier stage. An unpleasant vaginal discharge containing fetal remnants may have been seen. Treatment of such animals (see also Chapter 2) is often unsatisfactory and affected animals are usually culled. The cause of fetal death may be detected by laboratory examination of the placenta and vaginal discharges. Other ewes in the flock may have aborted and a firm diagnosis of an infectious cause obtained.

True prolonged gestation with a living fetus is usually associated with a defect in the hypothalamic–anterior-pituitary–adrenal axis in the developing lamb. Viral causes include border disease virus in Europe and akabane virus in other parts of the world. Exposure to these and other viruses in pregnancy may result in pituitary aplasia and hydranencephaly. Similar fetal lesions are produced by a number of plant toxins. The affected fetus is unable to produce sufficient ACTH and cortisol to initiate its birth process. Pregnancy may be prolonged beyond 200 days.

Ultrasonographic examination of affected animals may demonstrate cranial defects in the living fetus within the uterus. Affected lambs are unlikely to be viable and are of no economic value. Their ewes may be culled or an attempt can be made to induce parturition. Birth can be induced in such animals by an intramuscular injection of dexamethasone (16 mg) and cloprostenol (125 µg). Parturition normally commences 24–72 hours later. Assistance with fetal delivery is sometimes required and the ewe receives normal postparturient care.

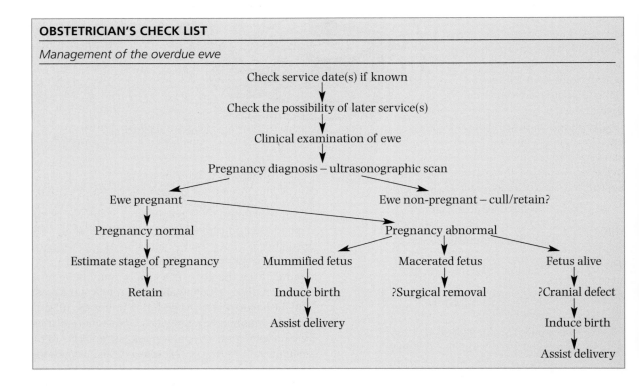

OBSTETRICIAN'S CHECK LIST

Management of the overdue ewe

Check service date(s) if known
↓
Check the possibility of later service(s)
↓
Clinical examination of ewe
↓
Pregnancy diagnosis – ultrasonographic scan
↙ ↘
Ewe pregnant   Ewe non-pregnant – cull/retain?
↓
Pregnancy normal   Pregnancy abnormal
↓   ↙   ↓   ↘
Estimate stage of pregnancy   Mummified fetus   Macerated fetus   Fetus alive
↓   ↓   ↓   ↓
Retain   Induce birth   ?Surgical removal   ?Cranial defect
                     ↓   ↓
                    Assist delivery   Induce birth
                                                      ↓
                                                     Assist delivery

Chapter 7

DYSTOCIA IN THE DOE GOAT

The goat is a small ruminant and in many ways the problems of dystocia encountered and their treatment resemble those seen in the ewe. The more important differences are discussed below but the overall approach to the investigation and treatment of dystocia is the same in the two species. Experienced goat owners may be unhappy to have the two species discussed as one and the obstetrician should, if possible, avoid comparisons between the species during obstetric work.

Although a number of large surveys of parturient ewes have noted the relative incidences of the different causes of ovine dystocia there are few accounts concerning goats. Failure of the cervix to dilate – ringwomb – appears to be less common than in the ewe.

INCIDENCE

The exact incidence of dystocia in goats is not known. In general they are kept in smaller herds than sheep and problems at parturition are less concentrated over a short period. Many goat herds are quite small and are not supervised by an experienced shepherd.

CAUSES OF DYSTOCIA

In a survey of 51 cases of dystocia in doe goats treated in Saudi Arabia (Rahim and Arthur 1982) the causes were found to be as shown in Table 7.1.

Uterine inertia

This condition is rarely seen as a primary cause of caprine dystocia. Periparturient hypocalcemia in goats may, however, lead to primary uterine inertia. In the Saudi Arabian survey (Rahim & Arthur 1982), secondary

Table 7.1 Causes of dystocia in the doe goat	
Cause	**%**
Fetal maldisposition	56
Fetopelvic disproportion	20
Obstruction of the birth canal	12
Uterine inertia	10
Uterine torsion	2
Modified from Rahim & Arthur 1982.	

uterine inertia was a frequent complication of cervical obstruction. In cases of uterine inertia the presenting fetus should be delivered manually. Further fetuses in the uterus should also be delivered. Postparturient uterine contraction should be stimulated by the intramuscular administration of 5–10 IU oxytocin.

OBSTRUCTION OF THE BIRTH CANAL

Although obstruction may involve any part of the birth canal the failure of the cervix to dilate (ringwomb) was the most common problem encountered in the Saudi Arabian survey. Five cases of ringwomb were seen and, of these, four required cesarean section to achieve delivery, as did the single case of uterine torsion. Treatment of ringwomb by drug therapy can also be attempted (Matthews 1999). Prostaglandin F2α (10 mg dinoprost or 125 µg cloprostenol) given by intramuscular injection has been used successfully and may be followed by kidding in 4 hours. Vetrabutine hydrochloride (2 mg/kg body weight) given by intramuscular injection may promote cervical dilation. The cervix and kids should be carefully evaluated as in the ewe (see Chapter 6) before treatment is commenced. Cesarean section should be performed if fetal life is thought to be at risk and in cases in which drug therapy has been unsuccessful.

FETAL MALDISPOSITION

This is the most common cause of dystocia in the goat. In the Saudi Arabian survey by Rahim & Arthur, deviation of the head and carpal flexion were the most frequently seen maldispositions. Shoulder flexion was seen in five animals but only one case of posterior presentation with hock flexion was seen.

Simultaneous presentation was a complication of 11 cases of dystocia and the proportion of animals carrying twins and triplets was high. One or more of the simultaneously presented kids may also have a malposture involving the head or limbs (Fig. 7.1).

The majority of cases in the Saudi Arabian survey were dealt with by manual correction of the maldisposition and then delivery by traction. Partial fetotomy was required in a few cases in which the maldisposed fetus was dead and not readily moveable. Cesarean section was performed in one case of shoulder flexion that could not be corrected manually.

FETOPELVIC DISPROPORTION

This abnormality was seen in nine cases in the Saudi Arabian survey. Pelvic size was considered small in two-thirds of the cases and fetal size excessively large in the remaining third. Two of the large kids were single males.

SIGNS OF DYSTOCIA

Any departure from the normal pattern of parturition can indicate the existence of dystocia and should be investigated. Non-productive straining is also a frequent sign. This may be accompanied by loud bleating, which often coincides with straining. The doe quickly tires and may appear exhausted quite rapidly if her attempts at fetal delivery are unsuccessful. The appearance at the vulva of a single fetal extremity, such as a head without either foreleg or a single hindlimb is – as in the ewe – an indication of possible fetal maldisposition.

The escape of allantoic fluid – if observed – may indicate the commencement of birth but in goats sudden loss of watery fluid (or 'cloudburst') may also indicate the end of pseudopregnancy. The presence of pseudopregnancy (hydrometra) rather than pregnancy may have been detected earlier by ultrasonographic scan or the presence (from day 45 of pregnancy) of estrone sulfate in the blood or milk of the genuinely pregnant doe. In some cases, however, no pregnancy diagnosis will have been performed and the obstetrician should bear pseudopregnancy in mind. The occasional doe showing signs of restlessness, mild straining, and the loss of quantities of watery fluid from the vagina may not actually be kidding, or indeed be pregnant at all. In the pseudopregnant doe there will be no placenta and no fetus. The fluid-filled uterus is readily detectable when a transabdominal scan is performed. Echogenic lines caused by the superimposition of the uterine horns cross the non-echogenic fluid and are visible in the pseudopregnant doe

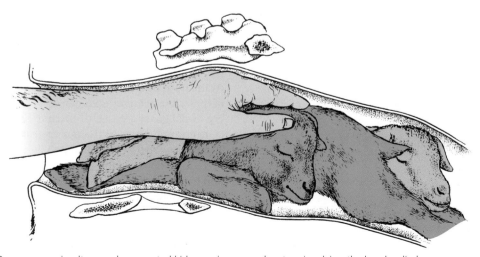

Figure 7.1 One or more simultaneously presented kids may have a malposture involving the head or limbs.

when the uterus is scanned. These lines are caused by superimposition of the image of one uterine horn on the other.

Some goat owners are very inexperienced and, where possible, advice concerning normal kidding and the signs of dystocia should be discussed in advance of the event.

APPROACH TO A CASE OF DYSTOCIA IN THE DOE GOAT

The basic approach is as in the ewe. History taking may be unrewarding if the owner is inexperienced. A general clinical examination should always be carried out before the obstetric evaluation. Some does may be in poor condition if feeding and management during pregnancy has not been satisfactory. The patient is normally examined in the standing position being restrained by a collar held by the owner. Many does will lie down when vaginal examination is attempted. The caprine uterus is very fragile and easily damaged by the fetal horn buds and displaced extremities.

Vaginal examination of the doe seems to cause great discomfort, even when the utmost gentleness is employed. The owner should be warned of this in advance. The apparently piteous cries of the doe are very unpleasant for owner and obstetrician. They probably do not indicate the severe discomfort that their volume suggests. Routine sedation of the doe is not necessary or advisable.

The vagina should be explored carefully to determine whether the cervix is open and whether one or more fetuses are palpable. Additional lubrication greatly facilitates the examination. If the cervix is not fully dilated, an attempt should be made to dilate it manually. If further dilation proves difficult or impossible, the cervix and uterine contents should be assessed in detail as in the ewe (see Chapter 6). In many such cases a cesarean section to deliver the litter will be necessary. The operation in the doe goat is discussed in detail in Chapter 11.

The presentation, position, and posture of any palpable fetuses should be ascertained, along with their living state. The size of the bony pelvis should be assessed and a decision made as to whether vaginal delivery is likely to be possible. If fetal maldisposition is present this should be corrected manually after repelling the fetus if necessary. In cases of simultaneous presentation it is easier to deliver a fetus in posterior presentation first as only two extremities (rather than three in anterior presentation) have to be dealt with. Once a fetus is in the correct posture for delivery it should be delivered by traction. Traction is applied in a caudal direction initially, and then downwards towards the maternal hocks. One leg should be advanced before the other and the fetus is eased through the birth canal. Help from the obstetrician aids the natural expulsive forces.

Multiple birth, especially of twins and triplets, is extremely common in goats. Great care must be taken to ensure that the uterus is searched methodically for further kids after each delivery.

Retention of a kid after the apparent cessation of kidding should be suspected in does in which the placenta is retained (Matthews 1999). Some animals give birth to a kid unaided up to several days after kidding appears to have been completed. In other cases of fetal retention the doe is lethargic and anorexic as she becomes progressively more toxemic and septicemic. A careful vaginal examination should be made in such cases. If a kid is found in the uterus it should be removed manually after generous application of lubrication. The doe should receive supportive therapy including antibiotic and non-steroidal anti-inflammatory treatment.

Resuscitation of the kids (using the same techniques recommended for lambs) may be necessary, especially if there has been any delay in recognizing and dealing with the dystocia.

AFTERCARE OF THE KID AND DOE

After delivery, each kid should be placed near its mother's head. Navel hygiene and supervision of colostral uptake are very important. Does kidding for the first time may be aggressive with, or apparently frightened of, their offspring. Patient assistance may be required to help establish the fetomaternal bond. The milk supply and teat patency of the doe should also be checked.

The risk of postparturient infection in goats is quite high, especially if there has been much lay interference or if the case has been neglected. Antibiotic cover for 5 days (with a broad-spectrum agent such as ampicillin) is advisable in all cases of assisted delivery.

THE OVERDUE BIRTH – PROLONGED GESTATION

This condition is less well documented in the doe than it is in the ewe. The general approach to the problem is the same in both species (see Chapter 6 for a detailed account of the management of prolonged gestation in the ewe). Although the date of service may have been recorded it is not uncommon for a doe to be served again. A later service may not have been observed but a new later kidding date is now in prospect.

As in the ewe, it is essential to determine by pregnancy diagnosis if the overdue doe is in fact pregnant. In goats, the quite common condition of pseudopregnancy should be kept in mind. Pseudopregnancy does not normally persist beyond the length of a normal pregnancy.

REFERENCES

Matthews JG 1999 Diseases of the goat, 2nd edn. Blackwell Science, Oxford, p 48–50

Rahim AT, Arthur GH 1982 Obstetrical conditions in goats. Cornell Veterinarian 72:279–284

Chapter 8

DYSTOCIA IN THE SOW

The shape of the porcine fetus and its small size in relation to that of its mother combine to make the incidence of dystocia in sows lower than in other farm animals. Litter size is normally in the range 8–14, but can be as small as one piglet or as large as over 20 piglets. The two long uterine horns resemble those of the dog and cat and, as in those species, the incidence of uterine inertia is quite high. Any delay in the birth process can lead to a high level of stillbirth and for this reason farrowing is normally closely supervised. The danger of injury to the piglets by their mother either as a result of aggression or through crushing injuries is also high. Much simple obstetric assistance is given by farm staff and induction of birth is widely practiced to ensure that farrowing occurs during working hours.

INCIDENCE

Dystocia occurs in 0.25–1.0% of all farrowings and may be higher in young, inexperienced gilts or very old sows. Many commercial sows are hybrids but among purebred herds some variation in the incidence of dystocia may be seen. Welsh gilts have particularly small pelvises while the Large White seems to be particularly prone to uterine inertia. As in other species, the apparent incidence of dystocia may be high in herds supervised by a particularly zealous herdsperson.

CAUSES OF DYSTOCIA

There have been relatively few surveys of the causes of porcine dystocia but in one study of 200 cases (Jackson 1972) attended on farms, the findings were as shown in Table 8.1.

Table 8.1 Causes of dystocia in the sow

Cause*	%
Uterine inertia (all types)	37.0
Obstruction of the birth canal	13.0
Deviation of the uterus	9.5
Maternal excitement	3.0
Fetal maldisposition	33.5
Fetopelvic disproportion	4.0

*In some cases more than one causal factor is present. From Jackson (1972).

Uterine inertia

The most common cause of dystocia in sows. Three forms are recognized and in the above survey their relative incidence was as follows:

- primary uterine inertia: 20%
- secondary uterine inertia: 49%
- idiopathic uterine inertia: 31%.

Primary uterine inertia

Although in the larger, monotocous species primary uterine inertia is usually accompanied by non-delivery of the fetus, in the case of the polytocous species, including the pig, one or more piglets may actually be delivered. Two forms of primary uterine inertia are seen in sows: that in toxemic sows (approximately 60%) and that in non-toxemic sows (approximately 40%).

Primary uterine inertia in toxemic sows   In these animals there may be some signs of illness before farrowing and a foul-smelling vaginal discharge with a characteristic sour 'dead pig odor' may have been noticed. The cause of the problem is not always clear, but may be associated with infections such as porcine parvovirus.

In the survey by Jackson, over 90% of the piglets in these cases were stillborn but it was not always clear whether fetal death had preceded uterine infection or vice versa. Vaginal examination in most cases reveals that the vaginal mucosa is dry and fibrous. The fetal membranes are usually separated from their uterine attachments and are dry; the vagina is distended and air filled. Response to oxytocin therapy is variable and the prognosis for affected sows is very poor.

Primary uterine inertia in non-toxemic sows
Affected sows are usually bright and alert. The cervix is dilated or easily dilatable and fetuses are palpable but no uterine contractions are present. Up to 20% of piglets may be stillborn. The exact cause of the condition is unclear; maternal calcium status is normal and hormone insufficiency may be implicated.

Secondary uterine inertia

This is the most common form of porcine uterine inertia. In all cases some primary factor has delayed parturition, resulting in tiring of the uterine musculature. Usually, a number of piglets have already been delivered and there may have been a history of unsuccessful straining. Common primary factors include a dead maldisposed piglet, simultaneous presentation of two or more piglets, or an obstruction of the birth canal. The stillbirth rate can be quite high, at approximately 40%.

Idiopathic uterine inertia

In this condition farrowing appears to commence normally but then stops with apparent cessation of uterine contractions. The condition may be more likely to occur in fat sows and in some sows serum calcium levels are slightly depressed. The precise cause is unknown but the condition is responsive to oxytocin. The stillbirth rate is quite low at about 10%.

OBSTRUCTION OF THE BIRTH CANAL

Obstruction may be caused by bony or soft tissue abnormality, the latter being the more common.

Bony tissue abnormality

The bony pelvis may be small in poorly grown gilts and is a particular problem when litter size is small and individual piglet size is large, with resultant fetopelvic disproportion. Although it is usually possible for the obstetrician's hand to pass through the sow's pelvis it may occasionally not be possible in those animals, especially gilts, with a small pelvic canal. An unusual bony tissue pelvic obstruction may be caused by the presence of a bony tuberosity on the dorsal surface of the pubic symphysis.

Soft tissue abnormality

The most common cause of this is distension of the urinary bladder. Other abnormalities include vulval constriction, vulval scar tissue, vulval hematoma, persistent hymen, non-dilation of the cervix, and obstruction of the uterine lumen.

Distension of the urinary bladder

In most cases the sow has had three or more litters and no history of previous dystocia. Litter size is often but not always greater than ten piglets. Farrowing may be slow in affected animals, with urine accumulating in the bladder. In some cases excessive relaxation of the birth canal and neighboring tissues is present. Vaginal examination reveals that when the sow strains the vaginal floor is pushed upwards and backwards in the form of a mound (Fig. 8.1). The bladder is palpable beneath this mound, which blocks the birth canal like a ball valve, preventing passage of piglets unless assisted. The hand may be readily passed over the obstruction and presenting piglets removed with ease. Catheterization or spontaneous emptying of the bladder will enable further piglets to be delivered without aid.

Vulval abnormalities

The vulva is occasionally small and not fully relaxed, especially in gilts. Scar tissue caused by previous injury (often the bite of another sow) may obstruct the vulval orifice. Gentle stretching by the obstetrician's hand may cause relaxation of the tissues but occasionally episiotomy is required. Vulval hematomas are seen frequently in periparturient gilts and sows but are rarely the cause of dystocia. They are mostly caused by the patient rubbing her hindquarters against the bars of her farrowing crate. One vulval lip is usually affected and is enlarged by the presence of a quantity of blood released into adjacent soft tissues, which may block the exit from the birth canal. Piglets can normally be removed manually past the obstruction but sedation may be required if the sow is in discomfort. Vulval hematomas in pigs should never be opened and drained

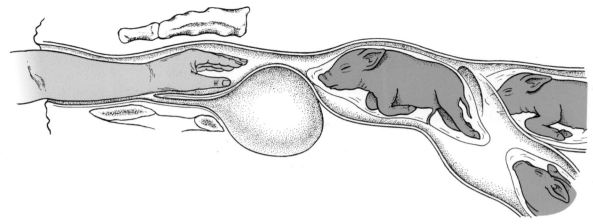

Figure 8.1 Obstruction of the birth canal in the sow caused by distension of the urinary bladder.

because profuse hemorrhage may ensue. Self-resolution normally occurs after farrowing. If the hematoma is accidentally ruptured, any bleeding vessels should be ligated to prevent chronic hemorrhage.

Persistent hymen

This is an occasional cause of dystocia in gilts. The vagina is obstructed just anterior to the external urethral orifice by a band of fibrous tissue, which almost completely occludes the lumen. In most cases the obstruction can be broken down with modest digital pressure or careful incision. Failing this, cesarean section may be required.

Non-dilation of the cervix

This is a rare condition in sows and in most cases the cervix can be dilated by gentle digital pressure. If this fails, cesarean section may be required.

Obstruction of the uterine lumen

This unusual cause of dystocia may be caused by pressure from distended intestinal loops, constriction due to scar tissue caused by previous damage to the uterine wall, or an apparent underdevelopment of a portion of the uterine body or horn. In some cases, manual removal of the piglets is possible after breaking down the obstruction or relieving external pressure but in other cases cesarean section may be required.

Downward deviation of the uterus

This condition is usually seen in sows beyond their third parity, with a 'deep' conformation and carrying a large litter, usually in excess of ten piglets. The sow may pass one or two piglets and then strain unproductively. Vaginal examination usually reveals no piglets within the vagina or uterine body. About 15 cm anterior to the pelvic brim the uterus deviates sharply downwards towards the ventral abdominal floor (Fig. 8.2). A piglet may be just palpable in the uterine body or horns vertically below that part of the vagina containing the obstetrician's arm. Uterine contractions are present but seem unable to move the piglets around the bends in the uterus caused by the deviation.

Manual removal of the piglets can be quite difficult. It may require insertion of the arm up to the shoulder so that the obstetrician's elbow may be bent within the sow and presenting fetuses grasped and removed. Encouraging the sow to adopt a standing position may aid delivery. Normally, after delivery of a few piglets the deviation straightens out and spontaneous delivery may ensue. Because the problem is normally detected and corrected early in parturition, the stillbirth rate may be as low as 6%.

MATERNAL EXCITEMENT

Maternal excitement is seen occasionally in gilts but rarely in older animals; it can delay or inhibit the farrowing process. Late movement into farrowing accommodation or innate nervousness may predispose to the problem. The condition may be accompanied by aggression towards the litter (see also Litter savaging, p. 140). Sedation may be necessary and azaperone given by intramuscular injection at 2 mg/kg body weight is effective and has little sedative effect on the unborn litter. Once sedated, uterine contractions are

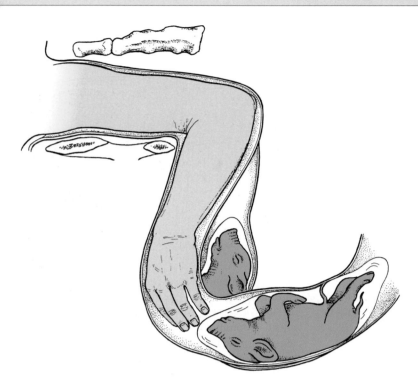

Figure 8.2 Dystocia in the sow caused by downward deviation of the uterus.

normally unaffected but supplementation with 20 IU oxytocin may be necessary.

FETAL MALDISPOSITION

This is a common cause of porcine dystocia, accounting for 33% of all cases. In larger animals fetal maldisposition may be caused or exacerbated by contact or engagement with the maternal pelvis. This can happen in the sow but dystocia can also arise by the fetus becoming maldisposed within the narrow confines of the uterine body or horns (Fig. 8.3). The short neck and limbs of the porcine fetus do not often predispose to malposture of the head or limbs but this may occur more readily if the fetus is small and poorly developed. Posterior presentation is regarded as normal in pigs, with up to 50% of piglets being in this orientation. The two most common maldispositions are breech presentation (bilateral hip flexion) and simultaneous presentation of two or more piglets at the pelvic inlet or at the junction of the uterine horns. Various combinations of anteroposterior orientation are seen, the most common being one piglet in anterior and one in posterior presentation. Small piglets may be born in an uncorrected breech presentation.

FETOPELVIC DISPROPORTION

The problem of small pelvic size was mentioned above and has a contributory role in this condition. Individual piglet size increases with decreasing litter size. Mean litter size in cases of fetopelvic disproportion was 4.3, compared with 10.8 for other causes of dystocia.

SIGNS OF DYSTOCIA

The boundary between normal birth and dystocia is not always clear cut. The following signs should be regarded as possible indications of trouble which should be investigated without delay:

- Foul discharge and decaying placenta at the vulva: a serious sign often indicative of fetal death and toxemia.
- Signs of imminent birth but farrowing has not commenced: may indicate primary uterine inertia in a non-toxemic sow. Vaginal examination required to ensure all is well.
- Straining but no piglets born: may indicate obstruction of the birth canal, fetal maldisposition, deviation

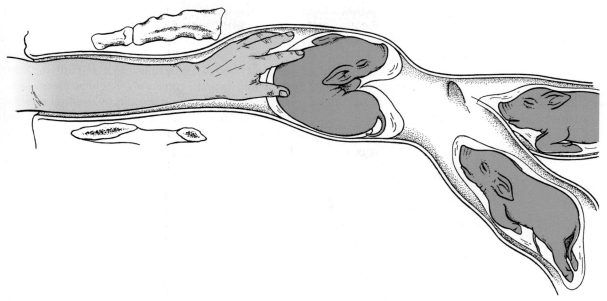

Figure 8.3 Dystocia in the sow can arise by the fetus becoming maldisposed within the narrow confines of the uterine body or horns.

of the uterus possibly complicated by secondary uterine inertia. Non-productive continuous straining lasting longer than 15 minutes should be investigated, as should intermittent straining lasting longer than 30 minutes.

- Premature cessation of labor: may be a natural break in farrowing or idiopathic uterine inertia. Cases should be examined without delay.
- Prolonged farrowing (normal duration of birth ½–4 hours, mean 2.5 hours): may indicate partial obstruction of birth canal or developing uterine inertia.
- Litter size unexpectedly small: farrowing may be complete or dystocia is present.
- Placenta not seen: it may have been eaten by sow. The placenta is seldom retained in sows unless one or more piglets has also been retained.

APPROACH TO A CASE OF DYSTOCIA IN THE SOW

The history of the sow is briefly ascertained. Details of any previous dystocia may be available. The number of piglets already born and their living state and the duration of labor are noted. If a number of dead piglets has already been born or if the duration of labor is prolonged the prognosis for further live deliveries is poor.

OBSTETRICIAN'S CHECK LIST

Call received

How many piglets already born?
↓
Previous history of dystocia
↓
Recent problems with dystocia in herd?
↓
Was the present birth induced?
↓
See the patient as soon as possible

A quiet and gentle approach must be adopted at all times and the presence of one assistant is all that is necessary. Most sows are docile at farrowing time but a careful watch for signs of aggression must be kept if the sow is loose in her pen and not confined in a farrowing crate. If a loose sow is attended, the obstetrician should always be protected by an assistant carrying a pig board. A brief general clinical appraisal of the sow should be carried out. In particular, the body temperature, the cardiovascular system, and the state of the udder should be checked. Hyperthermia can occur in animals suffering from dystocia confined too close to the heat of creep lamps and must be dealt with by cooling before obstetric treatment. Most cases can be dealt with using the hands and, apart from supplies of obstetric lubricant, no special equipment is required. A lambing snare can be useful to help deliver piglets in cases where pelvic size is small.

OBSTETRICIAN'S CHECK LIST

Arrive at pig unit

Update on number of piglets born alive/dead
↓
Inspect piglets already born
↓
Duration of labor?
↓
Safety considerations

OBSTETRICIAN'S CHECK LIST

Clinical examination of sow

General appearance of sow
↓
Temperature, pulse and respiration
↓
Check for signs of heat stroke
↓
Inspect the vulva
↓
Note presence of fetal membranes at vulva
↓
Check the udder for milk and milk let down

Vaginal examination

It is usually more convenient to encourage the sow to remain in lateral recumbency during vaginal examination except in cases of downward deviation of the uterus (see p. 131). Sedation should be administered to animals showing severe excitement. Gentle massaging of the udder will encourage most sows to remain in or adopt lateral recumbency, even when the hand is introduced into the vagina (Fig. 8.4). The obstetrician should nonetheless beware of sudden unexpected movements by the sow, which could injure the arms if they are trapped against the back of the farrowing crate.

Strict hygiene is essential before and during vaginal examination. The vaginal mucosa in the pig is especially fragile and excessive internal examination must be avoided. Generous lubrication is essential. The obstetrician's hand can be readily introduced into the birth canal and up to the cervix, which is immediately anterior to the pelvic brim. The external urethral orifice is recognizable on the vaginal floor within the pelvis and any hymenal remnants will be found just anterior to this. The fully dilated cervix is not palpable. The uterine body is short and the caudal extremities of the uterine horns are recognized by placing the thumb in one horn and the fingers in the other. Parts of each horn may be explored manually but it is impossible to explore the entire length of the long uterine horns.

The birth canal is checked for any signs of damage and any tears in the mucosa should be passed with great care to avoid further damage. The presence and disposition of any piglets or placenta within the birth canal is noted. Palpation of the uterine body and horns will allow assessment of uterine tone. If uterine tone is good the uterine walls may feel very hard and almost solid to the touch; in cases of uterine inertia they are soft and flabby. Palpation of the uterine walls may, however, induce spontaneous contractions. A diagnosis of the cause or causes of dystocia and a plan for resolution should be made. The obstetrician's hand enclosed in the uterine body will normally pass through the maternal bony pelvis and the dimensions of the pelvis are noted at this time.

Treatment   This is aimed at delivering any presenting fetuses – having first corrected any maldisposition – and then assisting the sow to complete the birth process as quickly as possible thus allowing a rapid return to normality for the sow and as low a stillbirth rate as possible in the litter.

Fetal delivery   This can normally be effected manually. A number of methods for grasping the fetus are illustrated (Fig. 8.5). The obstetrician's fingers should *never* be placed in the unborn piglet's mouth because injury by the latter's sharp teeth may be sustained. Occasionally, pelvic size is too small to allow passage of the fetal head enclosed in the obstetrician's hand although the hand alone, and the size of the fetal head, suggests it also will pass readily through the pelvis. The eye socket or nasal holds may be used in these circumstances and occasionally a lambing snare may be used to bring the piglet through the maternal pelvis. Placental tissue is grasped and removed by gentle traction. As soon as each piglet is born it should be held upside down by its hips or hind legs and gently shaken to remove

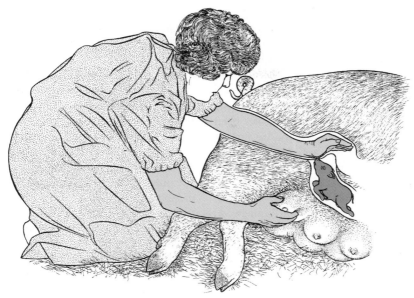

Figure 8.4 Gentle massage of the udder will encourage most sows to remain in lateral recumbency even when the hand is inserted into the vagina.

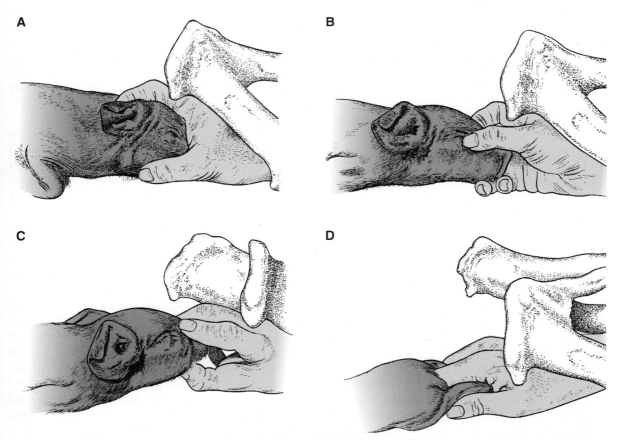

Figure 8.5 Holds for gripping the piglet to apply traction. (A) Head hold, (B) eye-socket hold, (C) nasal hold, (D) hindlimb hold.

mucus from the mouth and pharynx. The long umbilical cord usually breaks during the latter stages of manual delivery and is knotted approximately 5 cm from the piglet to reduce the risk of hemorrhage or access by infection. For details of piglet resuscitation, see p. 139.

If uterine contractions are strong, the obstetrician should wait for 10 minutes before re-examining the birth canal to determine if further piglets have been moved back within reach by uterine activity. Any further piglets and placenta should be removed. The temptation to make very frequent vaginal examinations must be resisted because the vaginal mucosa is easily damaged and may become swollen and edematous. Follow-up examinations must be made, however, and damage can be kept to a minimum by the use of generous amounts of obstetric lubricant. If uterine tone is low, ecbolic therapy is required.

Ecbolic therapy   This is used to stimulate uterine contractions if uterine inertia is present or if it is desired to hasten completion of the second stage of labor. Oxytocin is most commonly used and is the drug of choice. A dose of 20 IU into the muscles of the hindquarters should be given, this site being preferable and less disturbing to the sow than the muscles in the neck. The injection of oxytocin is painful and may cause the sow to jump to her feet with possible injury to the obstetrician or the piglets already born. However, gentle massage of the udder and careful insertion of the needle will often enable the injection to be given without disturbance. Before oxytocin is given the obstetrician must ensure that there is no obstruction of the birth canal or a fetus wedged in maldisposition. Ecbolic therapy may become less effective with increasing duration of labor. In cases of uterine inertia, a number of injections of oxytocin at approximately 30-minute intervals may be required until the whole litter has been delivered.

The obstetrician should remain with the case until it is believed that normal farrowing has resumed or is complete. If it is not possible to remain on the farm, the owner should be asked to telephone a progress report after 1–2 hours. The obstetrician should be prepared to revisit the case if progress has not been as anticipated.

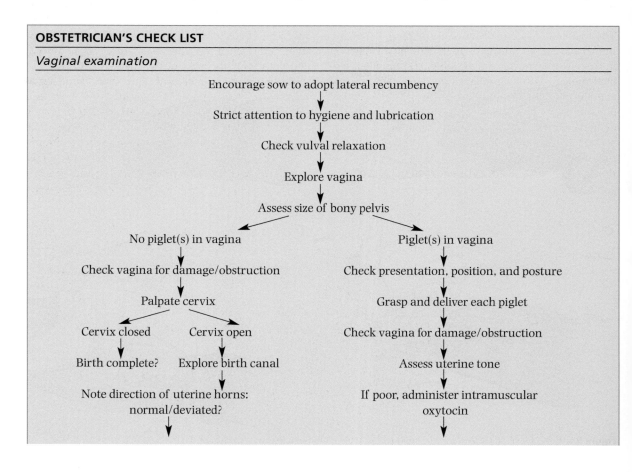

OBSTETRICIAN'S CHECK LIST

Vaginal examination

Encourage sow to adopt lateral recumbency

Strict attention to hygiene and lubrication

Check vulval relaxation

Explore vagina

Assess size of bony pelvis

No piglet(s) in vagina | Piglet(s) in vagina

Check vagina for damage/obstruction | Check presentation, position, and posture

Palpate cervix | Grasp and deliver each piglet

Cervix closed | Cervix open | Check vagina for damage/obstruction

Birth complete? | Explore birth canal | Assess uterine tone

Note direction of uterine horns: normal/deviated? | If poor, administer intramuscular oxytocin

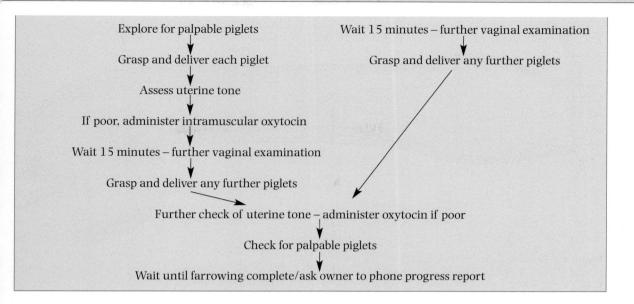

Explore for palpable piglets
↓
Grasp and deliver each piglet
↓
Assess uterine tone
↓
If poor, administer intramuscular oxytocin
↓
Wait 15 minutes – further vaginal examination
↓
Grasp and deliver any further piglets

Wait 15 minutes – further vaginal examination
↓
Grasp and deliver any further piglets

Further check of uterine tone – administer oxytocin if poor
↓
Check for palpable piglets
↓
Wait until farrowing complete/ask owner to phone progress report

DETERMINING THE END OF THE BIRTH PROCESS

The inability of the obstetrician to explore the entire uterus and the resentment of direct abdominal palpation in the sow may make recognition of the completion of birth difficult. Behavioral signs, such as standing to pass urine or feeding the piglets contentedly at the end of farrowing, are unreliable and misleading. The presence of living fetuses may be detected by auscultation or by Doppler or B-mode ultrasonography. X-ray examination of the abdomen will detect the presence of further piglets but is not normally practical under farm conditions.

Internal ballottement can enable the detection of unborn fetuses. If no piglets are detected by direct palpation the obstetrician's hand may be swept about the abdomen enclosed within one uterine horn. Unborn piglets may be balloted further along the same horn or within the opposite horn by this method (Fig. 8.6).

The most reliable clinical sign that farrowing is complete is if the maternal cervix has closed. In such cases the obstetrician can be 95% certain that farrowing is complete (Fig. 8.7). It is not uncommon for gilts to produce a single piglet followed by cervical closure, although it has been suggested that a minimum of four fetuses is required for recognition and maintenance of pregnancy. It is possible that dead unborn fetuses are

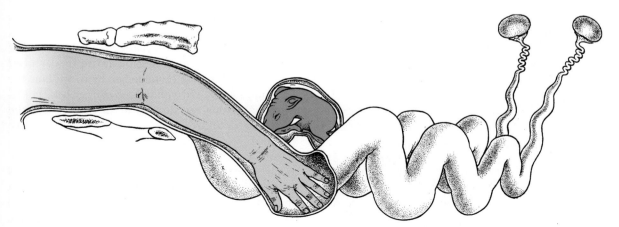

Figure 8.6 The technique of internal ballottement (see text) may help determine the end of the birth process.

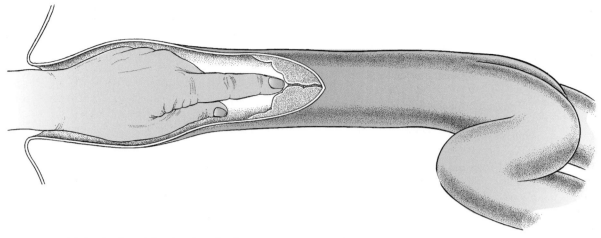

Figure 8.7 Digital palpation of the closed cervix of a sow.

occasionally left undetected in the uterus when farrowing appears complete. Provided no infection is present, such retained fetuses usually cause no harm. Their bodies become calcified and remain as inert intrauterine objects, probably not interfering with subsequent pregnancies. They may be noted within the uterus at the time of slaughter.

OBSTETRICIAN'S CHECK LIST

Determining the end of the birth process

Behavioral signs – unreliable

↓

Explore uterine horns as far as possible

↓

Terminal part of placenta seen?

↓

Internal ballottement negative?

↓

Ultrasonographic scan of abdomen negative?

↓

Cervical closure?

↓

Farrowing probably complete

The presence of dead piglets within the uterus

Individual stillborn and mummified piglets are often delivered without difficulty along with living members of litter. However, large numbers of dead and decaying piglets constitute a health hazard to the sow or gilt. This problem is seen in toxemic sows suffering from primary uterine inertia or in neglected cases of dystocia in which fetal death following placental separation has occurred. The sow may be severely ill and moribund. In such cases, emergency slaughter may not be possible and euthanasia may be necessary on humane grounds. Hysterectomy may be considered if the sow is well enough and the procedure considered economically viable. Fetuses within reach can often be removed from the uterus by gentle traction following introduction of generous amounts of obstetric lubricant. If the nose or feet only of another dead fetus are palpable it is best to leave the sow for about 12 hours and then re-examine her, by which time the fetus may have moved within reach and can be removed. Chronic metritis can develop in such cases and the prognosis for future breeding or even survival must be guarded.

Antibiotic therapy, for example 5 days of ampicillin, is advisable after any assisted delivery. In toxemic sows a non-steroidal anti-inflammatory drug such as flunixin may be beneficial. The farmer should be advised to monitor general health of sow and litter, including the milk supply.

AFTERCARE OF THE SOW AND LITTER

After manual delivery, each piglet is held up by its back legs and shaken gently to remove any mucus from the mouth and pharyngeal area. Piglets mostly gasp and wriggle while this is being done. Breathing starts almost immediately. The umbilical cord is knotted and then severed about 5 cm from the piglet. If the piglet fails to breathe, 5–10 mg doxapram hydrochloride can be injected intramuscularly. The obstetrician can blow into the piglet's mouth and nose. Breathing can also be encouraged using a Cox piglet resuscitator, which has a pump action and face mask through which air can be blown into the lungs. The piglets are normally placed with the sow as soon as they are born and care must be taken to ensure that they do not suffer from hypothermia or injury. The piglets' sharp incisor teeth are clipped or filed level with the gums to avoid biting injuries to the sow's udder and to other piglets. Piglets are encouraged to take colostrum as soon after birth as possible. On some farms, severe problems with neonatal enteric disease occur. In such cases antibiotic therapy may be required soon after birth to provide additional protection against disease to that provided by the colostrum.

OBSTETRICIAN'S CHECK LIST

Postnatal care of the piglets

Hold each piglet carefully by its hindlegs

↓

Shake gently to dislodge fluids/mucus

↓

Check heart beat

↓

Check breathing

↓

If no breathing inject intramuscular doxapram HCl

↓

Artificial respiration/piglet resuscitator

↓

Knot umbilical cord if bleeding

↓

Advise owner *re* colostrum, tooth clipping/grinding

↓

Dip navel in weak iodine solution

The sow and litter are watched carefully for the first few days of life to ensure that the piglets are growing well and are healthy. Mastitis–metritis–agalactia (MMA) syndrome can cause problems with milk supply when the litter is 48–72 hours of age. The condition responds well to antibiotic, steroid, and oxytocin therapy. The piglets are given artificial sow's milk until their mother's milk production returns to normal. For further details of postparturient problems, see Chapter 13.

OBSTETRICIAN'S CHECK LIST

Postnatal care of the sow

Check birth canal for damage

↓

Check udder/milk supply

↓

Antibiotic cover

↓

Consider NSAID treatment

STILLBIRTH AND DYSTOCIA IN SOWS

Between 3 and 6% of piglets are stillborn in normal birth. The incidence of stillbirth rises rapidly with duration of labor and this increase is more pronounced with cases of dystocia. Farmers should be encouraged to report suspected cases of dystocia promptly and the obstetrician should attend without delay and complete delivery of the litter as soon as possible (Jackson 1975).

PROLONGED GESTATION – THE OVERDUE SOW

Sows are occasionally presented as having passed their farrowing date without giving birth. Their service date and the possibility of further service should be checked. On many farms, pregnant sows run with a 'sweeper boar' in case they return to estrus. A later and unnoticed service often occurs in such circumstances.

The sow should receive a full clinical examination. If dead piglets are present in the uterus the sow may be toxemic and very unwell. Abdominal distension may be caused by ascites rather than by pregnancy. Mammary development and the presence of milk in the teats may indicate that the sow is close to farrowing. Pregnancy

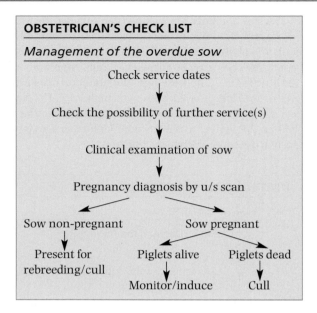

OBSTETRICIAN'S CHECK LIST

Management of the overdue sow

Check service dates

↓

Check the possibility of further service(s)

↓

Clinical examination of sow

↓

Pregnancy diagnosis by u/s scan

Sow non-pregnant   Sow pregnant

Present for   Piglets alive   Piglets dead
rebreeding/cull

Monitor/induce   Cull

diagnosis by ultrasonographic scan should be performed. If the sow is not pregnant she may be presented for rebreeding or culled. If she is found to be pregnant, the stage of pregnancy can be estimated chiefly by the size of the piglets seen in the uterine horns. The ultrasonographic scan should reveal whether the litter are alive or dead.

If the piglets are alive and birth appears imminent, induction of birth may be carried out (for details, see Chapter 15). If the piglets are dead and the sow appears unwell a vaginal examination with a gloved hand should be performed. Generous lubrication aids this examination. Dead and emphysematous piglets may be palpated and many others may be present further along the uterine horns. Fetal fluids have mostly disappeared in such cases. The prognosis is very poor for such cases and euthanasia may be the most humane and economic procedure. Hysterectomy may be considered but the guarded prognosis and small value of the sow after surgery usually rule it out.

LITTER SAVAGING BY SOWS

This is not uncommon, especially in first-litter gilts. There may be a hereditary predisposition to the problem and the abnormal behavior is occasionally repeated at subsequent farrowing. Gilts that are particularly friendly towards people may be especially aggressive with their litters. The problem must be dealt with urgently because the sow could quickly maim or kill her whole litter. The piglets must be removed immediately to a safe warm box. Sedation of the sow is best delayed until farrowing is complete to avoid sedation of the unborn piglets.

A number of drugs can be used, including acepromazine (0.5 mL of a 10 mg/mL solution per 50 kg body weight) by intramuscular or slow intravenous injection, azaperone (2 mg/kg body weight), or a combination of droperidol (5 mg/kg body weight) and midazolam 3 mg/kg body weight) given by intramuscular injection. Occasionally, anesthesia with pentobarbitone sodium by intravenous injection may be necessary. If intravenous therapy is given the sow must be restrained by a strong rope looped round the upper jaw behind the tusks and secured to a strong rail or wall. The ear vein is used and is raised by looping a rubber band round the base of the ear. The rubber band is gently removed before injecting the sedative. Sudden removal of the band by cutting will frighten the sow and often dislodge the needle.

Oxytocin is given to encourage milk letdown, the piglets' teeth are clipped, and they are placed to feed on the sow. When she recovers from sedation they are with her and she normally then accepts them. The sow is occasionally non-responsive to treatment and the piglets must be fostered onto other animals.

CESAREAN SECTION

Surgical delivery may be indicated in cases of fetopelvic disproportion, obstruction of the birth canal that cannot be delivered per vaginam and in cases of nonresponsive uterine inertia. The economics of the case must be discussed with the farmer before surgery is commenced. For details of the technique see Chapter 11.

FETOTOMY

This technique is not normally indicated or used in sows.

REFERENCES

Jackson PGG 1972 Dystocia in the sow. Fellowship Thesis, RCVS, London

Jackson PGG 1975 Incidence of stillbirth in cases of dystocia in sows. Veterinary Record 97:411–412

Chapter 9

DYSTOCIA IN THE DOG AND CAT

Fortunately, the incidence of dystocia in small animals is quite low but when cases are encountered it is essential that decision making and management are based on a thorough background knowledge of normal and abnormal birth. The obstetric knowledge of the small animal owner is extremely variable. An inexperienced breeder may have never witnessed animal birth and literally have no idea of what is involved; an experienced breeder may have witnessed many more births than the attending veterinary surgeon. A great deal of information can be gained from some breeders but others will have serious and sometimes long-standing misconceptions about the birth process. Such ideas and views may have to be diplomatically ignored and possibly corrected.

Much veterinary obstetric work is still of a 'fire brigade' nature with the parturient mother not having been seen prior to the emergency consultation. Clearly this is unsatisfactory and many problems could, with prior knowledge of the case, have been anticipated and prevented. Although it may be difficult to justify provision of the standard of antenatal care available to people, small animal and equine practice does offer the opportunity for some degree of antenatal care.

In some cases, contact is first made when the dog or cat is presented for pregnancy diagnosis but advice may be sought at an earlier stage regarding mating and other matters.

PREMATING CONSULTATION

The scope of this consultation will depend upon the owner's knowledge and the history of the patient. Advice regarding the patient's suitability for breeding from the breed-standard viewpoint or the show potential of progeny is probably best sought from experienced breeders. Veterinary input is, however, most important. A full clinical examination of both participants of the proposed breeding pair (if both are available) should be carried out to ensure they are fit and well. They should be skeletally mature as breeding from very small members of a breed may predispose to dystocia caused by fetopelvic disproportion. If there is any history of previous infertility then this must be investigated.

In addition to the clinical examination the following matters should be considered:

- The patient's medical and reproductive history.
- The patient's body weight: problems of obesity or malnutrition should be resolved before a decision to attempt breeding is made.
- Pelvic capacity: this should be large enough to allow the passage of fetuses of normal dimension. An external indication of pelvic size can be obtained by noting the distance between the wings of the ilia and between the tubera ischii. A digital rectal examination will allow further estimation of pelvic size. Suspected deformity possibly caused by an earlier road accident can be further evaluated by radiographic examination.
- Vaccination history of the patient: booster vaccination should be carried out *before* pregnancy. In the bitch, canine herpesvirus vaccination should be carried out during pregnancy, this is discussed on p. 145.
- Detailed examination of the genital system.
- Screening for specific problems: for example, hip dysplasia, feline leukemia virus.
- Bacterial investigation of the genital tract of breeding bitches may be necessary if there has been a history of previous infertility. Cultures may reveal the presence of mixed commensals only. In problem bitches, profuse growth of potential pathogens such as β-hemolytic streptococcus may be significant. Appropriate antibiotic therapy may be prescribed around the time of mating.

- Cytological and hormonal appraisal of the female.
- Hematological and biochemical appraisal if health is suspect.
- Genetic counseling.
- Monitoring the approach of ovulation with the aid of a progesterone profile and vaginal smears in the bitch.

Inherited malformations and diseases are relatively rare in the dog and cat. Selection for specific phenotypic qualities by inbreeding may increase the incidence of fetal abnormalities. However, the breeding of close relatives is quite frequently seen in pedigrees. Adverse consequences are fortunately not often encountered.

Where problems have occurred, evaluation of the pedigree for the degree of inbreeding may help to suggest a mode of inheritance of adverse factors. Test matings may be necessary and if a stud is suspected of carrying an abnormal gene a mating to a female also showing the trait is the quickest way of identifying the carrier, because the off-spring have a 1:1 chance of showing the abnormality.

Age of breeding

Male dogs are capable of breeding from around the time of puberty at 6 months and if the dog is to be used at stud in later life it is important not to suppress signs of potential libido during puppyhood. Regular stud use should be avoided until the dog is 1–2 years of age, and even then it should be introduced gradually.

Ideally, the mature stud should have not more than one bitch per week, allowing two or three services per bitch. There is some evidence that breeding in the female should not be delayed in either the bitch or queen much later than 3 years of age as it is claimed that subsequent fertility may be lower than in animals bred at an earlier age. The Kennel Club has recently prohibited the registration of puppies born to bitches that are over 7 years of age. Although bitch puppies can theoretically breed from the age of puberty, breeding is best delayed until the bitch is skeletally mature at about 18 months of age. The tomcat should not be used at stud until he is able to dominate his partner at successful coitus. It is advisable not to present a queen for breeding until her weight reaches at least 2.5 kg and she is at least 1 year old.

Selection of sire

This is chiefly influenced by pedigree and showing considerations, but with novice owners or where there has been a history of previous infertility, ease of access to the sire is very important. Wherever possible, a stud animal near to home should be selected. Good temperament is an essential quality in both members of the breeding pair. In the cat disparity of size between the sexes should be avoided because a short-bodied male may have difficulty in mating a long-bodied female.

Place of mating

In both dog and cat some degree of male aggression is necessary to allow coitus to occur. Taking the female to the male's established territory will normally encourage this. Time may be needed – especially in the cat – for dominance to be established. Where the male and female partners have lived together for some time before estrus there may be some reluctance to breed – especially in the dog – and it is wise to separate the pair before estrus is expected. The animals can be reintroduced for breeding once estrus has started.

Time of mating

Despite the longevity of canine spermatozoa, studies of infertility cases and the estrus behavior of bitches suggests that correct timing of mating is important. The most reliable indicator in normal animals is the willingness of the bitch to allow mating. Other indicators of potential receptivity include:

- Cessation of proestral bleeding (but this does not cease in 5% of bitches).
- Vulval relaxation.
- Vaginal cytology: the point of maximum cornification of superficial cells.
- Electrical resistance of the vaginal mucosa (unreliable).
- Second negative glucose test in vaginal mucus.
- Response to perineal stimulation.
- Rise in plasma progesterone, indicating approaching ovulation.

In the cat, estrus usually lasts 4–6 days with mating followed by reflex ovulation being permitted by the queen on the third day. There is no proestral bleeding in the queen cat.

Frequency of mating

In the dog, the pair will naturally mate up to five times daily. In controlled breeding mating should normally be allowed every 48 hours as long as the bitch remains receptive. More than one mating is undoubtedly beneficial because studies have shown that conception rate following a single mating may be approximately 60%, rising to >80% with two matings. Despite this, many stud owners and breeders claim excellent results over many years following a single mating on a specified day of the estrous cycle.

Ovulation in the queen cat is induced by coitus and several matings may be required before ovulation occurs. Estrus often ends abruptly 24 hours after coitus, thus allowing no further breeding to occur.

Mating behavior

When the bitch is fully in estrus she will stand to be mated after a period of play and mutual interest during which sniffing of the genitalia and attempts at mounting may occur. The bitch raises her tail and should show no objection to being mated. Coitus in dogs is prolonged as a result of the canine tie phenomenon, which can last up to 1 hour but is not absolutely essential for successful conception. Partial penile erection is seen as attempts to gain intromission are made with thrusting movements as the bitch is mounted. Further erection is stimulated by tight contraction of the vestibular muscles of the bitch. The dog's penis is trapped by the erection of the bulbus glandis held by the vestibular muscle and the tie commences. Ejaculation commences as the tie becomes more intense and the dog turns, still in the tied position, to stand facing in the opposite direction to his mate. Occasionally the tie is prolonged and causes concern to the owner. Sedation of both partners with acepromazine is effective in such cases, as is the traditional method of applying cold water to the pair!

In the cat coitus is brief and quite violent, and is often accompanied by noise and aggression. Signs of estrus include vocalization, posturing lordosis with the tail raised and treading movements of the hindlimbs, and frequent urination. Some of these signs may be intensified if the cat is grasped by her scruff. After some initial aggression mounting occurs, with the male grasping the female firmly by the scruff.

Treading movement with all four legs is displayed by the male and vigorous thrusting movements are seen as he attempts to achieve intromission. Mating is brief and the female shows signs of discomfort as the penis is withdrawn and she may turn and strike the male before vigorously licking her vulva. Occasionally the male does not release his grip on the female and mates her again before releasing her.

ANTENATAL CONSULTATION

The pregnant animal should be seen at least once during gestation or more frequently if necessary. Time must be allowed not only for a thorough clinical examination but also for the owner to ask questions and seek advice about matters of concern. Time can be saved by producing leaflets covering certain aspects of antenatal care and birth. The following points should be covered during the examination.

Case history

This should be reviewed in detail. Important points include the history of any previous parturition and of dystocia, infertility, metabolic disease, genital tract disease, clotting defects, etc. The management of bitches suffering from diabetes mellitus can be very difficult during pregnancy. Stabilization is difficult and puppies may be either markedly overweight or underweight at birth. If there is a history of road accident, pelvic patency should be checked by a digital rectal examination and radiography later in the consultation. Vaccination status should ideally be checked and brought up to date if necessary before mating. If booster vaccination is overdue it should be administered to the pregnant patient after careful consultation of the vaccine data sheets. Many of the infectious diseases of cats and dogs can have a devastating effect on pregnancy. Poor immunity in the dam can also result in suboptimal passive transfer of immunity to the litter. Vaccination against canine herpesvirus during pregnancy is recommended and details are given below.

Pregnancy diagnosis

Numerous methods of pregnancy diagnosis are available to confirm that the patient is really pregnant.

Abdominal palpation   This is best carried out at 3–4 weeks gestation when the firm amniotic vesicles of the fetuses may be palpated in the uterine horns. At this stage each vesicle has a bead-like consistency and is between 1 and 2 cm in diameter. Palpation may be difficult in tense or obese mothers. Palpation beyond 4 weeks of pregnancy is less satisfactory because the amniotic vesicles enlarge rapidly and become less tense after this stage of pregnancy. In late pregnancy – from 6 weeks onwards – individual fetuses may be palpable and fetal movement detected.

Ultrasonographic scanning of the abdomen
B-mode real-time ultrasonography provides a highly accurate method of diagnosing pregnancy in both dog and cat. At 5 weeks of pregnancy fetuses are readily detected, fetal hearts can be visualized, and the heart rate counted. Fetal numbers can be quite accurately assessed. If more than four fetuses are present the accuracy of estimation of fetal numbers is reduced. Owners should not be given a guarantee of the number of fetuses present in their animal. Some offspring may be lost through fetal resorption during pregnancy. The clarity of the amniotic fluid may also be observed and gross fetal defects may be seen. In some dogs, pregnancy may be detected as early as 14 days postcoitus, while in late pregnancy confirmation of fetal numbers becomes less accurate. Evidence of fetal life – through fetal heart beats and movements – may also be detected using Doppler ultrasound from approximately 21 days of pregnancy.

ELISA test   In both the bitch and queen the hormone *relaxin* is found in the blood of pregnant animals from day 25 of pregnancy. Relaxin can be readily detected by an ELISA test. As each fetus produces relaxin, it may eventually be possible to estimate fetal numbers by estimating the amount of relaxin present. The possibility of later fetal losses must be borne in mind. A further estimation of blood relaxin may be made later in pregnancy.

Acute-phase proteins   In the bitch, acute-phase proteins appear in the maternal blood – their presence in a healthy animal indicates pregnancy – between 27 and 35 days of gestation. Acute-phase proteins also rise in cases of pyometra, which may develop 21 days after estrus. The bitch must receive a thorough clinical examination when the blood sample is taken to ensure that she is free from inflammatory diseases that might cause elevation of the acute-phase proteins unrelated to pregnancy.

Abdominal radiography   Pregnancy can be confirmed by abdominal radiography, but only after 35 days of pregnancy when organogenesis is complete. Ossification of the fetal skeletons is demonstrable at about 40 days of pregnancy. Radiography of the entire abdomen will enable a count of fetal numbers to be made. It should be avoided if other methods of pregnancy assessment are available but can be used in safety during the management of a dystocia case.

Confirmation of whelping/kittening date

It is essential to check the owner's note of prospective whelping or kittening dates because miscalculations are often made. The gestation period for both species is an average of 63 days but if a number of services have taken place considerable variation from this figure may occur. In dogs it is known that acceptance of the male can occur up to 11 days before and up to 3 days after ovulation. The point of ovulation is indicated by the rising progesterone profile and the appearance of the vaginal cell cytology. The concentration of progesterone in the bitches' blood may rise to approximately 20 ng/mL just prior to ovulation. Vaginal smears stained with Shorr's trichrome stain will show the highest percentage of orange staining cornified cells just prior to ovulation.

A peak in the blood concentration of luteinizing hormone (LH) occurs 48 hours prior to ovulation. A study of 290 bitches showed that parturition was highly likely to occur 64–66 days after the LH peak. Frequent LH assays would be required to identify the timing of peak secretion and is not a practical proposition in most cases.

General clinical examination

A comprehensive health check should be carried out with special attention being paid to the genital system, the mammary glands, and pelvic capacity. If pelvic capacity is in any way doubtful it should be further assessed by digital rectal examination and radiography at an appropriate time. Fetal organogenesis is complete by 35 days of gestation and limited radiography can be safely used after that time.

Few problems should be found in the healthy breeding female but any abnormalities should be appropriately followed up and, if necessary, monitored throughout pregnancy. The animal should be in good bodily condition. Weight problems should ideally be recognized and addressed before pregnancy is contemplated. Obese animals should not be bred from – fertility is lowered and there is a greater risk of abortion, stillbirths, and dystocia in overweight animals. If the dam is malnourished her conception rate is reduced and the risk of pregnancy loss is increased. Any offspring born may be underweight and may also fail to thrive in later life. There is also a risk of hypoglycemia occurring in underweight bitches in late pregnancy and early lactation.

Canine herpesvirus vaccination

A vaccine is available for active immunization of bitches to prevent mortality, clinical signs and lesions in puppies arising from infection by canine herpesvirus in the first few days of life. Two doses (1 mL administered subcutaneously) are given to the bitch as follows: First dose: during estrus or 7–10 days after mating; second dose: 1–2 weeks before the expected whelping date. The vaccination program should be repeated each time the bitch is bred.

HEALTH DURING PREGNANCY

Pregnancy is not a disease but a natural reproductive function and health should be good throughout its duration. The desire for and the ability to take exercise become less and *in some bitches a period of mild illness may be seen about the third or occasionally as late as the fifth week of pregnancy.* The condition has been likened to morning sickness in people but does not share the same cause. Appetite may be reduced and some vomiting and increased thirst may be seen. The condition and the time that it occurs – about 3 weeks after mating – may raise suspicions that the bitch is developing *pyometra.* A careful clinical examination should differentiate the two conditions and ensure that no other disease process is present. In cases of pyometra, uterine enlargement may be palpable or demonstrable by ultrasonographic scan. The latter technique should enable positive signs of pregnancy to be confirmed even though a slightly later scan at 35 days is preferable. Radiography before 35 days of a possible pregnancy is best avoided because fetal organogenesis is incomplete. If the pyometra is open there may be evidence of a vaginal discharge and profuse bacterial growths, especially of *Escherichia coli,* may be obtained on culture. Other diagnostic features, such as a pronounced neutrophilia, may be of value. Acute-phase protein levels also rise in pyometra cases and may interfere with the pregnancy test which relies on estimation of these proteins between days 27 and 35 of pregnancy.

Although this form of illness is uncommon in bitches the obstetrician should be careful to ensure that it is not forgotten in bitches that show pyometra-like symptoms 3 weeks or so after service. *Hysterectomy should never be performed unless the obstetrician is quite sure that the patient is not pregnant.*

A transient anorexia may very rarely occur in the queen cat in early or very late pregnancy. The cat and its pregnancy should be evaluated carefully, as in the bitch, to ensure that no other health problem – including metabolic disease – is present. Normal eating usually returns within a few days without treatment.

Other problems may occur during pregnancy and the owner should be advised to seek help if the bitch or queen appears unwell at any stage of gestation. *Pseudopregnancy* in the bitch may be accompanied by quite unpleasant physical and psychological symptoms. Accurate pregnancy diagnosis is essential to confirm that such symptoms are related to pseudopregnancy rather than to pregnancy.

Pseudopregnancy lasting 35 days may occur in queen cats following a sterile mating. No external signs other than anestrus are normally seen.

Very occasionally, hypoglycemia, ketonemia, and ketonuria occur in late pregnancy in the severely undernourished pregnant bitch. The condition must be differentiated by plasma biochemistry from eclampsia (see Chapter 14), which is mainly caused by hypocalcemia but that can itself be complicated by hypoglycemia. In a confirmed case of hypoglycemia, immediate intravenous glucose therapy is indicated. Further treatment, including termination of pregnancy, may be required in severe cases.

MANAGEMENT DURING PREGNANCY

Feeding

Although most dogs and cats can 'manage' to survive pregnancy and lactation without major changes in their dietary regime – other than an increase in quantity – nonetheless the nutritional demands of pregnant animals are considerable. Optimal, balanced nutrition throughout pregnancy is very important in both dogs and cats. Trace elements such as iron and zinc are necessary for normal pregnancy and are available in commercial diets. In addition to food it is essential that fluids are available *ad lib* to both species. For convenience, nutritional needs in both pregnancy and lactation will be considered here, although the latter may best be discussed with the client after parturition has occurred. The adverse effects of obesity and malnutrition on conception and pregnancy have already been mentioned.

The dog

Pregnancy   Seventy per cent of the puppies' growth takes place in the last 3–4 weeks of pregnancy. For this reason, and to prevent excessive weight gain, the bitch should receive a well-balanced diet at maintenance level for the first 5–6 weeks of pregnancy. The energy intake of the bitch should only be increased for the last 4 weeks of pregnancy. The energy intake should then increase by 15% per week so that it is up by 60% at the time of whelping. Puppy foods may be used to provide the extra energy required. There may be a temporary drop in appetite during the fourth week of pregnancy (reason unknown) but in the last 3 weeks the food requirement rises to 25% above the maintenance level. Appetite may also be temporarily reduced at whelping time. The bitch should ideally return to her premating weight after whelping and maintain her weight during lactation.

Lactation   The energy demands of a litter of puppies that are to be supplied by the maternal milk are considerable. The bitch's diet must be adequate to support these demands. She will probably need 2.5 times her maintenance requirement of food to support herself and feed her litter.

Calcium supplementation   It is not known whether calcium supplementation during pregnancy in small animals causes reduced availability of calcium after birth as it does in the cow. Neither increased nor decreased levels of calcium should be fed during gestation. The diet should contain 1.0–1.8% calcium and 0.8–1.6% phosphorus. The calcium content should be greater than the phosphorus content.

During lactation the diet should contain 1.4% calcium, with a calcium : phosphorus ratio of 1 : 1.

Vitamin C supplementation   It is claimed that 250 mg vitamin C per day stops the bitch becoming 'disgruntled' during lactation but the reason for this is unknown.

The cat

Kitten growth and the queen's dietary needs rise on a more linear plane than in the dog and by the end of lactation the cat may eat at least twice her normal maintenance requirement. Energy intake in the pregnant queen should rise steadily from 60–90 kcal/kg/day in early pregnancy to 100–140 kcal/kg/day in late pregnancy. Fat reserves are laid down in early pregnancy and form a useful source of energy in lactation. Queens tend to lose weight in early lactation but should regain weight loss by weaning. The queen should receive normal cat food with 20–30% dietary protein with all the required amino acids, including taurine. A severe taurine deficiency during pregnancy may lead to fetal death or to the birth of deformed kittens. A short period of

anorexia may be seen at about 2 weeks into pregnancy and also in the last week of pregnancy.

Exercise

Active exercise should be maintained throughout pregnancy but exercise tolerance and agility are reduced towards the end of gestation. The heavily pregnant bitch may require help when jumping up into a car or climbing stairs. The heavily pregnant cat seldom needs assistance but her ability and willingness to climb trees may decrease as parturition approaches.

Worming

Dog   To reduce the risk of pre- and postnatal transfer of toxocara larvae, fenbendazole (25 mg/kg) given daily from day 40 of pregnancy to day 2 of lactation is recommended. This regime is thought to be 98% effective. Puppies should be given a 3-day course of fenbendazole at 2 and 5 weeks of age. A further dose is recommended when puppies leave their breeder's premises.

Cat   There is no evidence of transplacental transfer but transfer through the milk of *Toxocara cati* larvae to sucking kittens may occur. The pregnant queen should be given 100 mg/kg of fenbendazole as a single dose during pregnancy.

If no worm-control program has been put in place, puppies and kittens can be safely treated with fenbendazole from the age of 2 weeks.

External parasites

The bitch or queen must be carefully examined for any evidence of infestation by external parasites. It is essential that the pregnant bitch or queen, and the environment, should be free from external parasites. Infestations of fleas, lice, and ear-mites can, if present, readily spread to the puppies or kittens. Dosing for external parasites in puppies and kittens can be difficult as some preparations are unsuitable and too toxic for use on the young. If the mother is already on a flea-control program there should be no need for additional precautions during pregnancy.

If no flea-control program has been used, the following regime is recommended to control fleas on the mother and also in her environment: The egg and larval stages of fleas can be controlled by spraying the environment with cyromazine or methoprene. Permethrin controls emerging adults and also pupae. The bitch or queen should be treated at intervals with fipronil, imidacloprid, or selamectin at intervals prescribed by the data sheets.

Neonatal puppies and kittens with a flea infestation can be treated, if over 48 hours old, with fipronil spray. Permethrin can be used in puppies over 24 days of age but other products should not be used until the young are aged 6–8 weeks.

The bitch and queen should be checked for evidence of ear-mite infestation and treated if necessary.

Accommodation

Whelping accommodation

Ideally, a whelping box in a warm (29°C), quiet, but accessible room should be provided. The box should have raised sides and be of sufficient size to accommodate the bitch and pups until weaning. One side of the box – the entrance – should have a slightly lower wall to allow access by the bitch without repeated but minor trauma being caused to her mammary glands. Anti-crush puppy bars should be provided around all the walls. The box should be raised above ground level to prevent draughts and insulate the puppies from the cold floor. Strict attention to hygiene in the whelping quarters is essential. During birth, newspaper provides a useful and disposable floor covering and can be changed at intervals. After whelping, paper or a washable warm fabric may be used. Supplementary heating should be available – either underfloor or as an overhead heat lamp. The bitch should be introduced to her proposed quarters well before parturition is due.

Kittening accommodation

A cardboard or wooden box with a side entrance (above ground level) and a removable lid provides a useful kittening area. Floor covering is as for the bitch.

NORMAL BIRTH

The inexperienced owner should be given an account of normal birth and of the basic care of the mother and offspring during parturition (see Chapter 1).

Advising the owner when to seek veterinary help

If problems are anticipated or if there is a history of previous dystocia, the practice may wish to book the date of anticipated delivery. They may ask to be informed when birth commences and to be given updated reports by the owner at specified intervals. It is essential to make sure that the owner reports any abnormality or suspected abnormality. Abnormalities should be explained in as simple a manner as possible. A brief written account of normal birth may help the inexperienced owner. Specific signs of abnormality and hence possible dystocia include:

- Gestation prolonged beyond the expected date of parturition.
- Prolonged non-progressive preparations for birth.
- Vigorous straining for 20–30 minutes without fetal delivery.
- Weak, intermittent straining for 1–2 hours without fetal delivery.
- An interval of >2 hours between fetuses.
- Fetus apparently stuck in the birth canal and partially visible.
- Green vaginal discharge (in the dog), red–brown discharge (in the cat) but no fetus delivered.
- Delivery of dead puppies/kittens.
- Cessation of birth process but the owner thinks some fetuses remain undelivered.
- Owner uncertain whether birth process is complete.
- Signs of maternal illness, distress or unexpected blood loss.

In general terms, the owner should be advised to report any apparent abnormality and to contact the obstetrician immediately if he or she has any worries about their parturient pet.

INCIDENCE OF DYSTOCIA

There are few references to the true incidence of dystocia in cats and dogs. There is a reluctance on the part of some breeders to admit to problems in their reputable stock. There is also a lack of a central coordinating body taking the part of, for example the artificial insemination companies, which evaluate calving problems in their bulls. Occasionally, a breed society may comment on the high incidence of cesarean section among their breed or report that uterine inertia appears to be more common than it used to be. Following-up such claims and observations is difficult because there is often no definitive baseline with which to compare present trends. Dystocia may occur in about 5% of canine births but in the brachycephalic breeds this may be an extremely low estimate.

The incidence of feline dystocia in pet cats is probably lower than in dogs, although a higher incidence is seen in the 'exotic breeds' than in the 'ordinary' cat.

In a survey of dystocia reported by the owners of mainly pedigree cats, Gunn-Moore & Thrusfield (1995) noted that dystocia occurred in 5.8% of nearly 3000 litters. Dystocia occurred in 0.4% of litters of a colony of cats of mixed breeding but in 18.2% of litters of Devon Rex cats. The authors suggested that the low incidence of dystocia in the colony cats may have been related to the fact that they were not bred for 'breed type'. Those cats in the colony that suffered from dystocia were not kept for further breeding, thus reducing the possibility of a further dystocia. Their high health status and minimal interference during gestation and parturition may have also contributed to a low level of dystocia. The head shape of the cat's breed influenced the incidence of dystocia. Breeds with dolicocephalic and brachycephalic head shape had a higher incidence of dystocia than mesocephalic breeds.

Some years ago, a survey of canine dystocia was carried out by 12 practices in South Wales. Dystocia in 265 bitches presented for treatment was reported: 20% of the bitches had suffered a previous episode of dystocia; 37% were primiparous animals and 26% were smaller than the breed average; 24% of cases were in Yorkshire terriers, 8% in Corgis and 8% in Jack Russell terriers but the incidence of these breeds within the local population was not stated. It is interesting to note that 60% of cases of dystocia were resolved by cesarean section.

CAUSES OF DYSTOCIA

Causes of dystocia in the bitch

In the South Wales survey the causes of canine dystocia were distributed as shown in Table 9.1.

In another retrospective study of 182 cases of dystocia in Sweden (Darvelid & Linde-Forsberg 1994), the causes of dystocia were as shown in Table 9.2.

This survey found no relationship between the incidence of dystocia and the age or breed of the bitch; 42% of those bitches that had whelped before had suffered a previous episode of dystocia.

Table 9.1 Dystocia in the bitch (South Wales survey)

Cause	%
Uterine inertia	36
Fetopelvic disproportion	22
Fetal maldisposition	11
Abnormalities of birth canal	9
Other causes	22

Causes of dystocia in the queen cat

In a retrospective study of 155 cases of feline dystocia seen in Sweden (Ekstrand & Linde-Forsberg 1994), the causes of dystocia were as shown in Table 9.3. The

Table 9.2 Dystocia in the bitch (Swedish survey)

Cause	No. of cases	%
Maternal		
Primary complete uterine inertia	89	48.9
Primary partial uterine inertia	42	23.1
Narrow bony birth canal	2	1.1
Uterine torsion	2	1.1
Hydroallantois	1	0.5
Vaginal septum formation	1	0.5
Total (maternal)	137	75.3
Fetal		
Fetal maldisposition	28	15.4
Fetal oversize	12	6.6
Fetal malformation	3	1.6
Fetal death	2	1.1
Total (fetal)	45	24.7

From Darvelid & Linde-Forsberg (1994).

Table 9.3 Causes of dystocia in the queen cat

Cause	No. of cases	%
Maternal		
Uterine inertia	94	60.6
Narrow birth canal	8	5.2
Uterine obstruction	1	0.6
Uterine prolapse	1	0.6
Total (maternal)	104	67.0
Fetal		
Fetal maldisposition	24	15.5
Fetal malformation	12	7.7
Fetal oversize	3	1.9
Fetal death	7	4.5
Total (fetal)	46	29.6
Other causes	5	3.2

From Ekstrand & Linde-Forsberg (1994).

incidence of dystocia in Persian cats was believed to be higher than in other breeds.

Fetal maldisposition and primary uterine inertia were reported by Gunn-Moore & Thrusfield (1995) to be the main causes of dystocia in brachycephalic breeds. The flattened head shape of brachycephalic cats may predispose them to fetal maldispostion involving the head. The longer head of the dolicocephalic breeds may aid fetal entry into the maternal pelvis as birth commences.

FAILURE OF THE EXPULSIVE FORCES

Uterine inertia

This, the most common cause of dystocia, is divisible into the two main categories of primary and secondary uterine inertia.

Primary uterine inertia

In the polytocous small animals there may be a complete or a partial failure of the uterus to start contracting. In partial failure the uterus may bring the first fetus to the pelvic inlet from whence it is delivered by abdominal straining. No further fetuses are presented and uterine contraction ceases.

An idiopathic type of primary inertia has been described, in which delivery starts normally and several members of the litter are delivered normally. There is no evidence of obstruction to birth through maternal or fetal cause. The uterus stops contracting and does not resume unless ecbolic therapy is given. It could be argued that this could be classified as a partial rather than a complete primary uterine inertia.

The single pup syndrome This can occur in any breed but the highest incidence is said to occur in the Scottish terrier, in which breed fetal viability is also said to be low. It is believed that the single puppy fails to produce sufficient ACTH and cortisol to initiate the birth process. Having outgrown its placental supply of oxygen and nutrients the puppy dies in utero and becomes mummified or macerated. If the cervix remains closed the fetus becomes mummified. It may remain in the uterus and be discovered later during an examination unrelated to pregnancy. When infection enters the uterus via the dilated cervix the puppy becomes infected, emphysematous, and macerated. A life-saving hysterectomy may be the only way of resolving such cases. In some cases of the single pup syndrome the bitch is not known to be pregnant until there is evidence of fetal death.

If the bitch is known to be pregnant and the presence of a single fetus has been confirmed by ultrasonography both she and the puppy should be carefully monitored throughout pregnancy. An elective cesarean section or induction of birth may be necessary at term. A cesarean section would be the safest option.

The single kitten A single kitten can also fail to initiate its own birth but the problem is less well documented than in the bitch. Queen cats often continue to breed at least until teenage. Litter size decreases with advancing age. Special care should be taken of the queen cat known (for example through pregnancy diagnosis) to be pregnant with a single kitten. Approaching birth should be carefully managed and the kitten monitored if possible. An elective cesarean section may be needed if spontaneous birth fails to occur.

Calcium The role of calcium in small animals uterine inertia is not entirely clear. There are many anecdotal accounts of cases that have responded to calcium therapy. However, in a small trial by the author (unpublished data) no significant difference was observed in the calcium levels in the plasma in animals suffering from primary uterine inertia and those whelping normally.

Hysteria An extreme state of excitement at whelping is seen chiefly in the toy breeds but is also prevalent in some strains of Cocker spaniels. It may be predisposed by environmental disturbance, although the latter is not always harmful. There have been a number of reports of bitches taken to the surgery for cesarean section that have given birth in transit. In Bull terriers an acute state of hysteria has been reported in which aggression towards both pups and owners is seen. This condition appears responsive to calcium therapy.

Secondary uterine inertia

This type of uterine inertia is a consequence of another cause of dystocia, such as fetopelvic disproportion, in which uterine contraction ceases after a period of nonproductive activity.

Abdominal muscle tone This may deteriorate in old and fat animals, reducing the efficiency of the abdominal straining that is so important in the second stage of labor. This problem of inefficient abdominal musculature is also seen in elderly parturient cats. Damage to the tendinous attachment of the abdominal muscles to the pubis may be sustained by cats in road traffic accidents. Surgical repair may be possible to avoid various potential problems, including the animal having a reduced ability to strain.

OBSTRUCTION OF THE BIRTH CANAL

Obstruction of the birth canal can result from bony or soft tissue abnormality.

Bony abnormalities

Pelvic fracture is a common sequel to road traffic accidents in cats and the subsequent displacement of the bones can severely obstruct the birth canal. In some breeds of dog – notably the Scottish terrier – the pelvis is relatively small. Pelvic size is sometimes very small in members of the brachycephalic toy breeds of dog and also in the Welsh Corgi. Gross pelvic abnormalities should ideally have been detected and avoided at the prebreeding examination or during an antenatal consultation. The internal pelvic dimensions can be evaluated by a digital rectal examination before birth or to a limited extent by vaginal examination during birth. A radiographic examination of the pelvis may be useful in cases where a pelvic abnormality is suspected but cannot be palpated.

Soft tissue abnormalities

Congenital stenosis may affect any part of the soft tissue component of the birth canal and the other abnormalities listed are seen occasionally. Vaginal stenosis in the vestibular region appears to be particularly common in Cavalier King Charles spaniels (author's unpublished data). Affected animals may be unable to mate and in any case should not be used for breeding.

Deviation of the uterus

Deviation has been described in the Boxer and occasionally in other breeds. In affected animals the heavily gravid uterus falls steeply away from the pelvic inlet and cervix. The steep ascent to the cervix and the partial obstruction caused by the deviation appears to interfere with fetal passage. Very rarely a portion of one uterine horn containing a fetus enters the sac of an inguinal hernia. The growing fetus becomes too large to pass into the abdomen and surgical removal is necessary.

Torsion of the uterus

Torsion has been reported in both the dog and cat. One or both uterine horns may be involved. Cesarean section is necessary to resolve (and possibly to diagnose) the problem.

FETAL MALDISPOSITION

The basic reason for the development of such maldispositions is not known. Abnormal maternal hormone levels have been blamed but it is possible that there may be some abnormality in the fetal nervous system. Prior to birth the small animal fetus is normally in the ventral position ('upside down') and rotates through 180° just before entering the pelvis. Failure to achieve this rotation may result in the fetus being born in a lateral or ventral position. Maldisposition of the fetal head appears to occur most frequently in the brachycephalic breeds.

Posterior presentation

In small animals this is not considered abnormal, with up to 40% of offspring being born in this manner. This presentation is often erroneously described as a 'breech birth' by owners – true breech birth is a posterior presentation with bilateral hip flexion.

Deviation of the head

Deviation of the head either laterally or downwards is one of the most common fetal malpostures in small animals (Fig. 9.1). Lateral deviation appears to be

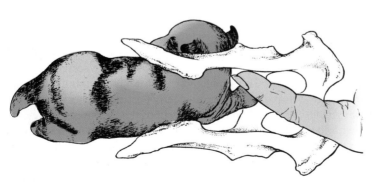

Figure 9.1 Fetal malposture – lateral deviation of a puppy's head.

most common in the 'long-necked' breeds such as collies. Downward deviation is seen chiefly in the brachycephalic breeds in which the dome-shaped cranium of the puppy or kitten so easily enters the pelvic inlet with the fetal muzzle catching on the pelvic brim. It is also seen in the 'long-headed' canine breeds, e.g. Sealyham and Scottish terrier, and in the dolicocephalic feline breeds.

FETOPELVIC DISPROPORTION

This is chiefly seen in the small breeds where litter size is numerically small and individual fetal size is large. In Welsh Corgis, considerable variation in the size of litter mates has been reported, with some fetuses passing easily through the pelvis whereas others are unable to do so. Yorkshire terriers seem particularly prone to fetopelvic disproportion.

Fetal monsters

Those causing dystocia in small animals include hydrocephalus, schistosomus reflexus, anasarca, and conjoined twins. In most cases the abnormal fetus is too large to enter the maternal pelvis. Vaginal delivery is impossible and delivery by cesarean section is necessary. The exact nature of the deformity may only become apparent when the fetus is delivered.

DYSTOCIA CAUSED BY FETAL DEATH

Up to 5% of the members of small animal litters may be stillborn. Stillbirth rates increase with the duration of labor and may rise to substantially above 5% in cases of dystocia that are not dealt with quickly. Stillborn fetuses may be either prepartum or intrapartum deaths. Some fetuses that die before birth become mummified and are usually passed without difficulty between the delivery of normal living members of the litter. Intrapartum deaths are often the result of asphyxia caused by inhalation of fetal fluids. Most occur as the result of delayed delivery, the loss of placental functional, and fetal hypoxia. Provided their presentation and size are normal they are often passed without difficulty. Fetal maldisposition may be predisposed and exacerbated by fetal death, the dead fetus being unable to make the small

spontaneous movements that can result in the correction of a minor maldisposition.

It may be possible to use transabdominal ultrasonography to determine whether a puppy at the pelvic inlet has a heart beat and is therefore alive. Spontaneous movements are a further indication of fetal life. Evidence of maldisposition may be detected by digital examination. If the presentation is normal, administration of oxytocin should encourage passage of the fetus into the pelvic inlet. Once in that position abdominal straining should result in fetal delivery.

Fetal death followed by maceration can be a life-threatening problem to the dam. The problem usually arises when parturition is unobserved and the patient fails to deliver all her litter. It is seen in both dogs and cats but especially in the latter species. The cat may attempt to deliver her kittens away from home or may be disturbed during parturition. One or more kittens are left in the uterus. Infection enters the uterus via the cervix. Fetal emphysema and partial maceration follow. The cat rapidly becomes toxemic and often severely dehydrated. Straining is not always seen but an unpleasant vaginal discharge is often present. Vaginal examination is difficult but with the aid of generous lubrication it may be possible to palpate a fetal part, often the head. An X-ray can be taken to confirm the diagnosis and the degree of fetal emphysema. Vaginal delivery is impossible as the fetal body is grossly enlarged (see Fig. 11.19). The cat should be given immediate fluid therapy and once the patient is well enough for surgery hysterectomy should be performed. For details of surgical treatment please see Chapter 11.

SIGNS OF DYSTOCIA

The signs of dystocia were discussed in the section 'Advising the owner when to seek veterinary help', see p. 147.

APPROACH TO A CASE OF DYSTOCIA IN SMALL ANIMALS

General points

Cases of dystocia must *always* be seen as a matter of urgency. Any delay can be dangerous, even if the owner's message suggests that the situation is not serious. The parturient animal is probably best seen in the surgery where full facilities, including X-ray and ultrasonography, are available.

OBSTETRICIAN'S CHECK LIST

Call received

Receive call concerning the dystocia case from the owner
↓
Take a brief note of the patient's immediate history and date of expected birth
↓
Arrange to see the patient as soon as possible – preferably in the surgery
↓
Check patient's case records for details of any antenatal visits and previous occurrence of dystocia

---

Case history

Although some information may be available from the antenatal consultation, the clinician should review the history of previous births and the general health record of the patient. Information about the present birth is obtained: Duration of gestation, history of illness or abnormal discharge in the last few days, duration and signs of labor, number of offspring born – live and dead, interval between births, intensity and pattern of straining, passage of placenta, lay interference.

Clinical examination

General clinical examination

This should be thorough and comprehensive and should result in an assessment of the animal's health status and signs of any adverse effects of parturition. The patient should be restrained gently but firmly either on a table or on the floor. Signs of toxemia or cardiovascular compromise must be sought and an examination of the mammary glands made to assess the level of milk production. The degree of abdominal distension and the shape of the abdomen may give some indication of the number of unborn offspring, although this observation is unreliable. Fetal movements may be felt when the hands are placed gently around the patient's abdomen (Fig. 9.2).

OBSTETRICIAN'S CHECK LIST

Owner and patient arrive at the surgery

Further assessment of case history: how many offspring already born, approximate time of births and living state of any fetuses delivered, passage of placenta?
↓
General clinical examination of the patient: visual inspection of the vulva, visual inspection of mammary glands
↓
Palpate contours of the abdomen: note any fetal movements, the degree of abdominal distension, and the presence of milk in the mammary glands

---

Examination of the genital system

Inspection of vulva   The quantity and nature of any discharge is noted. A foul smell may be indicative of fetal death and putrefaction. The presence of fetal parts, placenta, and their condition is noted. Quantities of fetal meconium passed into the amniotic cavity may be indicative of fetal anoxia. Vulval dimension and any obvious damage or constriction is noted.

Vaginal examination   Strictest attention to hygiene, gentleness, and careful restraint of the mother are essential prerequisites for this procedure (Fig. 9.3). In the average *bitch* the forefinger may be used but in the toy bitch or cat entry may be restricted to the little finger. In the bitch the vagina initially runs in an upward direction underneath the perineum before inclining anteriorly to pass through the pelvis. In the *cat* the vagina passes directly into the pelvis from its vulval opening. The vagina is assessed for moistness or dryness and for any sign of damage. The presence of any bony or soft tissue constriction or other obstruction is also noted.

The presence of a fetus in the birth canal – its location, presentation, position, and posture – is noted. Signs of life may include spontaneous or reflex movement and occasionally sucking of the operator's fingertip. The absence of these signs does not necessarily mean that the fetus is dead. In anterior presentation the fetal head with its ears and mouth, and occasionally one or both forelegs, may be palpable. The presence of covering amnion may make detailed palpation difficult. In posterior presentation the fetal hindlimbs and tail are

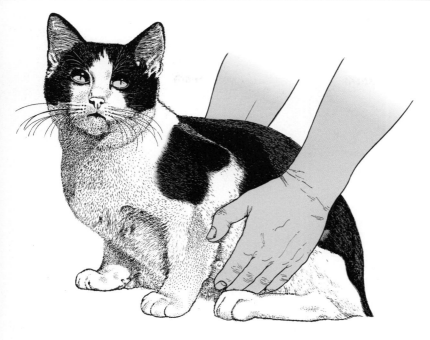

Figure 9.2 Fetal movements may be felt and assessed when the hands are placed gently over the patient's abdomen.

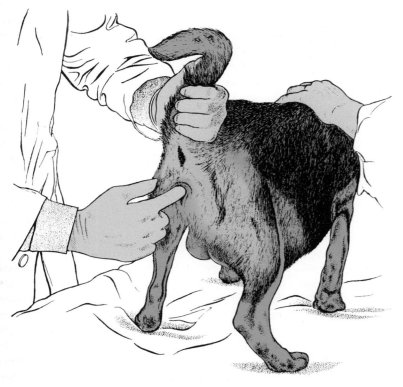

Figure 9.3 Vaginal examination in the parturient bitch.

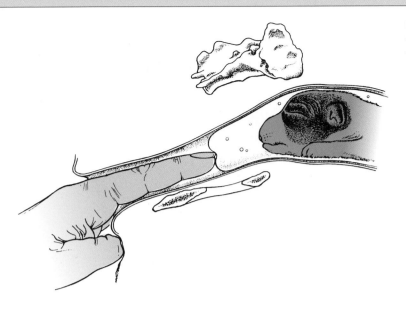

Figure 9.4 Palpation of the gossamer-like amniotic vesicle, which may herald the approach of a fetus (see also Fig. 9.5).

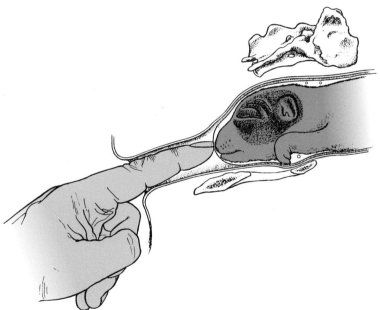

Figure 9.5 The fetal head may be palpable shortly after the amniotic vesicle (see also Fig. 9.4).

recognized but in true breech presentation only the tail and the hindquarters are palpable. Lateral deviation of the head may be difficult to recognize, especially in the long-necked breeds. Although a limb – possibly recognized as a forelimb – may be palpated, the head may be so deviated that only the base of the fetal neck can be palpated as a second landmark.

Quite frequently an amniotic vesicle can be palpated (Fig. 9.4), although its gossamer-like thinness can cause it to be easily missed unless the fetal head is immediately behind. The presence of an approaching amniotic vesicle normally means that a fetus is also approaching. Palpation a few minutes later will often reveal the fetal head (Fig. 9.5).

The fetus is usually palpable within the amnion but if the fetus has not fully engaged in the pelvis it is wise to avoid excessive interference at this stage. Touching the fetal head at this stage can cause the fetus to move back vigorously from the pelvic inlet and occasionally result in the establishment of a malpresentation.

A

B

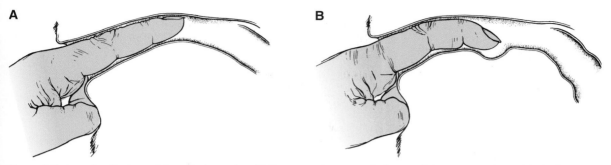

Figure 9.6 Assessing the tone of the anterior vagina. (A) Pronounced tone may indicate satisfactory muscular activity in the uterus. (B) Flaccidity may indicate uterine inertia.

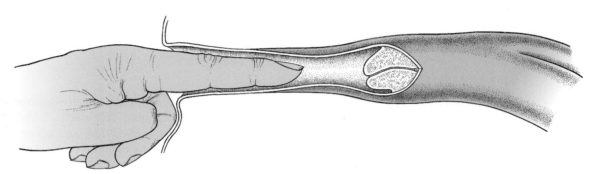

Figure 9.7 Palpation of the anterior vagina may indicate whether the cervix is dilated. Here there is little space in the anterior vagina and the cervix is closed.

In the 'average patient' the cervix and uterus cannot be palpated per vaginam but the palpable characteristics of the anterior vagina in the bitch *may* give some indication of what is happening at the cervix and within the uterus (Fig. 9.6). A dilated anterior vagina may indicate that the cervix is dilated – and indeed some obstetricians are convinced that they are actually palpating the cervix and beyond. Pronounced tone in the wall of the anterior vagina may be indicative of satisfactory activity in the uterine musculature. The presence of the finger just caudal to the cervix may provoke uterine activity via Ferguson's reflex. Flaccidity of the anterior vaginal wall and failure to stimulate the reflex may indicate the presence of uterine inertia. If the cervix is closed (either before or after whelping) the walls of the anterior vagina are slightly constricted and press on the obstetrician's finger (Fig. 9.7).

In the cat the obstetrician is mostly able to palpate the caudal parts of the vagina. Palpation of the anterior vagina and indirect assessment of cervical dilation or uterine tone in the cat is seldom possible unless the obstetrician has very small fingers. Movement of the

finger against the dorsal wall of the vagina in the bitch (sometimes termed 'feathering') may provoke straining and assist fetal delivery.

OBSTETRICIAN'S CHECK LIST

Gynecological examination: digital vaginal examination

Check for presence of an amniotic vesicle or fetus
↓
Check presentation of fetus
↓
Assess tone and dimensions of the anterior vagina
↓
Determine the presence and nature of vaginal fluids
↓
Assess dimensions of the bony pelvis

Abdominal palpation   A careful, gentle, and systematic examination of the abdomen is carried out. In the obese or tense animal this can be difficult and often

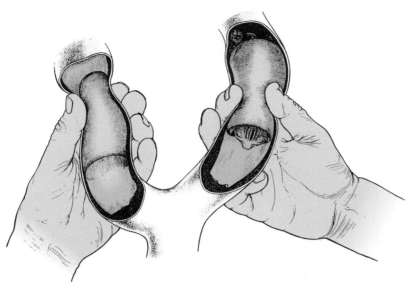

Figure 9.8 Careful palpation of the uterus may enable a fetus to be differentiated from a portion of retained placenta.

unrewarding. If a single fetus is present its size, its position in relation to the pelvic inlet and – if possible – its presentation should be determined. Two fetuses, if present, may be identified. If a larger number of fetuses are present it may be impossible to be sure of their number.

It is very easy to mistake the firmly contracted empty uterus for a fetus. The slightly more flaccid uterus containing portions of placenta can also be mistaken for a retained fetus. It may be possible to recognize with certainty the characteristic head–neck–thorax sequence of the fetus (Fig. 9.8) but if there is any doubt an X-ray must be taken.

Abdominal auscultation/ultrasonographic evaluation   Fetal heart beats can often be heard through a clinical stethoscope in quiet surroundings and can also be appraised with a Doppler or real-time ultrasound instrument. Although fetal cardiac activity is easily detected in pregnancy, during parturition it can be frustratingly more difficult. The difficulty may arise through air entering the uterus and interfering in particular with ultrasound waves. With Doppler and B-mode instruments, fetal limited movement may be appreciated – as it may by direct palpation. Excessive fetal movement may ominously suggest the presence of severe fetal hypoxia. Normal fetal heart rate in puppies and kittens is in the region of 150–220/min. Severe bradycardia or dysrhythmia also suggests developing anoxia and fetal distress. The rate and vigour of fetal cardiac activity and the degree of fetal movement can be particularly well demonstrated using real-time ultrasound. Loss of amniotic fluid – already relatively small in quantity in dogs and cats – may result in less effective differential acoustic impedance. Thus once birth is actually underway in these and other species, ultrasonographic evaluation of fetal viability may actually become less rather than more reliable. The presence of fetal hearts beating at a regular rate is a reassuring sign of fetal life. The absence of detectable heart beats may not necessarily (for the reasons mentioned above) be a certain sign of fetal death.

Radiographic examination of the abdomen

A single radiographic exposure of the gravid canine or feline abdomen to the diagnostic beam is unlikely to prove harmful to the unborn litter at term. This examination is essential if there is any doubt about the nature of the abdominal contents. The number and position of any unborn fetuses can be detected immediately. Signs of gross fetal maldisposition – such as transverse presentation at the pelvic inlet – may be seen radiographically. Signs of fetal death, including overlapping of the cranial bones – Spalding's sign (Fig. 9.9) – gas shadows in the fetal heart and stomach and in advanced cases fetal emphysema may also be seen. The spine of the dead fetus may be in a more tightly flexed position than that seen in the living fetus. In recently dead fetuses no radiographic abnormality is visible. An indication of the number of remaining fetuses can sometimes also be obtained by real-time ultrasonography subject to the limitations mentioned above.

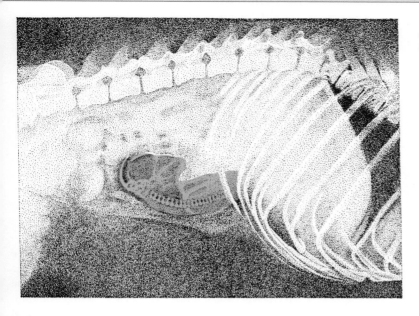

Figure 9.9 Radiography of a dead puppy showing overlapping of the cranial bones (Spalding's sign).

OBSTETRICIAN'S CHECK LIST

Gynecological examination: examination of the abdomen

Auscultation of patient's abdomen: assess fetal hearts if audible
↓
Systematic manual palpation of the whole abdomen: can further fetus(es) be palpated?
↓
Ultrasonographic examination of patient's abdomen to confirm presence, possible number, viability, and well-being of any further fetus(es)
↓
Radiographic examination of abdomen: as for ultrasonographic examination, evidence of fetal death or gross maldisposition

---

Diagnosis of the cause of dystocia and formulation of a tentative plan of treatment

The case history and clinical examination of the case should enable the cause or causes of dystocia to be established and a tentative plan of treatment to be drawn up. Treatment is aimed at assisting in the delivery of any fetuses within the birth canal and encouraging the uterus to deliver any further fetuses in an orderly fashion at the pelvic inlet. It is important that the planned course of treatment can be completed in a reasonable time so that fetal survival is not compromised. If there is evidence on clinical examination that fetal life is already at risk, emergency treatment such as an immediate cesarean section may be required.

Most planned courses of action in obstetrics are inevitably tentative and alterations to the plan may prove necessary from time to time. It may be anticipated that a case of fetal malposture may be corrected by manual manipulation. If attempts to achieve this do not prove possible, to protect both mother and offspring from further damage, surgical treatment may now be the only option. Treatment may: (1) be conservative – when a period of limited delay is thought likely to allow delivery to proceed; (2) involve ecbolic therapy; (3) be assisted delivery, possibly preceded by correction of a malposture; or (4) be surgical treatment.

It is essential that the treatment plan and any changes to it are discussed fully with the owner at every stage.

OBSTETRICIAN'S CHECK LIST

Diagnosis of the cause(s) of dystocia and tentative plan of treatment

Evaluate case history, health check, and the results of vaginal and abdominal examinations
↓

> ↓
> What is the cause(s) of the dystocia?
> ↓
> The basic plan of treatment will be to deliver any presenting fetuses and encourage the uterus to present the remaining puppies at the pelvic inlet
> ↓
> Is the litter at immediate risk?
> ↓
> Is immediate emergency delivery by cesarean section necessary?
> ↓
> Tentative plan of treatment – explain/discuss with owner
> ↓
> Report any changes of plan as the case progresses to the owner

TREATMENT OF DYSTOCIA

Conservative treatment

In some circumstances – such as the presence of an amniotic vesicle approaching the pelvic inlet and when uterine tone is thought to be satisfactory – it may be decided to advise a period of controlled waiting. Such periods should always have a time limit after which – if the anticipated event has not occurred – a further period of waiting or alternative treatment will be used. It is essential that whenever such conservative treatment is used, and especially when the client leaves the surgery, arrangements are made for a report to be given to the obstetrician concerning progress within a finite time interval. Contact must be maintained with the owner until there is a successful termination of the case.

Ecbolic therapy

Drug therapy to stimulate uterine contraction may be used to treat uterine inertia and to hasten the presentation of the next fetus at the pelvic inlet. It will also encourage passage of the fetal membranes and post-parturient uterine involution. Ecbolic drugs must *never* be used in cases of obstructive dystocia and their use should *always* be preceded and followed by vaginal examination.

Oxytocin (dose: dog 2–5 IU; cat 2–5 IU) is normally given by intramuscular injection. It can cause pain on administration and make the patient attempt to bite the obstetrician. After injection the patient should be left quietly for 10–15 minutes. The temptation to make more frequent vaginal examinations must be resisted. Excessively large doses of oxytocin may cause uterine spasm and occasionally signs of maternal distress.

If a single dose of oxytocin fails to produce the desired effect a further dose may be given after 20–30 minutes. Sometimes a single dose will be sufficient to achieve the desired object. In some cases of uterine inertia a number of injections given at strategic intervals may be required. Provided a reasonably rapid response to oxytocin is obtained, further doses can be used. The author has often used as many as five doses of oxytocin in cases of uterine inertia before the whole litter has been delivered. Occasionally, further doses are used but each dose must be preceded by evaluation of the progress of the case and the response to previous doses. Each dose should be preceded and followed by a digital vaginal examination of the patient. The presence of the obstetrician's finger in the anterior vagina may provoke straining and also stimulate further uterine contraction. If there is no response at all to oxytocin within 30 minutes and further fetuses remain in utero, surgical intervention is likely to be required.

The role of calcium in the treatment of uterine inertia is somewhat controversial (see p. 149) but undoubtedly some cases which have failed to respond to oxytocin are responsive to calcium. Calcium borogluconate 10% (dose: dog 5–15 mL; cat 2–5 mL) is given by slow intravenous injection with careful monitoring of heart rate. A 10% solution of calcium borogluconate is not commercially available but can be produced by dilution of a standard 20% solution used for treating milk fever in cows.

Assisted delivery of the fetus

Attempts to deliver the fetus should not be made until it is at the pelvic inlet and in the correct position and posture for delivery. Before any attempt at fetal delivery the whole perineal area must be cleaned. The obstetrician must scrub the hands and may choose to wear gloves. In cases presented early in dystocia where the fetus is malpresented it may be possible, using the finger tip and aided by external manipulation, to correct the displaced fetal part. In longer-standing cases the 'log jam' of fetuses building up behind the obstruction may not allow any fetal repulsion and loss of fetal fluid may prevent any attempt to correct the malpresentation. Lubrication using KY jelly or an obstetric lubricant should be introduced into the birth canal whenever natural fluids have been lost. Lubricant can be gently introduced into the more anterior parts of the vagina using a syringe and wide-bore male dog catheter. Correction of fetal malpresentation using instruments in the form of hooks or Rampley's sponge-holding forceps has been described but lack of space and difficulty of access may limit their use.

The arrival of a fetus in the maternal pelvis usually stimulates straining, causing the fetus to pass along the vagina and be delivered. The presence of the obstetrician's finger in the vagina and stimulating the roof of the vagina ('feathering') may encourage straining. The strength and success of straining can be assessed by fetal movement along the birth canal. The finger may also stimulate uterine contraction encouraging the presentation of the next fetus.

Episiotomy – to relieve tightness of the vulva that is preventing fetal passage – is seldom required in small animals. In cases of severe stricture there is a risk that the vulva may tear and a small incision in the vulval lip in a dorsolateral direction is made using scissors. The wound should be repaired immediately after parturition is complete.

Manual delivery

If fetal parts are visible or palpable just within the vulva they may be gently grasped and cautious traction applied in a caudal and ventral direction. Adequate lubrication is again essential and lubricants can be introduced into the birth canal and alongside the fetus using a syringe and wide-bore male dog urinary catheter. If the fetus is in anterior presentation, a grip may be obtained just behind the head (Fig. 9.10). In posterior presentation, the fetal hindlegs, or preferably the hindquarters, are grasped. Whenever even modest traction is applied to the fetal limbs, the grip of the obstetrician's finger should be softened by enclosing the fetal part in surgical gauze

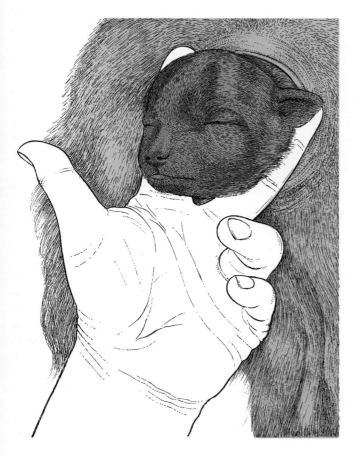

Figure 9.10 Gentle traction is applied to the fetal head.

before traction is applied. Severe fetal damage can be sustained by excessive pressure being placed on the distal portions of the fetal limbs. Passage of the fetus through the vulva is aided by moving the fetus gently from side to side while traction is carefully applied (Fig. 9.11).

If resistance to delivery is encountered, further lubrication should be instilled alongside the fetus and the fetus should be rotated through 45° before a further attempt at delivery by traction is made. If the fetal head is too far anterior to the vulval lips for a grip to be applied, it may be possible – in the bitch, where the vagina has a long perineal section – to apply external pressure via the perineum and ease the fetus closer to the vulva and delivery as described above.

An obstetrical vectis or a small teaspoon may be placed over the crown of the fetal head with counterpressure

being applied upwards between the fetal mandibles by the obstetrician's finger. Using this grip upon the head the fetus is delivered. A snare made of bandage is an alternative.

Assisting the efficiency of straining

This technique can be particularly useful if the fetus has just entered the pelvic inlet but progress through the pelvic canal is slow. Maternal straining is normally stimulated by the fetus passing the cervix and may be further stimulated by movements of the obstetrician's finger within the vagina. The efficiency of straining is increased by grasping the abdomen between the palms of the hands and gently but firmly compressing the abdomen when the animal strains. This ensures that

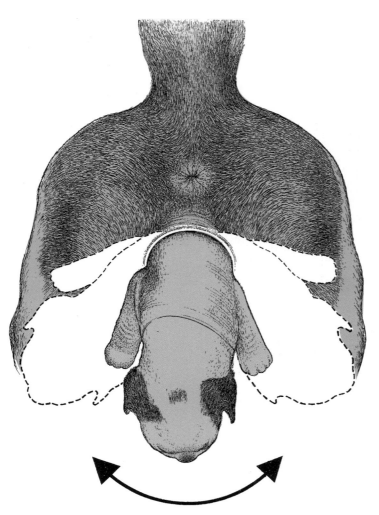

Figure 9.11 Passage of the fetus through the vagina and vulva may be aided by moving it from side to side while careful traction is applied.

all intra-abdominal pressure is exerted on the fetus at the pelvic inlet. Pressure can be exerted by wrapping the mother in a towel or – if she is recumbent – gentle downward pressure can be exerted on her uppermost side (Fig. 9.12). When the fetus is within reach, spontaneous expulsion may occur or assistance is given as described above.

Forceps delivery

This technique is used infrequently nowadays, probably because of the risks involved and the popularity and success of cesarean section in the treatment of small animal dystocia. However, forceps delivery can be indicated in dogs when it is thought that the delivery of the first fetus in the litter by forceps will allow spontaneous delivery of the remainder. Forceps delivery is particularly useful to deliver the last remaining fetus in a litter where the rest of the litter has been delivered successfully. The last fetus may be lodged in the pelvis and the only alternative to forceps delivery would be cesarean section. Access to such a fetus from the abdomen at cesarean section might be difficult. The small dimensions of the feline vagina make forceps unsuitable for use in cats.

Two main types of forceps are available: Hobday's rigid-jawed forceps, which come in various sizes, and soft-jawed forceps such as Rampley's sponge-holding forceps.

Hobday's forceps are very likely (as a result of the strong action of their jaws) to damage the fetus or cause its death when applied. They are usually applied to the head or hindquarters of the fetus, depending upon its presentation. Rampley's forceps have a much more gentle action. They can be applied to the upper jaw or even to the limbs of the fetus, and may be used singly or in pairs.

The forceps are guided into the vagina alongside the obstetrician's finger until contact with the fetus is made (Fig. 9.13). During introduction, the forceps are held in the closed position and are then carefully opened to grip the fetus. The fetus may be held in position by the operator's other hand outside the abdomen. Before gripping the fetus the forceps should be rotated to ensure that no portions of vaginal epithelium have become trapped within their jaws.

OBSTETRICIAN'S CHECK LIST

Treatment options for dystocia case

- These include one or more of the following:
  - Conservative treatment
  - Assisted delivery of a presenting fetus
  - Ecbolic administration – repeated as necessary – always preceded and followed by vaginal examination

---

Figure 9.12 Assisting the efficiency of straining (see text).

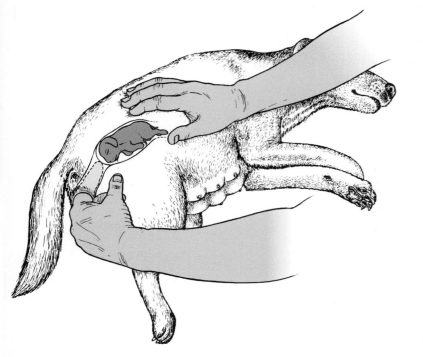

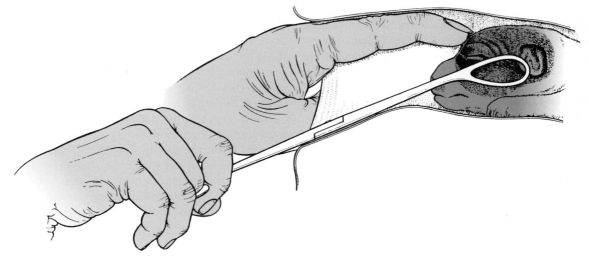

Figure 9.13 Forceps delivery (see text).

– Monitor the delivery of further offspring – assisted manual delivery as required
– Assisting the efficiency of straining

• Further possible options:
  – Forceps delivery
  – Surgical treatment – cesarean section/hysterectomy
  – Confirm delivery of the whole litter

FURTHER CARE OF THE PARTURIENT MOTHER AND OFFSPRING

After each fetus has been delivered it must be checked for vital signs. Excessive mucus is gently shaken out of the mouth or gentle suction applied. Traces of amnion are removed from the face and the umbilical cord is severed before the neonate is placed with its mother. If the mother is disinterested or distressed, the fetus should be carefully dried with a soft towel. Fetal skin is very delicate and easily damaged. After drying, the neonatal animal is placed in a warm box until it can be safely introduced to its mother.

Each fetus should be checked for evidence of cleft palate, which is one of the most common fetal abnormalities seen in the dog. Esophageal aplasia is less common but affected animals are unable to swallow and attempts to do so cause signs of great distress in the neonate. If this latter abnormality is suspected a lubricated soft tube should be gently passed into the esophagus. In normal fetuses the tube is easily passed into the stomach. If esophageal obstruction is confirmed the affected neonate should be euthanased. Gross defects of thoracic shape or limb deformity are usually immediately recognized. More subtle abnormalities may not be recognized until the litter is older.

OBSTETRICIAN'S CHECK LIST

Postnatal assessment of each fetus

Check for vital signs
↓
Remove amniotic remnants from face
↓
Shake very gently or use suction to remove mucus from the airway
↓
Blow into the fetal mouth
↓
Dry gently with fine towel
↓
Check for fetal anomalies
↓
Place with mother

Subsequent performance of the mother

The subsequent performance of the mother must be monitored carefully to ensure that help with subsequent fetal delivery or stimulation of uterine activity is given if required. In some cases, assistance with the delivery of one fetus only is required. This may be the last or only member of the litter. Sometimes the delivery of the first fetus allows the remainder of the litter to be delivered unaided. In other cases, assistance with the birth of several or all the fetuses may be required. Finally, the end-point of whelping or kittening must be identified. Observing the behavior of the mother should be used only as a guide. The end-point of parturition should be determined by careful clinical examination backed up by techniques such as ultrasonography or radiology, as required.

Has the whole litter been delivered?

If any doubt remains, a further vaginal and an abdominal examination must be performed to ensure that no fetus(es) remain either in the vagina or abdomen. Careful palpation of the abdomen will usually allow the presence or absence of further fetuses to be determined. The contracted uterus or a portion of placenta can be mistaken for a fetus (see Fig. 9.8). Ultrasonography or radiography are used if there is any doubt that further puppies or kittens remain in the uterus. Some obstetricians believe that a radiograph following assisted delivery in small animals should be mandatory to ensure beyond doubt that no fetus has been left in utero. Radiography may be preferable to ultrasonography at this stage. Air in the uterus reduces the clarity of ultrasonography. Special care must be taken to ensure that a fetus lying within the pelvis is not missed when an abdominal X-ray is taken. Some owners request an obstetric examination to be sure that birth is complete even when there have been no signs of dystocia. Antibiotic therapy after treatment of a dystocia case is advisable and should be given, for 3–5 days, to every animal in which birth has been assisted.

OBSTETRICIAN'S CHECK LIST

Is parturition complete?

Maternal behavior – unreliable indicator
↓
Vaginal examination
↓
Abdominal palpation
↓
Abdominal radiography/ultrasonography

Subsequent care of mother and offspring

The subsequent care of the litter is usually left in the hands of the owner. The dysmature state of the canine or feline neonate should be explained to the inexperienced owner. The neonate is particularly vulnerable to hypothermia, hypoglycemia, and dehydration. It cannot hear or see until 10 days of age. It is unable to shiver for the first 2 weeks of life and unable to control its glomerular filtration rate. It is unable to pass urine or feces without perineal stimulation. The transition from sleep to wakefulness is very rapid. Sleeping neonates respond immediately to touch and make searching movements with their heads as they seek a teat from which to drink. Their state of hydration can be immediately determined by gently pinching a fold of skin and watching it return to normal immediately in the healthy, well-hydrated neonate. Despite the absence of sight or hearing, the neonate's righting reflex is well developed and brisk in healthy animals from the time of birth onwards.

Growth rate is rapid in healthy puppies and kittens. The puppy should double its birth weight by 7–10 days of age. By 6 weeks of age the puppy should be 6–10 times as heavy as it was at birth. Socialization of puppies and kittens is considered very important and may contribute to a good temperament in later life. It is suggested that the neonates should be regularly exposed to human contact from the age of 2 weeks.

In very large litters the offspring may be offered supplementary artificial dog or cat milk. This is given using a small glass dropper or syringe – the neonatal animals will drink readily if hungry but refuse to drink if they are getting sufficient maternal milk.

Most bitches and queens settle rapidly into motherhood even after the birth of their first litter. They should be watched closely to ensure that they are feeding their offspring satisfactorily. They should also be encouraged to leave their litter regularly to feed and take exercise. Watch should be kept for the postparturient problems such as metritis and mastitis discussed in Chapter 14.

Late incomplete abortion

Adverse factors affecting the litter early in pregnancy often result in complete abortion. In late pregnancy abortion may be complete or incomplete. One or more fetuses are lost in cases of incomplete abortion but others remain in the uterus. Those fetuses remaining in the uterus may be dead or alive. Incomplete abortion occurs more commonly in the bitch than in the queen but overall management of the case is the same for both species. Ultrasonographic examination of the abdomen allows the living state of the litter to be determined and monitored in such cases. If the patient is within one week of parturition there is a chance that some of the retained litter may survive. The greater their maturity the better their chance of survival but the risk to the bitch – especially if the abortion was caused by infection – may increase. Any aborted fetuses should be submitted for laboratory examination and cultures taken from any vaginal discharge in the bitch. Antibiotic and supportive therapy should be commenced immediately. The antibiotic used may have to be changed later if sensitivity tests suggest another antibiotic might be more favorable.

The bitch should be seen as soon as possible. A full clinical examination of the patient should be performed and the litter examined by ultrasonographic scan. If the bitch is unwell, febrile and toxemic an immediate hysterotomy or hysterectomy may be required. It may be possible with care to rear any puppies delivered within one week of term. Similar surgical treatment is advisable if there is no sign of fetal life.

If the patient is well she and her unborn litter should be monitored by daily clinical and ultrasonographic examination. The prognosis for fetal survival should be guarded. The remainder of the litter may be carried to term or further abortions may occur. Daily examination of the patient and her litter is essential so that treatment can be adjusted to the health of the bitch and the litter. If the bitch or her litter deteriorate it may be necessary to terminate the pregnancy surgically. If the litter is carried to term they may be delivered spontaneously by the bitch. If pregnancy is prolonged the patient should be managed as an overdue patient (see below).

OBSTETRICIAN'S CHECK LIST

Management of late incomplete abortion in the bitch

See patient as soon as possible
↓
History of recent health. Expected whelping date – age of pregnancy
↓
Examination of aborted fetuses – laboratory investigation
↓

Clinical examination of mother – antibiotic and supportive therapy
↓
Culture any vaginal discharge
↓
Gynecological examination of the mother
↓
Ultrasonographic assessment of litter
↓
Litter alive – pulses >150/min – monitor daily taking pregnancy as near to term (63 days) as possible
↓
Litter dead – laparotomy – uterus compromised – hysterectomy – uterus healthy – further breeding desired – cesarean section

---

TREATMENTS GIVEN IN SURVEYS OF DYSTOCIA IN DOGS AND CATS

It is interesting to note the treatments given in the South Wales and Swedish surveys of dystocia in the dog and cat referred to above (see Tables 9.1, 9.2, and 9.3). Both surveys indicate the frequency with which cesarean section is used to treat dystocia in small animals.

The dog

In the South Wales survey, 60% of bitches were treated by cesarean section; 66% of the bitches in the Swedish survey were treated by cesarean section. One-third of those in the Swedish survey had no other treatment but in the other two-thirds treatment with oxytocin, calcium, and/or forceps delivery was attempted first. Digital manipulation including forceps delivery and/or ecbolic therapy without recourse to cesarean section was used successfully in 28% of cases.

Puppy deaths occurred in 53% of litters and the overall mortality rate in puppies was 22%.

The cat

Seventy-nine per cent of the queens were treated by cesarean section; 45% of these had no other treatment and in 55% treatment with digital manipulation and/or ecbolic therapy had been attempted before cesarean section. Dystocia was resolved by medical treatment in 20% of cats. Medical management was more likely to be successful in mesocephalic cats than in either dolicocephalic or brachycephalic breeds (Gunn-Moore & Thrusfield 1995).

THE OVERDUE PATIENT – MANAGEMENT OF THE OVERDUE BITCH OR QUEEN

The difficulty of predicting the likely birth date and the reasons for this difficulty, especially in the bitch, have already been mentioned. Any animal in which gestation goes over 63 or 64 days must be carefully monitored, and in particular efforts must be made to ensure that first-stage labor does not pass unnoticed. Ideally, the overdue patient should be examined daily, especially as day 70 approaches because this is regarded by many as the maximum safe duration of normal gestation. The general health of the patient must be monitored, with special attention being paid to body temperature and appetite. A temperature 1°C below normal may indicate imminent parturition. Real-time ultrasonographic evaluation of the litter is extremely useful. A steady heart beat, a fetal pulse of 150–220, lack of excessive movements, and clear amniotic fluid usually suggest that all is well with the litter. A fetal heart rate of <150/min may indicate the onset of fetal distress. The presence of a dark green (dog) or dark red (cat) vaginal discharge must be watched for and, if present, may indicate the need for immediate action to deliver the litter. Signs of fetal life and movement must be assessed and a check made for the presence of milk in the udder of the mother. Heavy lactation with evidence of let-down may indicate that birth is about to begin. Vaginal examination should be performed daily to assess the tone of the anterior vagina, which may 'mirror' cervical and uterine tone. Reduced tone in the anterior vagina may indicate a degree of relaxation of the cervix. Tightness in the anterior vagina may indicate that the cervix is still fully closed (see Fig. 9.7).

Plasma progesterone levels fall in the bitch as birth approaches and should be monitored frequently (ideally every 24 hours) in the overdue bitch. If plasma progesterone falls below 1 ng/mg, birth is imminent and could be safely induced. For details of methods used to induce birth in the dog and cat, see Chapter 15.

When day 70 is reached further action is usually advisable. If the anterior vagina is relaxed and milk is present an intramuscular injection of oxytocin (2–5 IU) may be given in an attempt to induce birth. If this fails,

an elective cesarean section should be performed, after again checking details of service date and the adequacy of milk supply. There is a risk that the offspring may be dysmature. This is probably outweighed by the risk to mother and offspring if pregnancy is allowed to progress further.

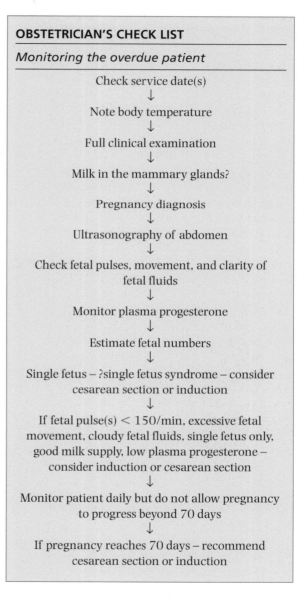

OBSTETRICIAN'S CHECK LIST

Monitoring the overdue patient

Check service date(s)
↓
Note body temperature
↓
Full clinical examination
↓
Milk in the mammary glands?
↓
Pregnancy diagnosis
↓
Ultrasonography of abdomen
↓
Check fetal pulses, movement, and clarity of fetal fluids
↓
Monitor plasma progesterone
↓
Estimate fetal numbers
↓
Single fetus – ?single fetus syndrome – consider cesarean section or induction
↓
If fetal pulse(s) < 150/min, excessive fetal movement, cloudy fetal fluids, single fetus only, good milk supply, low plasma progesterone – consider induction or cesarean section
↓
Monitor patient daily but do not allow pregnancy to progress beyond 70 days
↓
If pregnancy reaches 70 days – recommend cesarean section or induction

CESAREAN SECTION IN THE DOG AND CAT

See Chapter 11.

POSTPARTURIENT PROBLEMS IN THE DOG AND CAT

See Chapter 14.

REFERENCES

Darvelid AW, Linde-Forsberg C 1994 Dystocia in the bitch: a retrospective study of 182 cases. Journal of Small Animal Practice 35:402–407

Ekstrand C, Linde-Forsberg C 1994 Dystocia in the cat: a retrospective study of 155 cases. Journal of Small Animal Practice 35:459–464

Gunn-Moore DA, Thrusfield MV 1995 Feline dystocia: prevalence, and association with cranial conformation and breed. Veterinary Record 136:350–353

Chapter 10

DYSTOCIA IN OTHER SPECIES

From time to time the veterinarian is asked to deal with cases of dystocia in species other than the main domestic ones that are discussed elsewhere in this book. The species vary from the small, such as guinea pigs, gerbils, etc. to the larger species such as llamas and deer. Problems with egg retention may be encountered in birds and in the egg-laying reptiles. Such cases are usually presented as emergencies and require immediate action and care. If specialist help is unavailable, cases should be dealt with according to basic obstetric principles. Advice regarding treatment and anesthesia should always be sought if possible from experienced colleagues with specialist experience, or from appropriate publications.

The following comments are not intended to be comprehensive but it is hoped they will be of some guidance in dealing with cases of dystocia in unusual species.

SMALL MAMMALIAN SPECIES

History and clinical signs

Cases of dystocia are sometimes presented with an impacted fetus protruding from the vulva. In other cases signs of impending parturition or straining have not been followed by birth of the young. History-taking may be unrewarding as the secretive nature of some species at parturition makes observation by the owner difficult. Close observation can be contraindicated because in some species it may predispose the mother to eat her young. Details of any offspring already born and their living state may be available. This information is useful both when attempting to decide whether further fetuses remain in the uterus and also the prognosis for future live births. A bloody, green, or brown vaginal discharge may indicate that fetal death has occurred. A foul-smelling discharge may indicate that fetal death occurred some time ago and that a life-threatening septicemia and toxemia may be developing.

Treatment

The size of the patient prohibits either vaginal examination or manipulation other than extremely gentle traction applied to the fetus. The passage of an impacted fetus may be aided by the introduction – using a small syringe with a fine but smooth nozzle or a catheter – of small quantities of obstetric lubricant. If the patient is nervous or distressed, general anesthesia may be required.

Gentle abdominal palpation may indicate the presence of further fetuses within the uterus but if there is any doubt a radiograph or an ultrasonographic scan should be taken to identify and count fetal skeletons. Palpation and radiography or ultrasonography are also important diagnostic aids if a female, believed to be pregnant, is presented with an abnormal vaginal discharge.

Very small doses of oxytocin have been used, e.g. 1–2 IU by intramuscular injection in the guinea pig and other species when uterine inertia is suspected. The drug may stimulate uterine contractions and the delivery of further offspring. Oxytocin must only be used if the obstetrician is as certain as possible that no actual obstruction of the birth canal or fetal impaction is present.

In many cases, and especially if a number of fetuses are known to be present in the uterus, it is advisable to proceed to an immediate cesarean section. In most small mammalian species, satisfactory induction and maintenance of anesthesia can be achieved with isoflurane and oxygen using a face mask. A midline laparotomy provides the best access to the uterus. If the uterus appears viable it is opened and any fetuses are removed. The uterus is closed with fine absorbable sutures and the laparotomy incision is repaired. If the uterus is damaged, contains dead offspring, or is severely infected it is advisable to remove it at surgery. Postoperative analgesia

Table 10.1 Gestation length and litter size in the small mammalian species			
Species	Gestation length (days)	Litter size (range)	Average litter size
Chinchilla	111	1–6	2
Ferret	41–42	5–13	8
Gerbil	24–26*	3–7	5
Guinea pig	59–72	1–6	3–4
Hamster	15–18	4–5**	6
Mouse	19–21	8–12	8
Rabbit	28–33	4–12	7
Rat	20–22	6–16	10

* Gestation in the gerbil may prolong if conception takes place during lactation.
** Litter size may be up to 9 in the Syrian (golden) hamster.
Data from Meredith & Redrobe (2002).

should be provided. Pethidine at a dose of 5–10 mg/kg given at 2–4 hourly intervals has been used in guinea pigs, mice, rats, and rabbits. Non-steroidal anti-inflammatory drugs have been used in some species. For further information obstetricians are advised to consult Flecknell & Waterman-Pearson (2000).

Details of the normal gestation length and litter size of the small species are listed in Table 10.1.

Chinchillas Like guinea pigs, chinchillas produce young that are alert and can see and move about easily. Birth often takes place early in the morning without prior nest building. Although litter size is variable it usually consists of two members. Dystocia is relatively uncommon but may be indicated by a delay in completion of birth or an abnormal vaginal discharge. Fetal monsters – especially schisotomes – have been reported and may cause dystocia. Cases of uterine inertia, uterine torsion, and fetal maldisposition have also been reported (Hoefler & Crossley 2002).

Gerbils Gerbils may show signs of pseudopregnancy. Abdominal enlargement and an abnormal vaginal discharge can be associated with both pyometra and uterine and ovarian neoplasia. Ultrasonography using a 7 MHz probe and a stand-off technique has been found useful in the differential diagnosis of pyometra and abdominal masses (Keeble 2002). Implantation may be delayed and gestation prolonged if mating takes place during lactation. If the litter size is very small the offspring may be consumed by their mother. This can also happen if there is no suitable nesting area, birth is disturbed, or the mother has mastitis.

Guinea pigs Gestation length is quite variable and may be shorter if the litter size is small. Pregnancy can be readily confirmed by abdominal palpation or ultrasonography. The sow guinea pig often shows few signs of imminent parturition. Her pubic symphysis opens as parturition approaches and some movement between the bones is palpable. A gap of 2–3 cm between the pubic bones is palpable shortly before birth. Birth is often completed within 30 minutes with intervals of 3–10 minutes between the young. The sow adopts a squatting position during birth. The young are precocious when born and are fully mobile shortly after birth. They may not suckle for 12–24 hours after birth.

In older nulliparous sows the pubic symphysis may fail to separate, thus predisposing to dystocia caused by fetopelvic disproportion. Large fetuses may be produced by overweight sows. Dystocia requiring cesarean section should be anticipated in nulliparous sows bred for the first time over the age of 9 months. Signs of dystocia include non-productive straining and the presence of an olive-green vaginal discharge without the delivery of the first fetus. The prognosis for both mother and offspring following cesarean section should be guarded (Flecknell 2002).

Pregnancy toxemia has been reported in overweight guinea pig sows in late pregnancy and during the early postpartum stage. The condition is predisposed by overfeeding and possibly an insufficiency of drinking water. Affected sows become dull, anorexic, and may have ketones and high levels of protein in their urine. Untreated animals may suffer fits and coma; death may follow. Treatment involves the oral administration of glucose and corticosteroids. Glucose saline may be given by subcutaneous injection (Flecknell 2002). Cesarean section may be used to terminate the pregnancy in such cases although the prognosis for complete recovery must be guarded. Induction of birth may be attempted using 1–2 IU oxytocin given by intramuscular injection.

Mastitis has also been reported in lactating guinea pigs (Flecknell 2002). Poor hygiene and overcrowding predispose to the condition allowing access by opportunist pathogens. Affected glands may become filled with pus and ulcerate. Treatment with antibiotic therapy (enrofloxacin being safe and effective) and non-steroidal anti-inflammatory drugs should be prescribed along with local surgical care and cleaning of the affected glands.

Hamster Dystocia is very rare in the hamster after a very short gestation period. Cannibalism of the young may occur if the female is disturbed at or around parturition (Whittaker 2001).

Rabbits May show signs of pseudopregnancy, which is accompanied by bed-making and mammary development. For this reason, if a doe is suspected to be suffering from a prolonged gestation, care should be taken to ensure that she really is pregnant. Abdominal palpation and radiographic and ultrasonographic examination should provide an immediate differentiation between pregnancy and pseudopregnancy. In normal pregnancy, milk production and let-down may not occur until parturition. Disturbance at birth or a few days afterwards may result in the doe cannibalizing her litter. Similar problems can occur in the rat and the ferret. In these species, postcesarean management can be extremely difficult. In any case, successful artificial rearing of these species whose young are produced in a relatively immature state can be difficult. However, successful artificial rearing of rabbit kits using a cat milk substitute has been reported (Meredith & Crossley 2002).

Many rabbit does give birth in the early hours of the morning. Their offspring are hairless and unable to hear or see. Feeding on highly nutritious milk from the doe may occur only once or twice daily. The kits may not be seen by their owner until they leave their nest at 2–3 weeks of age. Dystocia is uncommon.

Endometrial hyperplasia and uterine adenocarcinoma occur quite frequently in unbred does. Clinical signs of these conditions may include abdominal enlargement and a blood-stained vaginal discharge. Similar signs may be encountered in cases of dystocia. Radiography and ultrasonography are useful diagnostic aids.

Mastitis has been reported in lactating does. Infective agents include *Pasteurella multocida*, *Staphylococcus aureus* and streptococci. Abscessation of affected glands may occur and surgical drainage may encourage resolution.

Prompt treatment with antibiotics and non-steroidal anti-inflammatory drugs should be effective.

Rats and mice Parturition in these species often occurs in the early hours of the morning. It is usually completed within 1–2 hours. Dead offspring may be eaten. Newborn offspring should not be handled as this may cause cannibalism by the doe. Does may be aggressive at this time and may bite their owner if handled. Mammary tumors are seen quite frequently in both rats and mice. In rats mammary tumors are mostly benign but in mice they are often malignant (Orr 2002).

EGG RETENTION IN CHELONIANS

Egg retention may occur when the female is unable to find a suitable place to lay her eggs. The eggs may become lodged in a uterine horn, the body of the uterus, or the cloaca. Developmental abnormalities in the reproductive system of the female herself or her offspring may predispose to dystocia. The presence of retained eggs can be confirmed by palpation of the cloaca and radiography or ultrasonography of the abdomen. Animals suffering from dystocia may strain and show anorexia, lethargy, and hindlimb paresis (McArthur, Wilkinson & Barrows 2002). Provision of a suitable nesting site may help. Oxytocin at a dose of 1 IU/kg body weight and repeated twice at 24-hour intervals may aid the passage of retained eggs. Surgical removal of retained eggs may also be attempted.

EGG RETENTION IN LIZARDS AND SNAKES

Egg retention in these species may occur as a result of calcium deficiency, renal disease, or an unsuitable environment (Wallach & Boever 1983). The condition is diagnosed by gentle palpation of the abdomen and confirmed by radiography or ultrasonic examination. Passage of retained eggs in response to 3–6 IU oxytocin may be seen. If this treatment fails, laparotomy may be required to remove the eggs.

EGG RETENTION IN CAGE AND OTHER BIRDS

Egg retention is occasionally seen in cage birds and domestic poultry. It may be caused by oviduct

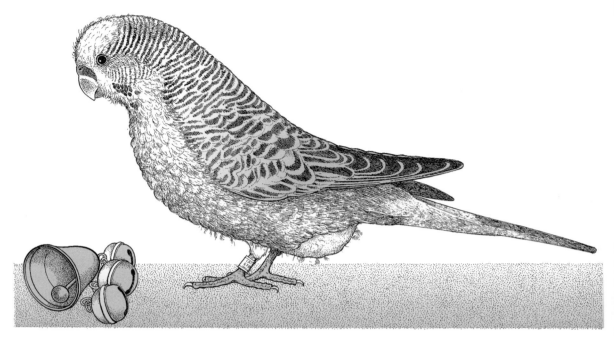

Figure 10.1 Budgerigar with egg retention. Note the dull demeanour and distension of abdomen and vent with loss of covering feathers.

malfunction or damage, repeated disturbance when the bird is trying to lay, oviduct infection, calcium deficiency, or tumor formation. If untreated it may lead to generalized fatal egg peritonitis. Affected birds are usually dull and progressively inappetant. The abdomen becomes enlarged and tense and tenesmus may be observed (Fig. 10.1). It may be possible to palpate one or more eggs through the abdominal wall. If the egg is within the cloaca it may be partly visible and palpable. Radiography and ultrasound may be used to confirm the number and position of retained eggs. The larger ones are normally brittle shelled.

Eggs within the cloaca can be removed with great care and the aid of lubrication. The egg shell may break or be broken and this may facilitate removal of the retained egg by reducing its size. An episiotomy-like incision may be made at the periphery of the cloaca to enlarge the exit from the cloaca. It is repaired after delivery of the egg. Sedation and local anesthesia or general anesthesia may be used. Eggs within the oviduct may be encouraged to pass towards the cloaca by intramuscular injection of small doses of oxytocin (0.1 IU) or dinoprost (0.02 mg). In non-responsive cases, laparotomy followed by removal of eggs from the oviduct may be attempted. Great care must be taken to avoid breaking an egg during its surgical removal from

the oviduct. Despite peritoneal lavage after such an accident there is a risk of egg peritonitis developing. Very early cases of egg peritonitis may respond to antibiotic therapy but in advanced cases the prognosis is grave and euthanasia may be necessary.

THE LARGER MAMMALS

Camels

According to Arthur (1996), the incidence of dystocia in camels is low, although the long neck and legs of the fetus predispose to fetal malposture. Birth is normally a rapid process with the second stage of labor being completed within 30 minutes. Like the llama, the camel does not lick her offspring after birth. In a recent study in Saudi Arabia (Al-Eknah 2001) found that maternal and fetal causes of dystocia accounted for 43% and 57% of cases, respectively. Uterine torsion was the cause of 50% of cases of maternal dystocia. Other causes of maternal dystocia included primary uterine inertia (20%), incomplete dilation of the cervix (20%), and vaginal stenosis (10%). Fetal maldisposition accounted for 90% of fetal dystocia cases. Cases of lateral deviation of the head, carpal flexion, hock flexion, and hip flexion have been observed. Repulsion of the fetus to enable the maldisposition to be corrected can be aided by lowering the anterior end of the camel. Under field conditions in Saudi Arabia this was done by digging a pit in the sand. In cases in which manual correction proves impossible, cesarean section or fetotomy are used. Fetal survival can be good in cases where manual correction of maldisposition proves impossible. Al-Eknah (2001) noted the case of a living fetus delivered by cesarean section 17 hours after amniotic rupture had occurred.

Cesarean section is performed by a left flank sublumbar laparotomy under xylazine sedation and local infiltration anesthesia. Fetotomy using standard bovine techniques (see Chapter 12) is used in cases where the fetus is known to be dead and the uterus readily accessible. Postoperative analgesia should be provided by the administration of non-steroidal anti-inflammatory therapy.

Deer

Occasional cases of dystocia are seen in deer, mostly as a result of fetal maldisposition or the simultaneous presentation of twin fetuses. In deer calving outside treatment can be difficult. Tranquilization of the hind by darting may be necessary to gain access to her. In some cases the calf may be dead by the time the hind is caught. Delivery is by traction following correction of any fetal maldisposition. If the calf is alive establishment of the fetomaternal bond may be difficult after assisted delivery. In such cases artificial rearing may prove necessary.

Llamas and alpacas

Gestation length is 335–360 days. Placentation is epitheliochorial and over 95% of pregnancies are within the left uterine horn. In late pregnancy and at birth the young llama (the cria) is enclosed in an additional membrane – the epidermal membrane – the function of which is unknown. The membrane is attached to the feet and at the mucocutaneous junctions of the cria. It dries and withers after birth. The newborn cria is not licked by its mother but gets to its feet and suckles within 2 hours of birth. Retention of the fetal membranes is rare. Birth is normally quite rapid and is completed within 1 hour of the appearance of fetal fluid at the vulva. Although normally born in anterior presentation with head and forelimbs extended, the cria can also be delivered without difficulty in a foot–nape posture.

Posterior presentation is rare but the risk of anoxia to the fetus in this presentation is higher than for the fetus in anterior presentation.

Dystocia in llamas is less common than in cattle and sheep. Although maternal causes of dystocia have been reported, fetal causes predominate. Cases of uterine inertia, uterine torsion, failure of the cervix to dilate, and vaginal stenosis have been reported. The pelvic inlet is quite small and is limited by the position of the sacrum and the ischiatic spines. Pelvic malformation has also been seen.

The long neck and limbs of the species do, however, predispose to fetal malposture. Lateral deviation of the head is reported as being the most common cause of dystocia (Fowler 1998). In a comprehensive account Fowler (1998) also reported that other malpostures, including downward deviation of the head, shoulder flexion, and breech presentation, were seen. Fetal malposition was uncommon. Fowler (1998) noted that the shape of the cria caused impaction of the shoulder girdle with the maternal pelvis to be more common than impaction of the fetal stifles or hips. Rotation of the fetus through 45° was usually sufficient to alleviate the problem and allow delivery. Fetal monsters, including schistosomus reflexus and hydrocephalus, have been seen. The small size of the llama makes internal manipulation in cases of dystocia difficult unless the obstetrician has very small hands.

If manual correction of dystocia proves impossible a cesarean section may be necessary. Access to the abdomen is via a mid-line or a high-flank laparotomy wound. A lower-flank incision is inadvisable as the muscles there are aponeurotic and suturing can be difficult and ineffectual.

Primates

According to Wallach & Boever (1983), calcium-deficient diets in some captive primates may lead to pelvic distortion. These authors reported that clinical signs of dystocia included non-productive straining and a serohemorrhagic vulval discharge. Treatment is normally by cesarean section. Primates normally give birth during the night and an animal found straining to pass a fetus in the morning should be considered an obstetric emergency. An immediate cesarean section is indicated in such cases. Fluid therapy should be commenced and analgesia (e.g. carprofen) is given prior to surgery.

If cesarean section is performed in primates, care must be taken to avoid allowing endometrial fragments to seed in the peritoneal cavity. If this happens the patient may develop endometriosis and show signs of abdominal pain during estrus. Good postoperative care, including observation of the wound for self-inflicted damage is essential. Postoperative analgesia can be provided by the administration of flunixin at a dose of 0.5–4.0 mg/kg given by subcutaneous injection. Pethidine at 2–4 mg/kg can be given at 3–4-hour intervals if additional analgesia is required.

REFERENCES

Al-Eknah MM 2001 Camels. In: Noakes DA, Parkinson TJ, England GCW (eds) Arthur's veterinary reproduction and obstetrics, 8th edn. WB Saunders, London, p 781–788

Arthur GH 1996 Camels. In: Arthur GH, Noakes DE, Pearson H, Parkinson TJ (eds) Veterinary reproduction and obstetrics, 7th edn. WB Saunders, London, p 659–666

Flecknell PA 2002 Guinea pigs. In: Meredith A, Redrobe S (eds) Manual of exotic pets, 4th edn. British Small Animal Veterinary Association, Gloucester, UK, p 52–64

Flecknell PA, Waterman-Pearson A 2000 Pain management in animals. WB Saunders, London, p 115–120

Fowler ME 1998 Medicine and surgery of South American camelids, 2nd edn. Iowa State University Press, Iowa, USA

Hoefler HL, Crossley DA 2002 Chinchillas. In: Meredith A, Redrobe S (eds) Manual of exotic pets, 4th edn. British Small Animal Veterinary Association, Gloucester, UK, p 65–75

Keeble E 2002 Gerbils. In: Meredith A, Redrobe S (eds) Manual of exotic pets, 4th edn. British Small Animal Veterinary Association, Gloucester, UK, p 34–46

McArthur SDJ, Wilkinson RJ, Barrows MG 2002 Tortoises and turtles. In: Meredith A, Redrobe S (eds) Manual of exotic pets, 4th edn. British Small Animal Veterinary Association, Gloucester, UK, p 208–222

Meredith A, Crossley DA 2002 Rabbits. In: Meredith A, Redrobe S (eds) Manual of exotic pets, 4th edn. British Small Animal Veterinary Association, Gloucester, UK, p 76–92

Meredith A, Redrobe S 2002 Manual of exotic pets, 4th edn. British Small Animal Veterinary Association, Gloucester, UK

Orr HE 2002 Rats and mice. In: Meredith A, Redrobe S (eds) Manual of exotic pets, 4th edn. British Small Animal Veterinary Association, Gloucester, UK, p 13–25

Wallach DJ, Boever WJ 1983 Diseases of exotic animals. WB Saunders, Philadelphia

Whittaker D 2001 Hamsters. In: Noakes DE, Parkinson TJ, England GCW (eds) Arthur's veterinary reproduction and obstetrics, 8th edn. WB Saunders, London, p 809–812

Chapter 11

CESAREAN SECTION

This procedure is widely and successfully used in veterinary practice, especially in the cow, ewe, and bitch. Provided the decision to go ahead with cesarean section is made early in the course of dystocia, and the technique is not used as a treatment of last resort, the prognosis for both mother and offspring should be good. The indications for the operation and the surgical techniques involved vary between the species and are described below. The operation is described in full detail in the cow, sheep, and small animals; comparative notes are provided for other species. Methods of anesthesia and analgesia are suggested for each species. Whenever possible, obstetricians should use a method of anesthesia with which they are familiar. Many agents cross the placenta and enter the fetus and small quantities of others may appear in the milk. Sedation is not required in every case but may be used in nervous animals or in some protocols prior to general anesthesia. Not all sedative drugs are licensed for use in every species:

- Lidocaine (lignocaine) hydrochloride: has been found to be a highly effective local anesthetic for use in ruminants. Although not currently licensed for use in farm livestock in the UK, it can be used under cascade legislation in preference to procaine.

Analgesia after cesarean section should be provided for all species. An example of one of these drugs is given in the text but in most cases alternatives known to work well by the obstetrician may be used. A single dose of a non-steroidal anti-inflammatory drug (NSAID) given at the end of the operation is thought to provide sufficient analgesia in most cases. Further analgesia using NSAIDs, if required, can be provided either by injection or by oral administration in some species. The onset of action of the NSAID analgesia is quite slow and once further safety data are available it may be possible to administer analgesia preoperatively. Details of the excretion of NSAIDs in the maternal milk of the cesarean

section patient are not available for all species. Prolonged administration is not advisable and might, in some species, predispose to gastric ulceration in the neonate. NSAIDs have been reported to cause premature closure of the ductus arteriosus in some species and thus use before surgery could be dangerous. If there is evidence of acute pain in the postoperative period, opioid therapy can be given safely in addition to the NSAID in most species. Opioids may, however, suppress the innate caring ability of the mother and the secretion of oxytocin. For further information on pain management the reader is recommended to consult Flecknell & Waterman-Pearson (2000). Drug data sheets should also be consulted.

CESAREAN SECTION IN THE COW

Indications

1. Resolution of existing dystocia

- Fetopelvic disproportion including cases of misalliance and postmaturity.
- Fetal maldisposition, which cannot be corrected by manipulation.
- Irreducible uterine torsion.
- Incomplete dilation of cervix or other parts of birth canal.
- Fetal monsters that cannot be delivered by other means.
- Uterine rupture or severe uterine hemorrhage.
- Damaged and severe vaginal prolapse where further damage might accompany vaginal delivery.

2. Elective cesarean section

- Surgical termination of prolonged gestation.
- To avoid existing or suspected fetopelvic disproportion.

- Termination of pregnancy in cases of life-threatening disease in the dam: for example, some cases of hydrops allantois and traumatic reticulitis or pericarditis. Induction of birth might be used as an alternative in such cases but the time required for the drugs to work may not be compatible with maternal life.

Prognosis

1. Resolution of existing dystocia

This should be discussed with the owner before surgery and depends on a number of factors. The prognosis for a successful outcome is proportional to the duration of existing dystocia. The bovine fetus may not survive more than 8 hours of second-stage labor. The mortality rate in the dam rises if surgery is not performed until more than 24 hours after the commencement of dystocia or if the fetus is dead and emphysematous. Prolonged attempts at delivery by traction will also reduce the chances of fetal and maternal survival. The availability of skilled assistance and the ability to maintain reasonable asepsis during surgery are also important factors. A maternal survival rate of 80–90% should be expected. Fetal survival should be good in cases of elective cesarean section but decreases with increasing duration of second-stage labor.

In some cases, fetotomy may be an alternative to cesarean section (see discussion in Chapter 12). Occasionally, if the fetus is dead and the cow is already suffering from toxemia, humane slaughter may be advisable.

2. Elective cesarean section

An elective cesarean section is more easily and safely performed in first-stage labor than during late pregnancy. The risks of an inadequate milk supply or retention of the placenta are smaller at this stage. Ideally, elective cesarean section should be performed when the cow's cervix is fully dilated. At this stage the calf has been subjected to some of the beneficial stresses of labor. As a result of the release of catecholamines that occurs in labor, the calf is better prepared for postnatal respiratory and metabolic adaptation. The release of adrenaline (epinephrine) by the mildly stressed calf produces more effective removal of lung fluids and better release of surfactant. Better gas exchange is promoted and better energy release helps to maintain body temperature in the neonate.

The location chosen for surgery

There is often little choice on farms, but a clean, well-lit location should be selected. A major sweeping and cleaning up of the location likely to stir up clouds of dust immediately prior to surgery is inadvisable.

Examination of the cow prior to surgery

The obstetrician will normally already have a good knowledge of the condition of both dam and fetus as a result of the examinations made before and during attempts at vaginal delivery. Further examination should determine, if possible, in which uterine horn the fetus is located, because this may influence the laparotomy site selected. The ability of the dam to remain standing if necessary during surgery, and her current state of well-being – including the need for fluid and other supportive therapy before or during surgery – should also be assessed. If the fetus is hyperactive or its residual amniotic fluid is stained green with meconium it may be becoming hypoxic. Surgery should be commenced with all possible speed to ensure delivery of a living calf.

Assistance required

If the operation is to be carried out on the standing cow, one attendant will be required to restrain the patient, but if a recumbent position is chosen at least two experienced assistants are necessary. Although cesarean section can be carried out single handed, skilled surgical assistance in the form of a colleague or veterinary nurse makes the procedure both simpler and safer. An additional assistant to help with removal of the calf and its care after delivery is advisable. If an emergency arises with either the cow or calf during surgery, the presence of skilled help will make resolution of the problem and maintenance of asepsis much easier.

Preparations for surgery

The obstetrician should ensure that everything necessary for surgery is to hand, make sure the patient is well prepared and that facilities are as good as possible. The obstetrician should also ensure that assistants – skilled or otherwise – are briefed on what to do in emergencies either involving the cow or calf. Once the operation is underway there should be no unnecessary delay – the longer the peritoneal cavity remains open on the farm, the greater the risk of infection.

Equipment should include:

- Appropriate drugs for sedation, local anesthesia, and analgesia.
- Electric clippers for removing hair from the surgical site.
- A portable halogen light if local illumination is poor.
- Resuscitation facilities, including arrangements to dry and warm the calf. Doxapram hydrochloride (50 mg) can be placed in a syringe with suitable needle prior to surgery in case it is needed urgently when the calf is delivered.
- Sterilized calving ropes or chains, which may be needed during removal of the calf.
- Solutions for skin preparation: severe contamination should be removed using soap and water. Skin disinfection prior to surgery can be achieved the aid of a surgical scrub solution of chlorhexidene, povidone–iodine, or 4% chlorhexidene gluconate followed by application of surgical spirit. Application of 10% povidone–iodine alcoholic tincture to the skin will enable a one-stage disinfection to be performed.
- Sterile drape, e.g. disposable paper type: useful to maintain asepsis but may frighten a nervous standing heifer.
- Surgical kit: scalpel, rat-toothed forceps, scissors, six hemostats, heavy-duty needle holders, suture scissors, selection of round bodied and cutting suture needles. A Robert's embryotomy knife should be included in case it is necessary to open the uterus deep in the abdomen.
- Suture material: an absorbable suture for closure of peritoneum, muscles, and subcutis. Monofilament or braided nylon for the skin.
- Antibiotics: antibiotic cover is given prophylactically, penicillin/streptomycin combination or ampicillin being useful. Treatment is preferably commenced prior to surgery. If infection of the peritoneum is likely, a water-soluble form of these drugs may be instilled into the peritoneal cavity before wound closure.

Position of the cow and selection of operation site

In most cases, a left-flank laparotomy is performed on the standing cow. Alternative sites include a right-flank, a ventrolateral, or a midline laparotomy. The advantages and disadvantages of the various sites are summarized as follows.

Flank laparotomy

Advantages   Only local anesthesia is required, the incision may be easily extended if necessary, the risk of postoperative soiling of the wound or herniation is small.

Disadvantages   The uterus is often difficult to exteriorize prior to opening, the peritoneum is readily contaminated with uterine contents especially if the calf is dead and emphysematous.

In left-flank laparotomy the rumen may occasionally make access to the uterus difficult but the risk of the small intestine falling out of the wound is normally small.

Right-flank laparotomy allows good access to a calf in the right uterine horn but the risk of loops of small intestine tending to slip out of the laparotomy incision is higher.

Flank laparotomy can be performed on the standing or laterally recumbent cow. Surgery on the standing patient is preferred by most obstetricians if the patient is likely to remain standing and not go down suddenly during surgery. Opening and closure of the peritoneal cavity is often a more straightforward procedure in the standing patient. There is less intra-abdominal pressure but exteriorization of the uterus can be difficult in some cases. If the cow is thought likely to go down during surgery it is probably better to sedate, cast, and restrain her in sternal or lateral recumbency with the upper hindleg pulled back.

Ventrolateral or midline laparotomy

Advantages   The uterus (even one containing an emphysematous calf) can more readily be exteriorized with less risk of peritoneal contamination.

Disadvantages   Heavy sedation or general anesthesia is required, the risk of postoperative soiling of the incision or herniation is higher.

Left-flank cesarean section in the standing cow

Restraint

The head should be secured with a halter, which should be fixed to a wall or other solid point but will permit the cow to lie down if she wishes. A length of rope should be attached to the patient's right hindleg so that it can be pulled forward – should the animal decide to lie down during the operation – thus ensuring continued access to the left flank.

Sedation

This may not be required in a quiet cow but is useful in nervous or aggressive animals. Xylazine is very useful. Dose: 2.5 mg/50 kg body weight by intramuscular injection or 0.05 mg/kg by intravenous injection – the latter is *not* a licensed route of administration for cattle in some countries. Xylazine may increase the tone of the uterine musculature, making exteriorization of the uterus more difficult during surgery.

Myometrial relaxation

Clenbuterol (300 μg) given by intramuscular or slow intravenous injection just prior to surgery will help to counteract the myometrial action of xylazine and may facilitate manipulation of the uterus during surgery.

Preparation of the surgical site

Hair is clipped from an area of the left flank extending laterally from the last rib to the tuber coxae and dorso-ventrally from the spines of the vertebrae down to the lowest part of the flank. If the patient is soiled the clipped site should be initially washed and scrubbed using liquid soap and water. The skin is then thoroughly scrubbed with a surgical scrub solution. Finally, surgical spirit is applied. (Alternatively, a 10% povidone–iodine alcoholic tincture can be used for one-stage disinfection.)

If local infiltration anesthesia is used the site should be prepared before the anesthetic is instilled, with a final preparation immediately prior to surgery.

Anesthesia

Epidural anesthesia is not essential but useful to prevent straining and tail movements during surgery; 5–8 mL 2% lidocaine (lignocaine) hydrochloride without adrenaline (epinephrine) is given epidurally into the first or second intercoccygeal space. A larger dose may cause the patient to become recumbent and is contraindicated.

Local anesthesia may be local infiltration, an inverted L block, or by paravertebral injection. Local infiltration anesthesia has the advantage of speed. It may occasionally interfere with wound healing and may be less effective than either of the other techniques if a muscle

splitting ('grid iron') approach to the abdomen is used. Approximately 80–100 mL of local anesthetic is needed for local infiltration. Paravertebral anesthesia is achieved by blocking the outflow from spinal nerves T13–L3. The nerves are found just behind the last rib and the first three lumbar vertebrae respectively; 20 mL local anesthetic is injected over each nerve. Figure 11.1 illustrates the sites of local infiltration, epidural, and paravertebral anesthesia. For further detailed discussion of anesthetic techniques, see Hall, Clarke & Trim (2003).

Surgical technique

Entry into the peritoneal cavity

Skin incision A vertical incision is made through the skin 25–30 cm in length commencing approximately 10 cm below the transverse processes of the lumbar vertebrae and halfway between the last rib and the tuber coxae. In fat animals, layers of adipose tissue

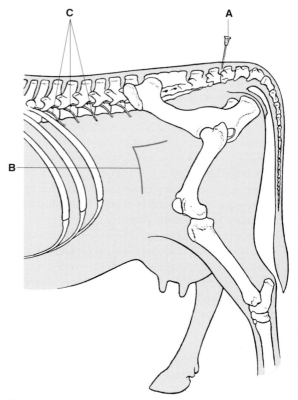

Figure 11.1 Bovine cesarean section – sites for anesthesia. (A) Epidural, (B) local infiltration, (C) paravertebral (see text for details).

may be found beneath the skin and between the muscle layers.

Muscle layers   Immediately below the skin and attached to it by fascia is the cutaneous trunci muscle, which is also incised. The external oblique muscle – a thick, fleshy structure whose fibers run downwards and backwards (Fig. 11.2) – is incised and a number of small and medium-sized arteries may be severed, to which hemostats are applied. Beneath this, the internal oblique – a thinner muscle, fleshy in its upper part and aponeurotic below, whose fibers run downwards and forwards – is incised with scissors to reveal the transverse abdominis muscle. This thin aponeurotic muscle, whose fibers run vertically downwards, is closely applied to the peritoneum. Before opening the peritoneum, the hemostats used to control bleeding points in the muscle layers should be removed after ligating any vessels still bleeding.

The peritoneum   A white, slightly opaque structure, is lifted up from underlying organs before being punctured with the tip of the scalpel; the incision is extended with scissors. As the peritoneum is incised a rush of air can be heard entering the peritoneal cavity. A small amount of peritoneal fluid is normally visible at this stage and may spill out of the wound. Great care

must be taken to identify the peritoneum and to avoid mistakenly incising into the rumen, which usually lies immediately beneath the laparotomy incision.

Locating the uterus

The uterus lies caudal to and below the rumen, but may occasionally be immediately visible as a gray-colored, fluid-filled muscular structure as soon as the abdomen is opened. If not visible, the uterus is located by pushing the rumen forwards and feeling downwards and backwards. The fetus is normally readily palpable within the uterus and fetal parts may be identified – the hindlimbs in an anterior presentation and the forelimbs and head in a posterior presentation. If the case has been ongoing for some time, most of the uterine fluids will have been lost and the uterus will be immobile and closely applied to the fetus. Although fetal parts may still be recognizable, it will not be possible to hold them or move them through the tight and tense uterine wall.

Opening the uterus

If the uterus is mobile, a fetal extremity is grasped within the uterus. It is used to bring the uterus up to

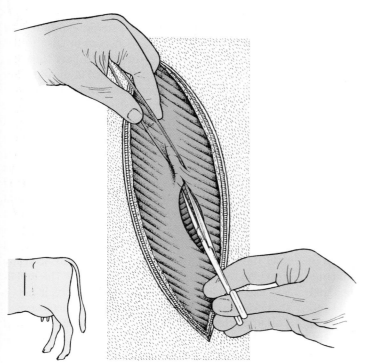

Figure 11.2 Bovine cesarean section – incising the external oblique muscle.

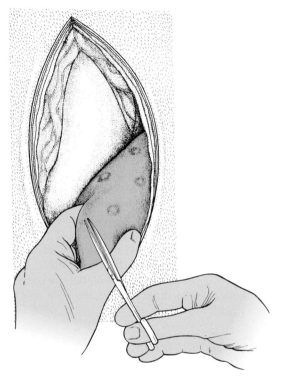

Figure 11.3 Bovine cesarean section – the uterus is opened over a fetal extremity along the greater curvature of the uterus.

and, if possible, just through the laparotomy incision so that it can be opened. The opening should be made over a fetal extremity in the greater curvature of the pregnant uterine horn using a scalpel or, preferably, scissors (Fig. 11.3). The incision should be approximately 20 cm long, should follow the direction of the longitudinal muscles, avoid cotyledons (from which profuse hemorrhage may occur) and be made towards the ovarian end of the uterine horn. If the incision is made caudally in the uterus towards the cervix, repair of the uterine incision can be extremely difficult. Care must be taken to avoid cutting into the fetus, which is still covered with the chorioallantois and the amnion. These structures are broken through using fingers or scissors to expose the fetus. Fetal fluids frequently spill from the uterus when the uterus is opened and when the fetus is removed. Spillage of uterine fluid into the peritoneal cavity should be avoided if possible. It should be of little concern provided fetus, placenta, and uterus are healthy. If the fetus is dead and

emphysematous the loss of such fluid – which may be infected and contain decaying fetal material – is extremely dangerous and may lead to peritonitis (see p. 184).

If, as frequently happens, the uterus cannot be brought to the incision, the obstetrician must open it – often unseen – deep within the abdomen. The uterine wall is smooth, hard, and immobile in such cases. It must be handled with care as it may easily puncture accidentally. The safest way to open the uterus is with the aid of Robert's embryotomy knife (Fig. 11.4). If this instrument is not available, a pair of scissors can be used – taking extreme care to ensure that only the uterine wall is being incised. The point of incision (as described above) is located and the uterine wall is penetrated with the tip of the embryotomy knife, closed scissors, or with the finger. The uterine incision is extended using the embryotomy knife. Some uterine fluid will inevitably be spilled into the peritoneal cavity. A fetal extremity is freed from the uterus and is brought up to the laparotomy incision.

Removal of the fetus

Calf in anterior presentation   The calf is removed caudal end first at cesarean section. The first hindleg to be retrieved is held while the second hindleg is located within the uterus, brought towards the laparotomy incision and is held by a sterile assistant. The size of the uterine incision is checked to ensure that there is enough room for the calf to pass through. If not, the uterine incision is extended in the direction away from the cervix. Preparations are made to remove the fetus. If it has been impacted in the maternal pelvis during attempted delivery an assistant may have to manually repel it per vaginam into the uterus before removal. The hindlimbs of the calf are handed to an assistant. The obstetrician must ensure that asepsis is not compromised at this moment. The calf is delivered by applying traction to the hindlimbs, first dorsally and laterally from the laparotomy wound (Fig. 11.5), and then caudally (Fig. 11.6) towards the hindquarters of the cow. During delivery, the obstetrician should hold the sides of the uterine incision and be ready to extend the incision further if necessary. The umbilical cord usually breaks during fetal delivery; if not, it should be severed by tearing between two hemostats.

Calf in posterior presentation   The calf is removed cranial end first at cesarean section. The first foreleg to be located is held while the head and second foreleg are

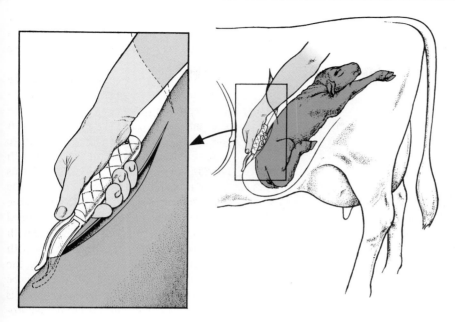

Figure 11.4 Bovine cesarean section – if the uterus cannot be brought to the laparotomy incision it is opened within the abdomen using a Robert's fetotomy knife.

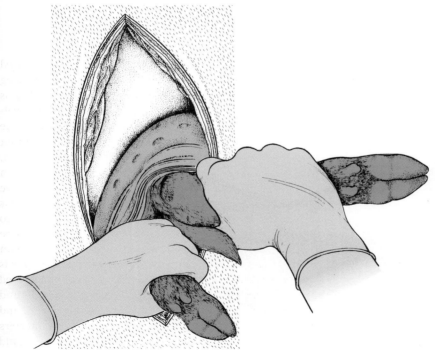

Figure 11.5 Bovine cesarean section – the calf is removed from the uterus by applying traction to the hindlimbs first dorsally and then laterally (see also Figure 11.6).

located and brought to the laparotomy incision. The limbs are passed to an assistant for application of traction. The obstetrician guides the head through the uterine wound and then holds the sides of the uterine incision as the calf is delivered. Traction is applied to the calf in a lateral and then caudal direction (Fig. 11.7).

Resuscitation is undertaken by a skilled assistant while the obstetrician completes the surgical operation (for details of resuscitation, see below).

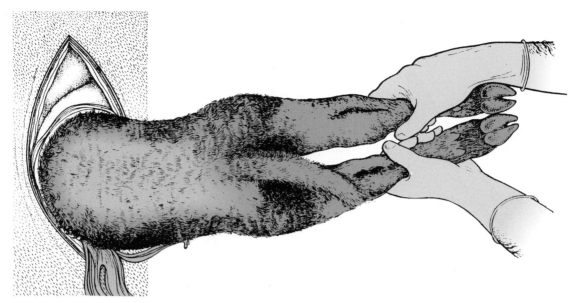

Figure 11.6 Bovine cesarean section – the calf is removed from the uterus by applying traction to the hindlimbs first dorsally and laterally (see Figure 11.5) and then caudally towards the cow's hindquarters.

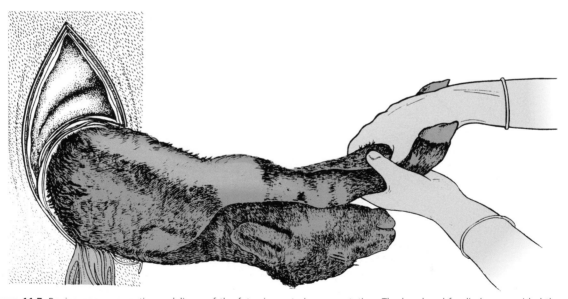

Figure 11.7 Bovine cesarean section – delivery of the fetus in posterior presentation. The head and forelimbs are guided through the uterine wound and traction is applied in a lateral and then a caudal direction.

Searching for a further fetus

Following delivery of the first calf, the uterus must be searched carefully, both inside and out, for evidence of further fetuses. The uterus must not be closed until the obstetrician is sure that no further fetuses remain.

Management of the placenta

If the placenta is readily and quickly separated from its cotyledonary attachments it should be removed carefully from the uterus. If it cannot be removed quickly it should be left in situ, even if the cervix is closed. Before

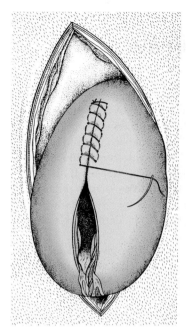

Figure 11.8 Bovine cesarean section – closure of the uterine wound with a layer of inversion sutures. Care must be taken to ensure that no pieces of placenta protrude through the wound.

closing the uterus the obstetrician must ensure that any remaining placenta is entirely within the uterus and does not become entangled with the sutures during closure of the uterine incision.

Repair of the uterine incision

The uterine incision is held by an assistant at or near the laparotomy incision for repair. A continuous single layer of inversion sutures is used with the suture line commencing at the cervical end of the uterus (Fig. 11.8). An absorbable suture is used for uterine closure. Uterine inversion often occurs rapidly after fetal delivery and, if repair is delayed or commenced at the ovarian end, the cervical end of the incision may contract back beyond reach of the obstetrician. This can make the placement of sutures extremely difficult. A second layer of inversion sutures may be placed over the first if there is any doubt that the uterus has been properly sealed. Any other small holes detected in the uterine wall should be carefully repaired using purse-string sutures.

Following repair, any visible blood on the uterus or elsewhere is gently removed using a damp, sterile gauze swab. This greatly lessens the risk of postoperative adhesions. If the uterus is involuting naturally no additional treatment is necessary. If uterine involution is poor, 20 IU oxytocin is given to the cow by intramuscular injection. Unnecessary use of oxytocin should be avoided because it can produce excessively strong uterine contractions with loosening of the uterine sutures. If contamination of the peritoneal cavity through leakage of uterine contents has occurred, further action should be taken to avoid peritonitis. The peritoneal cavity is lavaged with at least 5 liters of warmed sterile normal saline. The saline is removed by suction before closure of the abdomen.

Closure of the laparotomy incision

Before closure of the incision a quantity of crystalline penicillin (5–10 megaunits) or ampicillin (1–2 g) may be instilled into the abdomen as a soluble solution to minimize the risk of peritoneal infection. The laparotomy incision is closed in layers using an absorbable suture. A continuous suture is used for each layer. Muscle layers may be sutured individually or in groups. The following technique of suturing works well:

1. Peritoneum and transverse abdominis muscle.
2. Internal oblique muscle.
3. External oblique muscle.
4. The skin and cutaneous trunci muscle, using non-absorbable monofilament or braided nylon. Bovine skin is thick and suturing is greatly aided by very sharp suture needles and heavy-duty needle holders. Horizontal interrupted mattress sutures provide good skin closure.

Resuscitation of the calf

The following procedure should be followed:

1. Remove mucus from the fetal mouth, larynx, and pharynx either by holding the calf upside down and shaking it gently while slapping the chest or by suction, if available.
2. Check for the presence of fetal heart beat, check for vital signs including palpebral reflex.
3. If spontaneous respiration is not present it may be stimulated by pinching the fetal nose, tickling the nasal mucosa with straw, or by splashing cold water on the fetal head. If these methods are ineffectual, respiration may be further stimulated by giving 40–100 mg doxapram hydrochloride to the calf by intravenous injection or sublingually.
4. If respiration still fails to start but cardiac function is present, artificial respiration should be attempted. After clearing the airways the calf is laid on its side with neck extended. The upper chest wall is raised

and lowered holding it by the humerus and the last rib. This may help achieve the strong negative intrathoracic pressure required for the first breath. Excessive pressure must not be applied to the ribs because they are readily fractured and liver damage can also occur. If no spontaneous breathing occurs an attempt should be made to intubate the calf so that positive-pressure ventilation can be provided. A further method of attempting to inflate the lungs using the initial placement of an esophageal tube is described under resuscitation of the calf after an assisted calving in Chapter 4. Oxygen may be supplied via the endotracheal tube or by face mask.

5. Once spontaneous breathing is established the calf should be monitored to ensure that a normal pattern of respiration is established.

Further care of the neonatal calf

The calf must be dried and kept warm and, unless she is worried by its presence, within sight of the dam. Initial drying may be achieved with towels and later by application of a hair dryer. Warmth may be provided by placing the calf in a thermal blanket with a warm hot-water bottle or under an infra red lamp. Calves born by cesarean section are extremely susceptible to hypothermia and body temperature should be checked at 30-minute intervals until the calf is fully viable and united with its mother.

Respiratory distress is sometimes seen in calves born by cesarean section. This may be associated with fetal dysmaturity or a partial failure of surfactant production and release (for further details concerning the etiology of this problem, see p. 77). Affected calves are hyperpneic and dyspneic, with signs of respiratory distress being evident shortly after birth. Oxygen should be administered by face mask. Dexamethasone (6 mg) should be given by intravenous injection and antibiotic therapy should also be provided. The prognosis for affected calves is very guarded, especially if no improvement in their clinical condition is noticed within 1 hour of birth.

The calf should receive colostrum within the first 6 hours of its life. The fetal respiratory acidosis that accompanies delayed birth may interfere with absorption of colostral antibodies. Colostrum should therefore ideally not be given until an hour after birth. One liter of colostrum is given then by stomach tube (or if the calf will suck by bottle) with a further liter 2 hours later unless it can be ascertained that the calf has drunk colostrum from its mother in the meantime. The calf should be checked for evidence of congenital defects, including cleft palate and contracted flexor tendons. The navel should be dipped in weak iodine solution or sprayed with oxytetracycline, as after normal birth.

Postoperative care of the dam

Routine antibiotic cover (e.g. with penicillin and streptomycin) for 5 days following on-farm surgery is advisable. The cow should be observed carefully for signs of any of the complications mentioned below. Fetomaternal bonding may be weaker than normal following cesarean section. The owner should be advised to watch for complications such as hypoglycemia in the calf or mastitis in the dam in such cases, especially in beef heifers.

The cow should be given analgesia to avoid postoperative pain. A non-steroidal anti-inflammatory drug such as flunixin should be administered intravenously. The drug is given at a dose rate of 2.2 mg/kg. The treatment can be repeated 24 hours later if required.

Right-flank cesarean section in the standing cow

This approach can be useful if the fetus is known to be in the right uterine horn and is clearly palpable through the right flank of the mother. The operation is carried out as for the left-flank operation. The risk of escape of loops of small intestine through the laparotomy wound is greater than with the left-flank approach, which is why the latter approach is most frequently used.

Cesarean section via a ventrolateral or midline laparotomy

The special features of these approaches include the following.

Indications

Delivery of a dead emphysematous calf that cannot be delivered per vaginam or by fetotomy.

Restraint

The cow is sedated with xylazine and placed in lateral recumbency (for the ventrolateral approach) or dorsal recumbency (for the midline or paramedian approaches).

Anesthesia

For the ventrolateral approach the cow is sedated with xylazine. Local anesthesia is given by infiltration of lidocaine (lignocaine) around the proposed site of incision.

General anesthesia with endotracheal intubation is preferable for midline and paramedian approaches. Induction may be achieved using xylazine and ketamine and the animal is maintained on halothane or isoflurane. If possible, the cow should be starved (if she is eating) for 12 hours prior to surgery to reduce the risk of rumenal tympany. When surgery is urgent, as it is in most cases, starvation is seldom practical. If tracheal intubation is not available a stomach tube should be passed into the esophagus in an attempt to prevent inhalation of rumenal contents.

Sites of surgical incision and surgical techniques

Ventrolateral approach   The cow is placed on her right side with her left hindleg pulled backwards and fixed in this position by tying to a post or other suitable fixed object. The incision, 20–25 cm long, is made 8 cm lateral and parallel to the left external abdominal (milk) vein and the dorsal border of the udder (Fig. 11.9). The

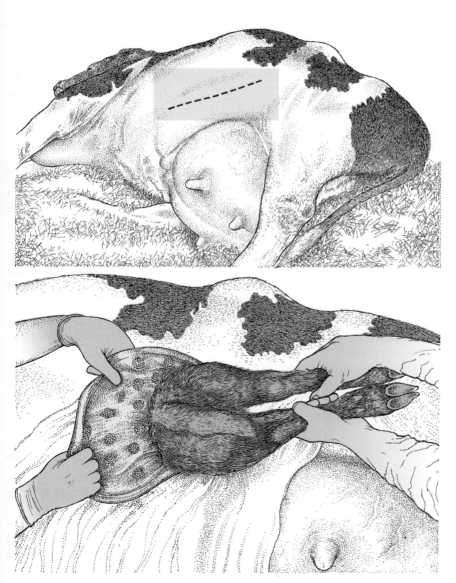

Figure 11.9 Bovine cesarean section – ventrolateral approach.

incision passes through the skin and underlying rectus abdominis muscle. The peritoneum is lifted and opened to expose the uterus, which is usually covered by omentum. The omentum is pushed forwards and the uterus exteriorized through the laparotomy incision. It is packed round with sterile drapes and opened. The fetus is removed, the uterus is closed with two rows of inverting sutures and, after lavaging with sterile saline, is returned to the abdomen. If the edges of the wound are contaminated by uterine contents they should be dissected off before closure to expose healthy, non-contaminated tissue. If septic material has accidentally spilled into the peritoneal cavity the latter should be lavaged with 2–3 liters of warm normal saline. This can be run in from a standard bag of saline and then removed by suction or baling. The abdominal incision is repaired with closure of the peritoneum, muscle, subcutis, and skin. Although an absorbable suture can be used for the internal layers, some obstetricians prefer to use a non-absorbable suture to lessen the risks of wound breakdown. Intensive antibiotic and supportive therapy is given. Intraperitoneal antibiotics, including crystalline penicillin, may help reduce the risk of infection. Fluid therapy during and after surgery is beneficial and the antiendotoxic and analgesic action of flunixin may be useful.

Midline approach   The cow is placed in dorsal recumbency with her hindlegs extended and secured. The midline incision extends 30–35 cm forwards from a point just cranial to the udder. The uterus is opened with great care, as in the previous technique, and the fetus is removed. Following fetal removal, the abdominal incision is closed with interrupted non-absorbable sutures in an attempt to avoid postoperative wound breakdown. Aftercare is as under the ventrolateral approach above.

A paramedian approach can also be used. The incision is made parallel and a few centimeters lateral to the white line.

Complications of bovine cesarean section

Peritonitis

This is always a major risk if there has been leakage of infected uterine contents, including fetal debris, during surgery. The cow may seem quite bright for up to 3 days after surgery when the signs of peritonitis develop. The cow becomes dull and pyrexic. The mucous membranes are dirty and have a toxic appearance. Appetite is absent or poor. The cow may have diarrhea and shows signs of pain and guarding when the abdomen is palpated. Respiration may be labored and accompanied by grunting. Generalized adhesions may be palpable on rectal examination. There may be a neutrophilia with left shift or a profound neutropenia as white cells are sequestered in the peritoneum. Peritoneal tap reveals profuse hypercellular fluid and sometimes frank pus. Aggressive antibiotic therapy should be prescribed. Non-steroidal anti-inflammatory therapy should also be given. Fluid therapy and peritoneal lavage may also be beneficial to the patient. Response to treatment is poor and further progressive debility requiring euthanasia may develop. Occasionally the cow is able to temporarily localize the peritonitis around her uterus. In such cases the animal may survive but chronic adhesions cause persistent inappetance, pyrexia, weight loss, and terminal debility. Infertility may be seen in cases where adhesions involving the ovary occur.

Uterine prolapse

Although uncommon after cesarean section, uterine prolapse has been seen in occasional cases. The clinical signs and treatment are as seen following a normal calving and are discussed fully in Chapter 13.

Wound breakdown

Dehiscence of tissues around the sutures, which may be caused by excessive tightening of the sutures, is another possible consequence of surgery. Breakdown occurs more commonly in the outer layers and the peritoneum normally remains intact. The animal may be bright but pyrexic for a few days prior to breakdown if infection within the abdominal wall is present. Treatment consists of local debridement of necrotic tissues and flushing any infected pockets with mild antiseptic solutions. Lavage with running water once or twice daily may also be used to clean the healing wound. Healing by second intention normally follows and resuturing is seldom indicated or desirable.

Subcutaneous emphysema

This may develop within 24 hours of surgery if the peritoneal incision has not been sealed effectively. Treatment is not necessary and spontaneous resolution normally accompanies a course of prophylactic antibiotic.

Seroma formation

This is one of the most common sequelae of cesarean section. A pocket of sterile serous fluid accumulates between muscle layers or under the skin. Its presence can be confirmed by ultrasonography when clear, non-purulent fluid is seen. Alternatively, a sterile needle tap will confirm that serum and not pus is present. Self-resolution usually occurs. The seroma should not be opened and drained as secondary infection will normally ensue. However, if the volume of fluid is very large, drainage may become necessary.

Retention of the fetal membranes

Spontaneous passage of the fetal membranes should follow within 12 hours of cesarean section even if the cervix was closed at the time of surgery. If the membranes are still present at this time manual removal later will probably be necessary as it normally is if the uterus was infected at the time of surgery. For details of fetal membrane removal, see Chapter 13.

Metritis

This condition may develop after removal of a decaying fetus or after retention of the fetal membranes. In neglected cases, metritis may already be developing before fetal delivery is attempted. The cow is usually pyrexic, anorexic, and has a foul-smelling vaginal discharge. Intensive antibiotic treatment possibly combined with non-steroidal anti-inflammatory therapy should be instituted. If the cow is toxic, uremic, or dehydrated, intravenous fluid therapy is indicated. The uterus should be explored carefully for any fetal or placental remnants, which should be removed. Uterine lavage or siphonage with warm saline may also be beneficial.

Vaginitis

Vaginitis may be caused by precesarean-section treatment of dystocia. The condition may produce straining and a foul vaginal discharge. Inspection of the vaginal mucosa will reveal severe inflammation of the mucosa and sometimes necrotic plaques. Gentle vaginal examination or rectal palpation should confirm whether concurrent uterine disease is present. Application of local emollient creams, e.g. udder cream, will reduce discomfort and encourage healing. In warm weather the possibility of blow-fly strike should be considered and prevented by application of insect repellents.

Infertility

Provided the calf was not infected and surgery was uncomplicated, a high proportion of cows that have had cesarean section will conceive again normally. Causes of infertility include chronic metritis and salpingitis with subsequent blockage of the oviducts. Uterine biopsy and oviduct dye tests can be used to confirm the diagnosis. Adhesions involving the ovary may arise if fibrosis occurs following spillage of blood at the time of surgery. Some adhesions are palpable on rectal examination and if detected early after surgery can be manually broken down. Removal of blood from the surface of the uterus and surrounding tissues at surgery is an important prophylactic action. A standard postnatal check of the cow 3 weeks after delivery of the calf is advisable.

Mastitis

This may occur after or at the time of any calving, including cesarean section. *E. coli* infection is particularly likely at this time and must be treated aggressively with intravenous antibiotic (e.g. oxytetracycline), non-steroidal anti-inflammatory and fluid therapy. Frequent stripping of the affected quarter(s) and intramammary antibiotic therapy are also used.

Sudden death

Death may occasionally and unexpectedly follow uneventful surgery. Causes include a major hemorrhage and endotoxic shock.

CESAREAN SECTION IN THE MARE

Indications

- Fractured pelvis in the mare: this may be an elective operation.
- Fetal malpresentation that cannot be manually corrected: e.g. transverse presentation, foal in 'dog sitting' position. Malpresentations in small ponies and miniature horses in which manual access to the uterus is severely complicated by lack of room.
- Torsion of the uterus, which cannot be corrected by other means.
- Fetal monsters that cannot be delivered per vaginam.

Prognosis

This is quite good for the mare if the decision to operate is made early in the dystocia and prolonged attempts at manual vaginal delivery have not been made. Other than in elective cases the foal is very likely to be dead at the start of surgery because survival during second-stage labor is short.

Anesthesia

General anesthesia is essential.

Position of the mare and selection of the operation site

A midline laparotomy is generally accepted as providing the best surgical approach to the pregnant uterus. Skilled anesthetic and surgical assistance are required. Standard preparation of the site is carried out.

Surgical technique

The skin incision and opening the abdomen

A midline incision is made from a point just caudal to the umbilicus and extending approximately 30 cm back towards the udder. The skin and subcutis may be edematous in late pregnancy. The mare's gravid uterus is fragile and must be handled with care to avoid rupture. It should be moved closer to the laparotomy incision, if necessary by the obstetrician holding a fetal part within the uterus. The uterus is opened on its ventral greater curvature over a fetal extremity.

Removal of the fetus

The fetus is removed carefully from the uterus and, if possible, held close to the mare as in normal birth so that the umbilical cord is not ruptured until 5 minutes after the establishment of fetal respiration. If (as if often the case) the foal is dead, the placenta can mostly be easily removed before uterine closure. If the placenta is still tightly attached it is left in situ but may be trimmed back to ensure it is clear of the uterine incision when this is sutured.

Closure of the uterus

Some hemorrhage from the uterine incision is to be expected and on occasion it may be profuse either during or after surgery. Any large bleeding vessels are clamped with hemostats. Before uterine closure the edges of the uterine incision are sutured to compress the layers of the uterine wall in an attempt to reduce the risk of hemorrhage (Fig. 11.10). The uterus is then

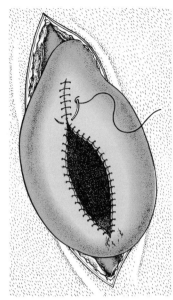

Figure 11.10 Cesarean section in the mare – before uterine closure the edges of the uterine wound are oversewn to reduce the risk of hemorrhage.

closed with a layer of inversion sutures. Any blood clots are removed from the abdomen. The peritoneal cavity may be lavaged with warm normal saline to assist in the removal of any small debris and reduce the risk of peritonitis.

Closure of the abdomen

This is carried in the standard way and non-absorbable sutures may be used to lessen the risk of postoperative herniation.

Postoperative management of the mare and foal

The foal should be dried and kept warm until the mare has recovered from anesthesia. Colostrum intake should be monitored and the navel managed in the normal way. The mare should be offered a light laxative diet and have limited but regular exercise for the first few days. Parenteral antibiotic therapy, using a broad-spectrum drug such as crystalline penicillin, should be prescribed for 5 days postsurgery. Tetanus prophylaxis should be provided for both mare and foal if there is any doubt about the mare's vaccination status or the foal's colostral uptake. Postoperative analgesia can be provided by an intravenous injection of

1.1 mg flunixin/kg body weight. If continuing analgesia is required further doses of flunixin can be given orally once daily for 2–3 days.

Postoperative complications

Ventral edema A degree of this occurs in almost every case and will usually disappear spontaneously within a few days.

Retention of the placenta Retention of the fetal membranes quite frequently follows cesarean section in the mare. If the placenta is retained at 6 hours after fetal delivery, 10–40 IU oxytocin may be given by intramuscular injection or, as an alternative method, 10–20 IU oxytocin by intravenous bolus. A further method of administration is to give 30–40 IU oxytocin in 1 liter of normal saline by intravenous drip therapy over a period of 1 hour. If the placenta is not passed within 12 hours despite this treatment, manual removal should be attempted (see Chapter 13). Antibiotic cover should be provided if this has not already been given. The use of the non-steroidal anti-inflammatory drug flunixin may also be advisable. In heavy horses placental retention must be especially carefully managed to avoid severe metritis and laminitis (for further details, see Chapter 13).

Postoperative peritonitis This is most likely to occur if the foal was dead and decomposed. The mare is extremely dull, toxemic, shows signs of colic, and abnormal fluid is found on peritoneal tap. Despite intense antibiotic therapy and nursing care the prognosis is grave. Adhesions may develop postoperatively and, if they involve the ovaries, may result in infertility.

CESAREAN SECTION IN THE EWE

Indications

1. Resolution of existing dystocia

This is as for the cow, especially in:

- Incomplete or non-dilation of the cervix (ringwomb) in which medical treatment has failed or was not attempted.
- Fetopelvic disproportion: especially in ewe lambs, which often carry a single large fetus that cannot pass the maternal pelvis.
- Fetal maldisposition that cannot be corrected by manipulation.
- Severe vaginal prolapse with traumatic damage.

2. Elective indications

These are as for the cow but especially in cases of pregnancy toxemia, which cannot be treated or are unsuitable to be treated by non-surgical methods.

Prognosis

This should be good for the ewe and lambs if the decision to go ahead with surgery is made early in the course of dystocia and prolonged attempts at vaginal delivery have not been made. In cases of pregnancy toxemia, the prognosis for survival must be very guarded if the ewe is in a moribund condition. Lamb survival is heavily influenced by their state of maturity. They are unlikely to survive if they are delivered more than 48 hours before their prospective birth date. The administration of 16 mg of dexamethasone up to 24 hours before surgery may encourage surfactant production and enhance fetal survival.

Location for surgery

In sheep-breeding areas, ewes suffering from dystocia are normally brought to the surgery for treatment, including cesarean section. In many surgeries a special treatment/operating room is available. This should provide much better facilities for good hygiene and aseptic surgery than are available on many farms. Great care must be taken when handling heavily pregnant ewes because the uterus is very fragile and can easily be ruptured.

Examination of the ewe prior to surgery

The general health of the ewe should be assessed before surgery and details of her history and the attempts at vaginal delivery by the shepherd should be ascertained. The obstetrician should always carry out a vaginal examination to ensure that the existing dystocia is still as described by the shepherd and that vaginal delivery remains impossible or inadvisable.

Evidence of fetal life can be assessed by external palpation of the abdomen, when spontaneous fetal movements may be evident, and by vaginal examination of the fetus if the cervix is open. Doppler and real-time ultrasonographic examination may also be used to monitor fetal life. They are less reliable during labor than in late pregnancy, possibly as a result of small amounts of air entering the uterus once the cervix is open.

If the fetus is dead fetotomy is very occasionally an alternative to cesarean section. The technique is only possible if access to the uterus and fetus via the cervix is possible and adequate lubrication can be provided. In neglected cases of dystocia the ewe may be moribund and unfit for surgery and euthanasia may be advisable on welfare grounds.

If the ewe is bright but toxic, supportive therapy prior to surgery may be helpful. Intravenous fluid therapy must be used carefully in sheep and goats because fatal pulmonary edema develops readily with even slight circulatory overload. Oral electrolyte fluid solutions by stomach tube at 40 mL/kg body weight per day are very effective especially if rumenal movements are present. Fluid therapy may be given to toxic animals together with antibiotic and non-steroidal anti-inflammatory therapy.

Assistance required

One person is required to restrain the sedated ewe during surgery and it is helpful to have a skilled assistant to help with surgery and lamb resuscitation.

Preparations for surgery and equipment required

Preparations and equipment are as in the cow.

Position of the ewe and selection of the operation site

Cesarean section via left-flank laparotomy with the ewe in right lateral recumbency is the technique commonly used (Fig. 11.11A) and is very satisfactory in most circumstances. A ventrolateral site can also be used (Fig. 11.11B). The advantages and disadvantages of each site are compared below.

Flank laparotomy site

Advantages   There is little risk of damage to the incision by feeding lambs and the risk of contamination is small. Healing of the skin incision is readily observed.

Disadvantages   Extensive clipping of fleece is required to expose the operation site. A full rumen may obstruct access to the uterus. Hemorrhage from the incised flank muscles may be quite heavy.

Ventrolateral laparotomy site

Advantages   Little preoperative clipping of fleece is required. Access to the uterus is not obscured by the rumen. The uterus is readily exteriorized at the time of surgery. This can play a major role in reducing peritoneal contamination at the time of surgery if infection is present within the uterus. There is very little hemorrhage from the aponeurotic muscles, which are readily repaired.

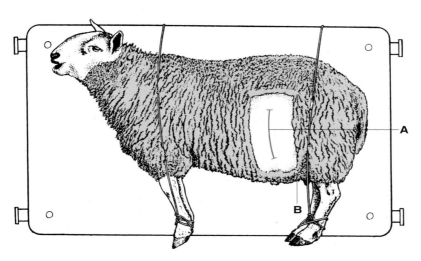

Figure 11.11 The sedated ewe is placed in lateral recumbency and is secured by tying her legs together and to the table using bale string. (A) Site of flank laparotomy, (B) site of ventrolateral laparotomy.

Disadvantages The incision is exposed to butting injuries inflicted by the feeding lambs. The wound is exposed to contamination from soiled bedding.

A midline laparotomy site can also be used but requires a general anesthetic. Access to the uterus at surgery is good. The healing incision cannot be readily observed and is at considerable risk of infection from contaminated bedding.

Restraint and sedation

Sedation is not essential but is helpful to relax the ewe during surgery, especially if help is limited. Xylazine at a dose of 0.05–0.1 mg/kg body weight by intramuscular injection has been shown to produce excellent sedation. Sedation can also be achieved using diazepam (0.1–0.2 mg/kg) either alone or with butorphenol (0.05–0.1 mg/kg). The ewe is placed in right lateral recumbency on a table and secured by tying her fore- and hindlegs together with bale string, the ends of which are used to tie her to the table (see Fig. 11.11).

Preparation of the surgical site

The wool is clipped from the whole of the left sublumbar fossa. Frequent cleaning and lubrication of the clippers may be necessary because of the high lanolin content of the wool. Plucking the wool is painful to the ewe and should not be used. The site is prepared for aseptic surgery as in the cow.

Anesthesia

Local anesthesia is normally used and may be given by local infiltration, inverted L block, or paravertebral techniques. Approximately 60 mL of 2% lidocaine (lignocaine) is required for the local infiltration technique in the average ewe. Epidural anesthesia is useful to prevent straining during surgery and 2–4 mL of 2% lidocaine (lignocaine) is injected using the space between the first and second coccygeal vertebrae.

Surgical technique

The skin incision and opening the flank

An incision approximately 15 cm long is made through the skin in the left sublumbar fossa. The incision commences approximately 10 cm below the transverse processes of the lumbar vertebrae and is equidistant from the last rib and the tuber coxae. The muscle layers (cutaneous trunci, external oblique, internal oblique, and transverse abdominis) are picked up in turn with forceps and divided with scissors. The muscle layers are thinner, have larger aponeurotic portions, and are often less vascular than in the cow. The peritoneum is opened, taking care to avoid the underlying viscera.

Locating and opening the uterus

The uterus lying behind and below the rumen is usually readily brought up to the laparotomy wound in sheep. Lambs are present in one or both horns. An incision with scalpel or scissors over a fetal extremity is made on the greater curvature of the pregnant horn (if only one horn contains a lamb). The left horn is opened if both horns are pregnant, taking care not to damage underlying fetal tissues. The exposed fetal extremity is held while its other extremities are retrieved, identified, and aligned ready for removal from the uterus. The fetus is removed from the uterus by gentle traction and is handed over to an assistant for resuscitation. If the lamb cannot be removed from the uterus with ease, the obstetrician should check again that the extremities belong to the same fetus. The uterine incision can be slightly enlarged if it is thought that fetal removal could tear the uterine wall. Any further fetuses within the first horn are delivered in a similar fashion.

Removing fetuses from the second horn

The septum between the two uterine horns in ewes extends so far caudally that it may initially seem difficult to locate the entrance to the second horn (Fig. 11.12). The hand is inserted into the now empty left horn and is directed caudally and medially behind the intercornual septum and then anteriorly into the second horn to locate any further lambs. The lamb is brought caudally and behind the septum into the left horn and is then removed from the uterus.

Ensuring that all lambs have been delivered

Multiple birth must be expected in ewes and before closing the uterus the obstetrician must ensure that no further lambs are left inside. The uterus (both horns and the body) is fully explored internally and is then – as an additional check – palpated externally from the cervix to the ends of each curved horn for evidence of any remaining offspring.

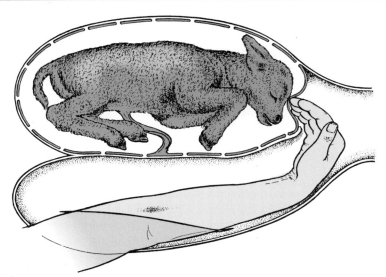

Figure 11.12 Cesarean section in the ewe – removal of a fetus from the second uterine horn (see text).

Repairing and closing the uterus

Any detached or readily detachable placenta is removed before uterine closure. Any attached placenta is left in situ, even in cases where cesarean section has been performed to alleviate dystocia due to ringwomb. In such cases, the cervix usually opens some hours after surgery and the placenta is delivered. The uterine incision is repaired with a single continuous layer of inversion sutures using absorbable suture material. Before wound closure, great care is taken to remove any blood or uterine debris from the peritoneal cavity.

The laparotomy incision

The incision is repaired layer by layer with continuous sutures using an absorbable suture. The skin wound is closed with interrupted horizontal mattress sutures using monofilament or braided nylon.

Resuscitation of the lambs

The general approach used is as in the calf (see p. 181). Immediately after delivery the lamb is suspended upside down and shaken to encourage loss of mucus from the mouth and pharynx. It may also be swung carefully to and fro, but the obstetrician must retain a tight grip to avoid dropping the lamb, which is often slippery from natural and artificial lubricants.

Artificial respiration, if required, must be applied gently and with great care. Fractures of the ribs and rupture of the liver are readily sustained. Mouth-to-mouth respiration must never be used in lambs because a number of unpleasant zoonotic diseases can be contracted in this way. Doxapram hydrochloride (5–10 mg) may be given by intravenous or subcutaneous injection, or sublingual placement to stimulate respiration. For further discussion of resuscitation of the lamb, see Chapter 6.

Postoperative management of the ewe and lamb

This is in many ways similar to the management that follows an assisted lambing. The lamb's navel is dressed with antibiotic spray or dipped in a weak iodine solution and the milk supply of the ewe, including teat patency, is checked. Sometimes, after cesarean section, the ewe seems reluctant to accept and mother its lambs. Gentle vaginal dilation of the ewe using the lubricated hand and smearing the lamb with maternal vaginal mucus immediately before it is presented to its mother may help establish the bond. Prophylactic antibiotic therapy with a long-acting preparation is normally given to the ewe and skin sutures are removed 14 days postoperatively. Postoperative analgesia can be provided by the intravenous injection of flunixin at a dose of 2.2 mg/kg.

Postoperative complications

Complications are relatively uncommon in ewes but those conditions affecting wound healing etc. (described in the cow, see p. 184) are occasionally seen and are treated in the same way. Manual removal of the retained placenta is not normally attempted but antibiotic cover is provided until natural separation occurs. Any trailing portions of placenta are cut off.

The placenta must be removed from the lambing pen to prevent the ewe from choking when trying to eat it. Observant management should enable any problems to be picked up quickly and dealt with effectively.

Wool break may occur within 1 to 4 weeks of surgery, probably as a result of stress. The entire fleece is cast leaving the ewe without any wool, but regrowth is evident within a few weeks.

CESAREAN SECTION IN THE DOE GOAT

Indications are as in the ewe and include failure of the cervix to dilate, fetopelvic disproportion – seen especially in first kidders – and cases of misalliance. The operation may also be indicated in selected cases of pregnancy toxemia in does.

A left-flank laparotomy with the doe sedated and placed in right lateral recumbency is a very satisfactory approach. Local anesthesia is used, as in the ewe. Xylazine provides good sedation but the goat is extremely susceptible to this drug and the dose is only 0.01 mg/kg body weight by intramuscular injection; diazepam and butorphenol may also be used as sedatives. The doe is less phlegmatic than the ewe and it may be helpful to have the owner or a familiar attendant restraining the patient's head as she lies in lateral recumbency. If the doe is very quiet she may be operated on while standing. Kids may occupy both horns of the uterus. It may be possible to remove all the kids through one uterine incision. In some cases, if entry to the second horn through the uterine incision is difficult, it is advisable to make a second incision into that horn after repairing the first.

As an alternative, general anesthesia can be employed. Anesthesia is induced with xylazine and ketamine, and maintained with halothane or isofluorane following endotracheal intubation. A midline laparotomy or a flank approach to the uterus may be used under general anesthesia. The midline approach is preferred if the kids are known or thought to be dead. In such cases, every effort must be made to avoid peritoneal contamination during surgery. Antibiotic therapy should be commenced prior to surgery. If any infected uterine contents are spilled accidentally they should be removed and peritoneal lavage carried out before abdominal closure.

Over 80% of goat pregnancies involve more than one fetus and great care must be taken to ensure that all fetuses are removed at the time of surgery.

Postoperative analgesia greatly aids recovery and is achieved by the intravenous injection of flunixin at a suggested dose of 2.2 mg/kg.

CESAREAN SECTION IN THE SOW

Indications

1. Resolution of existing dystocia

- Fetopelvic disproportion: especially in gilts with a numerically small litter. Previous pelvic fracture with healing exostoses may severely reduce the pelvic diameter.
- Uterine inertia that is not responsive to ecbolic therapy. In cases of toxemic primary uterine inertia, hysterectomy may have a slightly better prognosis than cesarean section. The prognosis for recovery is poor with both techniques and the economics of such cases should be carefully discussed with the owner before surgery.
- Obstruction of the birth canal that cannot be treated by other means.
- Severe vaginal prolapse, possibly complicated by rectal prolapse with existing mucosal damage.
- Damage to the birth canal caused by lay attempts at delivery.

2. Elective indications

Cesarean section may be used as an alternative to hysterectomy in the production of gnotobiotic piglets.

Prognosis and examination of the sow prior to surgery

The prognosis should be quite good if the piglets are alive and the sow appears well. If the piglets are dead and the sow is toxemic the prognosis should be extremely guarded and surgery should not be undertaken. A poor prognosis is likely in cases where the sow has been in labor for more than 12 hours. Toxemia is most likely to arise from the presence of dead piglets within the uterus or from a disease process such as acute mastitis. A careful clinical examination should be carried out before surgery to ensure that the sow is in good health. If toxemia is present the sow may have a subnormal temperature, be weak, have purple blotches on the skin of the ears, neck and perineum, and if stimulated to move may utter a thin reedy squeal.

Position of the sow and selection of the operation site

The sow is normally placed in lateral recumbency and a right or left laparotomy is performed.

Anesthesia

The temperament of the sow is such that general anesthesia is *essential* for cesarean section. Sedation prior to induction of anesthesia may be required in nervous patients. Unfortunately, most of the sedative and anesthetic agents available have a sedative effect on the unborn piglet. Induction by thiopentone and maintenance on isoflurane may be used in the field. If the sow is toxic, an epidural anesthetic can be used; 10–15 mL 2% lidocaine (lignocaine) is injected into the lumbosacral space.

Surgical technique

A skin incision approximately 20 cm is made horizontally in the flank about 5 cm above the lateral edge of the udder (Fig. 11.13). Alternatively, a vertical incision higher up in the flank may be used. The muscles of the flank wall are split carefully with scissors. There is often a layer of dense fat immediately outside the peritoneum and this should be separated carefully to expose and lift the peritoneum from the underlying viscera before opening the abdomen. In neglected cases, a considerable amount of peritoneal fluid may escape from the abdomen when the peritoneum is opened.

The bifurcation of the uterine horns is located and the nearest horn is gently pulled out of the laparotomy wound. Tearing of the fragile uterus is avoided by grasping a fetus through the uterine horn and using this grip to exteriorize the horn.

A longitudinal incision is made in the horn near the bifurcation and the first piglet is removed. Further piglets are brought back to the uterine wound by reaching inside the horn or by squeezing the uterus externally to push each piglet back to the wound. In some cases it may be possible to remove the fetuses in the second horn via the same incision. It is often easier to repair the first incision with a layer of continuous Lembert sutures using an absorbable suture. The first horn is replaced in the abdomen and another incision is made into the second horn. Fetuses are removed from this horn in the same way. Any placenta that is easily detached is gently removed by traction, taking care not to telescope the uterine horn. If the placenta cannot be detached it is left in situ.

Before closing the uterus the obstetrician must examine the uterine body and the vagina via the uterine incision to ensure that no piglets are present. The whole length of each horn from ovary to bifurcation must also be palpated before closure to ensure that it is empty. After closure the uterus is gently wiped to remove any blood before repairing the laparotomy incision.

The muscle layers are repaired in turn with an absorbable suture taking care to avoid trapping fat between the sutures. The skin is repaired with braided nylon.

Postoperative care of the sow and litter

The piglets must be kept warm, especially if they have been sedated by the anesthetic. Milk let-down should be encouraged using 20 IU of oxytocin given by intramuscular injection. In some studies up to 50% mortality has been recorded in the piglets after cesarean section and they must be monitored carefully to ensure

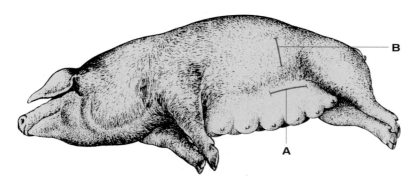

Figure 11.13 Cesarean section in the sow. The incision is made horizontally in the flank approximately 5 cm above the lateral edge of the udder (**A**). An alternative approach is via the flank (**B**).

they are warm and well fed. Any problems, such as *E. coli* septicemia in the piglets, or agalactia and mastitis in the sow, must be dealt with immediately. The sow should be given an injection of a long-acting preparation of an antibiotic such as ampicillin. Postoperative analgesia is provided by the intramuscular injection of ketoprofen at a dose of 3 mg/kg bodyweight.

CESAREAN SECTION IN THE DOG AND CAT

Indications

Cesarean section must be considered whenever other methods of treatment have failed to achieve fetal delivery. Specific indications include:

- Uterine inertia that fails to respond to ecbolic therapy.
- Fetopelvic disproportion failing to respond to other treatment methods.
- Obstruction of the birth canal.
- Fetal malpresentation that cannot be corrected.
- Evidence that fetal life is becoming compromised.

Other indications include:

- *Convenience for the practice*: convenience for the practice should not be a serious indication for surgery. Faced with a busy consulting period ahead and a slowly progressing case of uterine inertia, it is tempting to operate to 'bring the case to a conclusion' or to 'save time' by performing cesarean section. Of course, if there is evidence of fetal distress in a case of uterine inertia then immediate surgery is indicated. However, a number of cesarean sections are performed for reasons other than those indicated strictly by good obstetric practice.
- *Elective cesarean section*: elective cesarean sections are sometimes performed prophylactically when the mother has a history of severe dystocia accompanied by fetal death at her previous birth. Ethically, this type of operative interference is questionable. Attempting to breed from an animal that is unlikely to be able to give birth without help cannot really be justified. However, the decision not to breed should have been taken before permitting mating and, unfortunately, the obstetrician is often presented with a *fait accompli* and may have to agree to operate in the interests of the patient.

Timing of surgery

Once a decision has been made to deliver the litter by cesarean section the operation should be carried out without delay. It is essential, at all times, to ensure that an adequate surgical team is available to cope with any emergencies that may arise during the operation.

Preferably, surgery should not be performed before late first-stage or early second-stage labor because operating before this time can result in excessive placental-site hemorrhage and in the delivery of dysmature offspring. However, in cases where whelping is overdue, an elective cesarean section may be necessary.

Prognosis

The following guidelines for prognosis have been suggested in relation to the duration of second-stage labor when surgery is performed in the bitch (they are also generally applicable to the cat):

- *Before 6 hours*: good for bitch and pups, although placental separation may have occurred in the first puppy.
- *6–12 hours*: good for bitch and pups but the first pups are unlikely to survive.
- *12–24 hours*: good for bitch, some pups may be dead.
- *24–36 hours*: fair to good for bitch, poor for most pups.
- *36+ hours*: guarded for bitch, very poor for pups.

In practice, it may be difficult to establish exactly when second-stage labor started in a dystocia case. In these circumstances the prognosis – especially for puppy survival – should be guarded.

Anesthesia

Although local and epidural anesthetic techniques can be used for cesarean section, general anesthesia is more satisfactory in most respects. Almost all anesthetic and sedative agents will cross the placenta and have some adverse effect upon the fetus. The barbiturates are excreted by the liver, which, being poorly supplied with enzymes in the neonate, is slow to remove these drugs. The problem of delayed excretion is especially severe in those fetuses that were somewhat anoxic before surgery. It must be said, however, that some authors report excellent results with barbiturate anesthesia. However, the longer the puppies or kittens are exposed to the anesthetic agent, the more they are affected by it.

Preparations for surgery such as clipping are better done before induction of anesthesia to reduce the exposure time of the fetuses to sedative and anesthetic agents before delivery.

Fluid therapy is advisable if the bitch or queen is toxic and has been in prolonged labor. Fluid therapy also helps support the maternal circulation during and after surgery.

Gaseous anesthetics are excreted rapidly via the respiratory system in both kittens and puppies and are probably the safest anesthetic agents for cesarean section. In amenable patients, masking down with isoflurane followed by intubation and maintenance with isoflurane and oxygen produces satisfactory anesthesia.

In large bitches or excitable animals, induction with thiopental at minimum dose may be used followed by isoflurane maintenance. Saffan (a steroidal preparation of alphaxalone and alphadolone acetate) can be used for induction in the cat. Propofol is also a valuable intravenous agent for anesthesia in both the dog and cat. Halothane may reduce the activity of uterine muscle and postoperative administration of oxytocin to encourage uterine involution is advisable.

A good supply of oxygen must be maintained throughout surgery, and during the induction period, to ensure that fetal life is not compromised. Intubation is helpful in the heavily pregnant mother, in whom the tidal volume of respiration may be reduced by the large uterus pressing on the diaphragm.

In neglected cases, appropriate fluid therapy may be required before, during, and after surgery.

The weight of the pregnant uterus may compromise venous return via the caudal vena cava during surgery. The risks of this problem are avoided by not having the mother lying completely on her back during surgery. She should be tilted 30° to one side of the vertical.

Recovery from general anesthetic must be monitored carefully. Vomiting may occur in the recovery phase – as it may during induction – if the stomach was full at the time of surgery. Preoperative starving is seldom possible in emergency cesarean section cases.

For a fuller discussion on anesthesia for cesarean section, readers are referred to Hall, Clarke & Trim (2003).

Surgical technique

A midline approach to the abdomen is generally favored and, on opening the abdomen, the uterus is

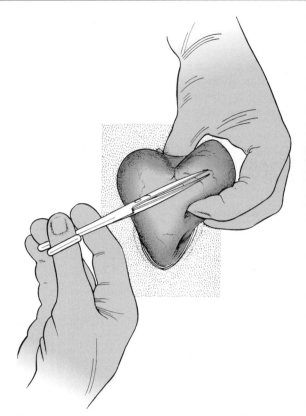

Figure 11.14 Cesarean section in the bitch – the uterus is opened at the junction of the body and one horn.

wholly or partially exteriorized and is packed off to ensure minimum contamination of the peritoneum by uterine contents.

The uterus is opened on the ventral surface of its body or at the junction of body and one horn (Fig. 11.14). Great care must be taken when opening the uterus that an underlying fetus is not also accidentally incised. The first fetus is gently withdrawn from the uterus within its amnion (Fig. 11.15) after entering its chorioallantoic sac. The amnion is then removed from the fetal head and body. The umbilical cord is clamped and severed 2 cm away from the navel with artery forceps and the fetus handed to an assistant for further care and resuscitation. Mucus is gently shaken from the mouth or removed by suction (Fig. 11.16). The fetus is dried in a towel – this activity can stimulate respiration and movement and almost immediately, in the healthy fetus, a cry is heard. Gently blowing into the mouth, which raises the carbon dioxide level in inspired air,

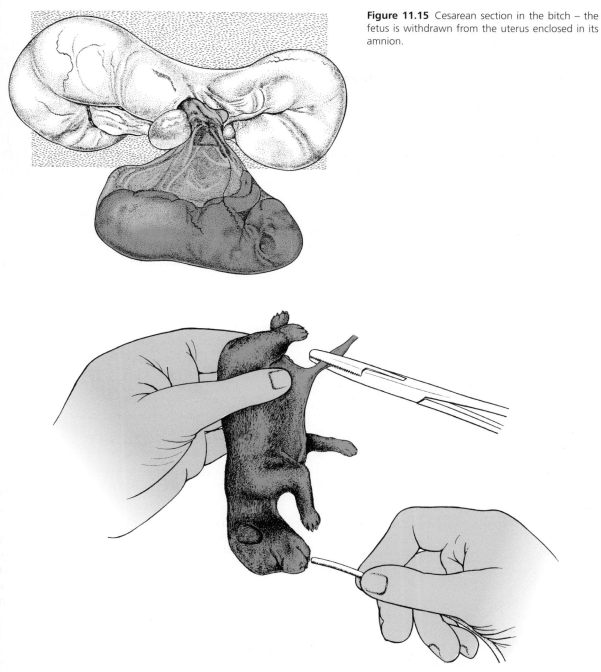

Figure 11.15 Cesarean section in the bitch – the fetus is withdrawn from the uterus enclosed in its amnion.

Figure 11.16 Cesarean section in the bitch – clamping the cord and resuscitating the puppy.

also has a stimulatory action. In difficult cases, drug therapy may be needed; 1–5 mg of doxapram hydrochloride can be placed under the tongue of each fetus to stimulate respiration.

Attempts are made to remove each placenta of each fetus by careful traction (Fig. 11.17), but if difficulty is experienced or fresh hemorrhage is provoked the placenta should be left in situ to be expelled later – possibly assisted postoperatively by ecbolic therapy. Subsequent fetuses from each horn are gently pushed along towards the uterine incision from whence they are removed. In most cases, all fetuses can be removed from a single uterine incision. Occasionally the obstetrician may find it easier to gain fetal access by making an incision into the second uterine horn after closing the first.

Before the uterus is closed it must be checked to ensure that no offspring have been left behind. The whole genital tract must be checked, including the caudal uterine body and intrapelvic vagina. Inverting Lembert sutures of an absorbable suture material are used to close the uterus, ensuring that any small portions of placenta do not compromise the wound edges (Fig. 11.18). Any traces of blood must be removed from the outer surface of the uterus in an attempt to prevent postoperative adhesions. The abdomen is closed in the normal way and a small gauze pad may be affixed onto the skin wound to protect it from direct contact with the offspring.

Postnatal care of the bitch and queen and their litters

Antibiotic cover and analgesia should be provided and preferably commenced prior to surgery. The bitch or queen should be allowed to recover from anesthesia before the litter is introduced. Full recovery from surgery is normally rapid and uneventful.

Postoperative analgesia can be provided by the administration of an NSAID after recovery from anesthesia. A range of NSAIDs is available for the dog and cat. Preoperative administration is safe in most cases. Carprofen can be used in both species (dose: 2–4 mg/kg by subcutaneous injection). The drug may be administered orally if further treatment is required. If the patient is experiencing severe pain, the obstetrician should try to ascertain the cause and deal with it. Opioids can be used to provide additional analgesia. Butorphanol at a dose of 0.2–0.6 mg/kg can be given by intramuscular or subcutaneous injection in both cats and dogs. Pethidine and morphine can be used in both cats and dogs.

The owner should be encouraged to monitor the animal's progress closely, and to monitor that of her litter postoperatively. The bitch or queen should initially be offered small quantities of good-quality food at frequent intervals and should be encouraged to leave the litter for moderate exercise at intervals during the day.

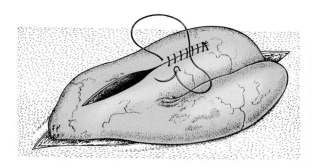

Figure 11.18 Cesarean section in the bitch – the uterus is closed using inverting Lembert sutures.

Figure 11.17 Cesarean section in the bitch – an attempt is made to remove each placenta by careful traction.

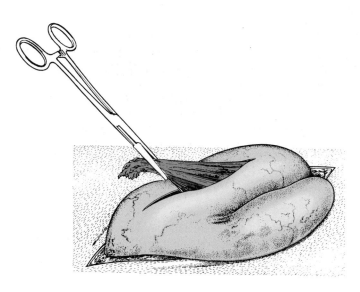

Water should be available on an *ad lib* basis. The laparotomy incision normally heals rapidly and is not damaged by the activities of the feeding litter. The postoperative problems that occur after normal birth can also occur following cesarean section (see Chapter 14).

The litter should be dried carefully and completely before being placed in warm box (optimum ambient temperature is 29°C) to await the recovery of their mother. The umbilical cords should have been crushed or ligated at the time of delivery; they should be observed at intervals for signs of hemorrhage and further ligation applied if necessary. It is not normally necessary to feed the puppies or kittens before they receive their mother's colostrum. Artificial milk can be offered by dropper if recovery of the dam is delayed. The offspring should be introduced carefully to their mother, in case she shows unexpected signs of aggression towards them. Crushing injury to the offspring can be caused if the dam is unsteady on her legs. Milk production after cesarean section is normally good. Supplementary feeding should be introduced if there is

evidence of hunger or poor growth among the offspring. Owners should be advised to report any problems in either mother or offspring without delay.

Hysterectomy

This may prove necessary if the uterus is found to be damaged or if the uterine contents are putrefied. Owners who do not wish to breed from their animal again may request an ovarohysterectomy, which is performed at the time of cesarean section. This procedure is well tolerated by most healthy animals and the patient's milk supply is normally maintained. However, some obstetricians prefer to limit surgery to cesarean section, to be followed – after the litter has been weaned – by ovarohysterectomy.

In a cat in which dystocia has not been observed, a fetus may be found impacted in the body of the uterus and cervix. Fetal death and decay may have occurred and hysterectomy is indicated. The presence of the

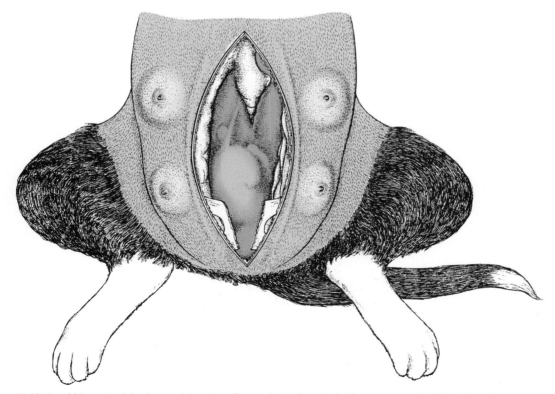

Figure 11.19 Dead kitten stuck in the caudal vagina of a queen cat (see text). The queen's pubic bones have been removed for clarity of illustration.

kitten makes normal cervical ligation impossible. Fluid therapy prior to and during surgery is essential. In such cases the fetus, despite its state, *must* be removed and the uterus must be opened to allow this, with great care being exercised to prevent peritoneal contamination (Fig. 11.19). When the kitten has been carefully removed the cervix can be ligated and the stump omentalized. The uterus is removed after ovarian artery ligation. Despite the difficulties, such cases usually have a favorable prognosis, if the cat is helped – when necessary – by appropriate fluid therapy. A program of antibiotic cover and non-steroidal anti-inflammatory therapy should be commenced prior to surgery.

REFERENCES

Flecknell PA, Waterman-Pearson A (eds) 2000 Pain management in animals. WB Saunders, London

Hall LW, Clarke KW, Trim CM 2003 Veterinary anaesthesia, 10th edn. WB Saunders, London

Chapter 12

FETOTOMY

'Fetotomy' (often termed 'embryotomy') is the term used to describe methods of dividing a fetus, which cannot be delivered, into small pieces that will more readily pass through the birth canal. The technique should be used only when the fetus is known to be dead. Fetotomy is used most commonly in cattle, occasionally in horses, rarely in sheep and goats, and almost never in pigs and small animals. Fetotomy can be complete, when a whole fetus is divided into smaller pieces, or partial, when a small part of the fetus, such as a leg, is removed.

Two techniques of fetotomy are available – percutaneous and subcutaneous:

- In *percutaneous fetotomy* a tubular embryotome is used, through which a flexible wire saw is passed. The wire saw is used to cut through the fetus while the embryotome protects the maternal tissues from damage.
- In *subcutaneous fetotomy* parts of the fetus are dissected out from within its skin, thus reducing fetal bulk and allowing delivery of the remainder through the birth canal.

Percutaneous fetotomy is the preferred method unless the fetus is in a very decomposed state and can readily be broken up by hand.

INDICATIONS

- The relief of dystocia caused by fetal maldisposition that cannot be corrected by manipulative means.
- The relief of dystocia caused by fetopelvic disproportion in which the fetus is dead and cannot be removed by traction. The fetus may be normal but oversized or it may be abnormal as a fetal monster.
- The relief of dystocia caused by the fetus becoming stuck during delivery – for example in the cow when stifle lock (sometimes termed 'hip lock') occurs after the head and part of the fetal thorax have been delivered.
- During cesarean section when the dead fetus is either too large to remove from the uterus in the normal way, is deformed, or is in a maldisposition that cannot be corrected.

THE FETOTOMY/CESAREAN SECTION DEBATE

The obstetrician must decide which of these two techniques to use:

- Fetotomy should be considered only when the fetus is known to be dead.
- Cesarean section *must* be used when the fetus is known or believed to be alive.

The extent of the fetotomy likely to be required is another very important factor, as is the accessibility of the fetus to the obstetrician. If a moderately sized dead fetus has a lateral deviation of the head that cannot be corrected manually and the birth canal is sufficiently dilated for the obstetrician to gain easy access to the base of the fetal neck, then fetotomy is indicated. The fetal neck is sectioned to allow delivery of the deviated head followed by the remainder of the fetus. If the fetus is in the same maldisposition but the cervix is only partially dilated – making access to the fetus extremely difficult – fetotomy may be impossible. In such circumstances cesarean section, even though the fetus is dead, may be the best or even the only solution.

Other considerations include the experience of the obstetrician and the availability of equipment. A complete fetotomy in a restricted space can be an extremely demanding and time-consuming procedure for even the experienced obstetrician. The longer and more complicated the fetotomy, the greater the risk of maternal damage and infection. It has been suggested that, ideally, a fetotomy should involve no more than six cuts with the embryotome and should not take more than an hour to complete. If it is thought that these limits cannot be observed then cesarean section may provide the best course of action.

The inexperienced obstetrician may feel happier to embark on the more familiar technique of cesarean section, although the prognosis of this technique is poorer when the fetus is dead. If the obstetrician is unsure of his or her competence to embark on either technique, further professional assistance should be sought. A partial fetotomy is normally quite a simple procedure and having successfully completed a number of such cases the obstetrician may feel happier to take on more complicated cases.

A good tubular embryotome with all its accessories is essential for successful fetotomy. Although in an emergency fetotomy can be performed without an embryotome, the risk of damage to the mother is much greater.

In some circumstances there may be no alternative to fetotomy. An example of this – which is probably the most common indication for bovine fetotomy – is when the obstetrician must deliver a bovine fetus stuck in stifle lock. In most cases the calving has been unattended and the dead fetus is found with its head and part of the thorax protruding from the cow's vagina (see Fig. 4.22). It cannot be delivered by traction and it cannot be repelled into the uterus so that cesarean section could be performed. Fetotomy provides the only answer and, in most examples of this problem, can be completed without difficulty even by the inexperienced but well-equipped obstetrician.

In all cases the condition of the mother is of paramount importance. In both fetotomy and cesarean section the prognosis of a successful outcome is closely related to the duration of the dystocia. The longer an animal suffers from dystocia before treatment is commenced, the poorer the prognosis.

A number of surveys have compared the success of fetotomy and cesarean section, with somewhat conflicting results in terms both of recovery from the procedure and future fertility. The best results are likely to be achieved by a skilled obstetrician who has made an early decision to proceed with either technique in a healthy patient in a clean environment.

EQUIPMENT

It is essential to have all the necessary equipment available before embarking on a fetotomy (Fig. 12.1). The following items are required:

- Standard parturition equipment for the species: including protective clothing for the obstetrician, ample supplies of obstetric lubricant, and facilities to administer epidural anesthesia.

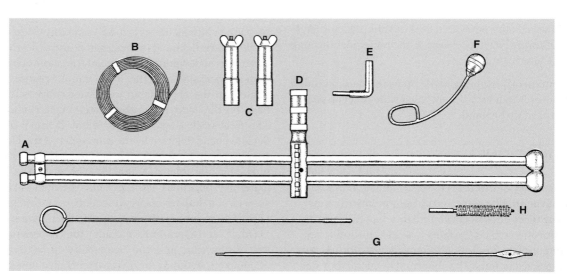

Figure 12.1 Fetotomy equipment. (A) Tubular embryotome, (B) fetotomy wire, (C) handles for wire, (D) handle for embryotome, (E) screw to tighten handle, (F) introducer, (G) threader, (H) cleaning brush.

- A tubular embryotome: the double-tubed 'Danish' embryotome is the most popular but other models may be available in some practices. The embryotome plays a vital part in protecting the birth canal from the cutting action of the wire saw. Two pieces of strong rubber tubing can be used in an emergency, but are much less satisfactory than the embryotome.
- A roll (and a spare) of fetotomy wire.
- A pair of wire-cutting pliers to remove the required length of wire from the roll.
- Handles to attach to the ends of the wire: either special metal handles supplied with the embryotome or, if these are not available, two short lengths of broom handle.
- A threader to pull the wire through the tubes of the embryotome. This is a vital piece of equipment – it may be impossible to thread the flexible wire through the embryotome without it.
- A metal introducer to attach to the end of the fetotomy wire while it is passed around the part of the fetus to be sectioned. A number of introducers are available but any fairly heavy small object to which the wire may be readily attached will be satisfactory.
- One or more fetotomy hooks. Among the most useful are Krey's self-tightening hooks, which grip fetal tissues more tightly as traction is applied using a rope or chain attached to the hooks.

All equipment must be cleaned thoroughly before and after use and should be sterilized if it is to be used during cesarean section. The perineal area of the patient is thoroughly washed before commencing fetotomy and every effort must be made throughout the procedure to keep contamination to a minimum.

ASSISTANCE REQUIRED AND RESTRAINT OF THE PATIENT

At least one person, and ideally two, is required to restrain the patient and to assist the obstetrician. The patient is secured as for normal assisted delivery. Fetotomy is more easily carried out in the standing patient but if she is unable or unwilling to rise the obstetrician must deal with her in the recumbent position. An epidural anesthetic is useful to stop the patient straining. A larger dose of epidural may be helpful in the recumbent patient and in such animals access to the uterus may be facilitated by slightly raising the hindquarters. Relaxation of the uterine musculature may be achieved by the use of clenbuterol. Sedation may be required in

some animals and a general anesthetic may be necessary in some mares, especially if a prolonged procedure is anticipated.

THE TECHNIQUE OF PERCUTANEOUS FETOTOMY

The use of the embryotome

The fetotomy wire must be threaded through one or both tubes of the instrument before use:

- If the fetal part to be sectioned is directly accessible (e.g. the head of a calf in normal anterior presentation) both tubes are threaded, the handles are attached and the loop of wire at the end of the tubes is placed around the part in question.
- If the fetal part to be sectioned is not directly accessible and the wire cannot be looped around it (e.g. a forelimb in shoulder flexion), only one tube of the embryotome is threaded. The other end of the wire is attached to the introducer, which is passed around the part to be sectioned and pulled out of the birth canal before being passed through the second tube of the embryotome.

Placement of the wire in all cases is facilitated by generous use of obstetric lubricant. Two liters or more should be instilled into the uterus and topped up as required. Once in position, the wire is pulled tight and the obstetrician carefully checks its position. Sawing is commenced by the assistant using long strokes. The embryotome is held firmly in position by the obstetrician. Initially the wire may take a little time to engage in the skin of the part being sectioned and short sawing strokes are used at this stage. Muscle is readily sawn through but more effort is required for bony tissue. The efficiency of sawing is increased if the part to be sectioned is under a little tension and if the embryotome can be held still as the wire is engaging. If the fetal head is being removed by sectioning the neck this tension can be supplied by applying moderate traction to the head using a calving rope applied in the normal way or using self-tightening hooks engaged in the flesh of the fetus.

Occasionally the wire breaks as it is being used, especially if it has been used before. In such cases the embryotome must be re-threaded and the process started again. The risk of breakage is reduced by using a length of wire in good condition and avoiding the development of kinks in the wire by keeping it under slight tension at all times once it is threaded through the embryotome.

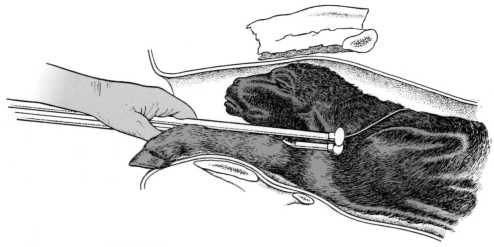

Figure 12.2 Fetotomy – removal of the head.

Progress may be checked manually by the obstetrician at intervals, who must ensure that the assistant does not move the wire saw while checking is taking place. If possible, the obstetrician should ensure that the fetotomy wire does not come in contact with the uterine wall. This may be done by trying to hold the uterine wall away from the head of the embryotome.

Once the fetal part has been cut through the movements of the wire will suddenly encounter much less resistance. The embryotome is then removed and the sectioned fetal part is retrieved and removed. In most cases bone will have been sectioned and great care must be taken during removal to ensure that the birth canal is not damaged by sharp bony fragments.

Complete fetotomy

Fetus in anterior presentation

Removal of the head

- If protruding from the vulva: attach a rope to the head and simply cut the head off with a stout knife or scalpel by disarticulating the neck as low down and close to the shoulders as possible.
- If within the vagina: loop the fetotomy wire over the head and back along to the base of the neck. Saw through as close to the shoulders as possible (Fig. 12.2).

Removal of a foreleg   A loop of fetotomy wire is passed along the leg to be removed. The loop is guided over the top of the scapula. The threaded embryotome is brought up on the medial aspect of the leg (Fig. 12.3). Sawing is commenced, with frequent checks that the position of the wire and progress are satisfactory. The wire is sometimes difficult to keep in position over the top of the scapula – making a small incision in the skin between the scapula and the withers with scalpel or knife may help.

An alternative technique using acute-angle sawing with the embryotome can be used to remove a foreleg. The threaded embryotome is passed forwards along the lateral aspect of the limb to be removed to just beyond the dorsal edge of the scapula. The loop of the wire is on the medial aspect of the limb. The wire is tightened and sawing is commenced holding the embryotome firmly in position just dorsal to the scapula. The wire saws through the tissues between the limb and the chest wall. With this method there is less risk that the embryotomy wire will fail to cut between the scapula and the fetal chest wall. There is a slightly increased risk that the embryotomy wire may break.

Further fetotomy   Having removed one forelimb and the head it may then be necessary to remove the other forelimb. The procedure already described is repeated on the second leg.

Removal of the thorax   The next stage is to remove the thorax of the calf by sawing the body across caudal to the ribs in the lumbar region. A generous loop of wire threaded through the embryotome is worked carefully over the thorax using plenty of lubrication and easing it forward a little bit at a time. The embryotome is introduced into the vagina and the wire tightened. The point of section must be caudal to the last rib

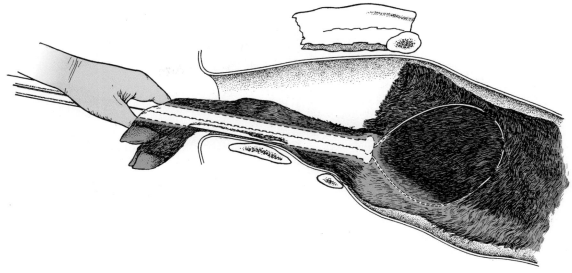

Figure 12.3 Fetotomy – removal of a forelimb.

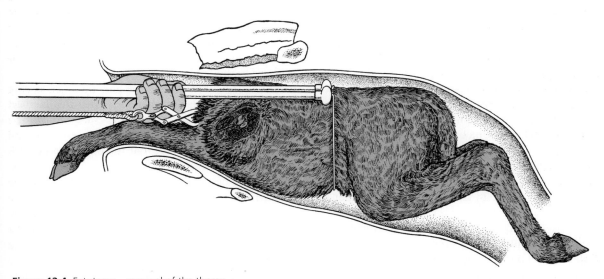

Figure 12.4 Fetotomy – removal of the thorax.

(Fig. 12.4). Once the body has been sectioned the thorax can be gently removed. The fetal abdominal viscera will have been exposed and are removed manually.

If the fetus is large it may be necessary to remove the fetal thorax in two parts. The first transverse incision is made just caudal to the attachment of the forelimbs and the second caudal to the last rib. If the fetal rib cage separated by the two transverse incisions is too wide to pass through the pelvic canal it may be partially collapsed by making a longitudinal incision with the embryotome at the junction of the ribs and the thoracic vertebrae on one side.

Division of the pelvis   The rear end of the calf remains in the uterus after removal of the thorax. The severed lumbar vertebrae are sharp and care must be exercised to prevent them damaging the uterus. Although it may occasionally be possible to remove the remainder of the calf without further section,

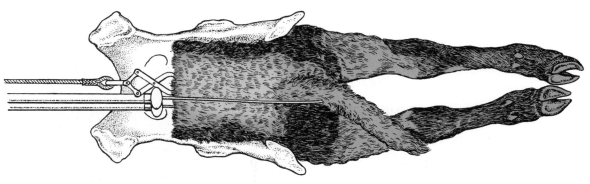

Figure 12.5 Fetotomy – splitting the pelvis (dorsal view).

it is mostly necessary to divide the pelvic girdle longitudinally so that the caudal part of the calf may be removed in two smaller parts.

A length of wire is threaded through one tube of the embryotome and is attached to an introducer. The introducer is carried into the uterus and is dropped over the dorsal aspect of the rear end of the fetus as near to the fetal midline as possible. The obstetrician seeks the introducer beneath the ventral aspect of the rear end of the calf. The hand is introduced between the hindlegs of the fetus as they extend anteriorly in the uterus. Once the introducer with wire attached is located it is pulled out with its attached wire placed between the hindlegs of the calf. The introducer is removed from the end of the wire, which is then pulled through the embryotome using the threader. The wire is tightened and the embryotome is placed against the anterior surface of the fetal pelvis (Fig. 12.5). Sawing is commenced, having made certain 'by checking at intervals' that the wire is going to cut between the ischial tuberosities of the pelvis. This will ensure that the pelvis is divided into two roughly equal parts. Sectioning the pelvis may be helped by holding it in position by applying traction to it through a pair of self-tightening hooks. When the hind end is divided, one half at a time is removed, taking care to protect the dam from damage from the exposed sawn-through and pelvic edges.

Fetus in posterior presentation

Hindlimb removal   A loop of fetotomy wire is passed up the limb so that the end of the loop lies anterior and medial to the wing of the fetal ilium. A small incision in the skin with a scalpel will help the wire saw to become embedded here. The head of the embryotome is placed between the fetal ischial tuberosities and the loop

arranged so that the cut includes the tail – a procedure that will stop the tendency for the wire to slip down the leg.

An alternative method using acute-angle sawing with the embryotome may be used to remove the hindlimb. The threaded embryotome is passed along the lateral aspect of the limb to be removed to just beyond the tuber coxae on that side. The wire loop passes up the medial aspect of the limb. Sawing is commenced and the embryotome is held firmly just anterior to the fetal tuber coxae (Fig. 12.6). The wire sections the fetal pelvis and the limb attached to part of the pelvis is carefully removed. With this method it may be easier to ensure that the embryotomy incision is on the medial aspect of the tuber coxae. There is a slightly increased risk that the embryotomy wire may break.

Should it be necessary the other hindlimb can be similarly removed. The body of the calf can then be divided in the lumbar region or further forward by passing a loop of wire forward as already described for anterior presentation. Forelegs can be removed with the aid of the introducer to put the wire over the shoulder joint, i.e. between the neck and the forelimb. Alternatively, the anterior part of the body can be divided longitudinally.

Partial fetotomy

This technique may be required to facilitate delivery of a dead fetus in which manual correction of maldisposition has proved impossible.

Deviation of the head   The fetotomy wire is passed around the base of the neck using an introducer. The base of the neck is sectioned as low down as possible and the head and part of the neck are removed (Fig. 12.7).

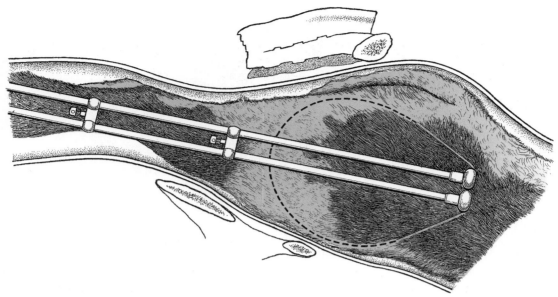

Figure 12.6 Fetotomy – acute-angle sawing to remove a hindlimb.

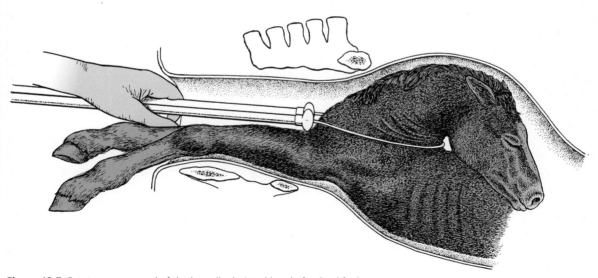

Figure 12.7 Fetotomy – removal of the laterally deviated head of a dead foal.

Shoulder flexion The fetotomy wire is passed between the fetal thorax and the medial aspect of the retained limb using an introducer. The skin between thorax and limb is incised to assist placement of the fetotomy wire. The aim is to cut through the muscular attachment between forelimb and body wall.

Breech presentation (bilateral hip flexion) The fetotomy wire is passed between the medial aspect of retained thigh and the fetal abdominal wall using an introducer. The second tube of the embryotome is threaded and the wire tightened. If possible, a skin incision is made in the fetus to ensure that the

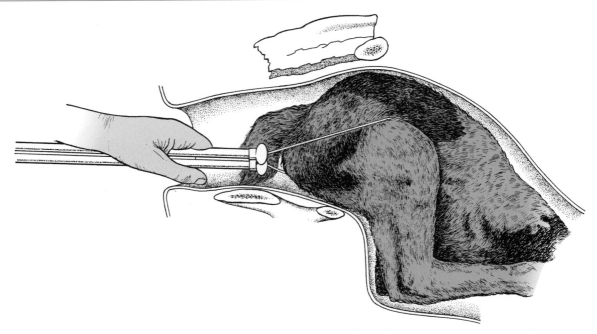

Figure 12.8 Fetotomy – removal of a hindlimb from a calf with irreducible bilateral hip flexion (breech presentation).

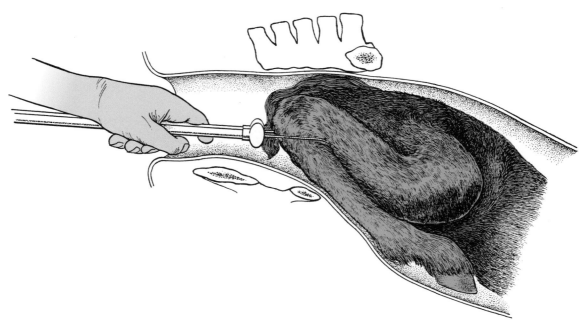

Figure 12.9 Fetotomy – removal of a portion of a hindlimb with irreducible hock flexion.

cut is made on the medial aspect of the fetal tuber coxae (Fig. 12.8). The limb is removed after section. The space now available may allow retrieval of the second limb and its conversion into a posterior presentation with delivery by traction. If this is not possible, the second limb is removed by fetotomy in the same way as the first. The remainder of the fetus is then delivered by traction. Self-closing hooks may be attached to the fetus so that traction may be employed.

Posterior presentation – hock flexion   The fetotomy wire is passed around the limb using the introducer. The limb is sawn through just below the hock (Fig. 12.9). The prominence of the hock joint is thus preserved and may be a useful point to which to fix a rope so that traction may be applied.

Fetal monsters   Fetotomy may be useful in this type of dystocia if the deformed fetus is accessible. Parts may be removed by directly looping the fetotomy wire round them if this is possible or by using the introducer to encircle the part to be removed with the wire. Fetotomy may also be required when a fetal monster is delivered by cesarean section. In some cases, for example when fetal joints are ankylosed, it may prove impossible to deliver the fetus through the normal-sized uterine incision. In such cases the sterilized embryotome is introduced through the uterine incision. The embryotomy wire is passed around the monster either directly or by using the introducer. The fetal monster is divided into sections which can be readily removed through the uterine incision.

AFTERCARE OF THE DAM FOLLOWING FETOTOMY

The vagina and uterus of the dam should be examined manually after fetotomy for evidence of soft tissue damage. Local and parenteral antibiotics should be administered. Non-steroidal anti-inflammatory therapy may be useful to supply analgesia and combat toxemia. If the placenta is readily detachable from the uterine caruncles it should be removed. Careful nursing for a few days is indicated.

FURTHER READING

Bierschwal CJ, de Bois CHW 1972 The technique of fetotomy in large animals. VM Publishing, Bonner Springs, KS

Chapter 13

POSTPARTURIENT PROBLEMS IN LARGE ANIMALS

HEMORRHAGE

Some degree of blood loss is inevitable at birth. A trickle of blood is almost always seen at the vagina after fetal delivery. Some blood may originate from minor trauma to the walls of the birth canal during parturition. If the umbilical cord ruptures within the uterus some of the blood appearing at the vagina may be fetal blood from within the placenta and not from the maternal circulation. Obvious blood loss does not normally continue for more than a few minutes after birth of the fetus.

Serious postparturient bleeding can occur into the uterus or other parts of the birth canal, and some may be seen at the vulva. Bleeding can also occur – internally and unseen – into the broad ligaments, peritoneal cavity, or the retroperitoneal part of the pelvis. In the latter cases the general signs of hemorrhage may be seen, but not the actual blood loss.

Hemorrhage into the birth canal

Etiology   Caused by accidental damage to the soft tissue walls of the birth canal, especially the uterus and vagina. The damage may be caused by an unguarded sharp fetal extremity or by excessive obstetric force, especially if the birth canal is not fully dilated. The parturient birth canal is hyperemic and mucosal damage can easily be complicated by laceration of arteries, with resultant blood loss. Clotting defects are uncommon in large animals but, if present, may result in persistent bleeding from an otherwise minor injury.

Clinical signs   Mostly blood coming through the vulva. Normal blood loss should not occur at a greater rate than a fast drip and this should slow down within a few minutes. A stream of blood should always be regarded as being potentially serious and must be investigated. A pulsating stream of bright red blood

may indicate arterial damage. Whenever bleeding occurs the animal should be monitored for general signs of blood loss, including pallor of the mucous membranes, weakness, and shock.

Detection of the bleeding point   The vulval lips are parted and examined for signs of damage and the caudal part of the vagina is also inspected. If no source of blood is found, the anterior vagina and palpable parts of the uterus are examined systematically by hand. Laceration of the mucosa or the discovery of a pulsating artery may indicate the site of hemorrhage.

Treatment   Visible and palpable bleeding points are subjected to pressure with damp cotton wool. If a spurting artery is located it is clamped with artery forceps. Ligation of the vessel should follow but, if impossible, the artery forceps (preferably an inexpensive or disposable pair) should be left in place for 24 hours. If the bleeding point is not detected, an injection of oxytocin will cause uterine contraction and possibly some pressure onto the bleeding point. If blood loss continues despite this the vagina and uterus may be packed with towels soaked in cold water.

Vulval hematoma in sows

Unilateral or bilateral enlargement of the vulval lips may follow farrowing, especially in gilts. In many cases the swelling is caused by a hematoma forming within the vulval lips. The affected lip may have a purple discoloration. Hematoma formation may be caused by the pressure of a fetus passing through the vulva or by the patient rubbing her hindquarters against the bars of the farrowing crate. Vulval hematomata should never be opened deliberately because many contain a bleeding artery. If left, they usually regress within a few days of farrowing. Occasionally spontaneous rupture of the thin wall of the hematoma occurs. In such cases blood loss is controlled by local pressure and ligation of any bleeding vessels.

Hemorrhage into the broad ligament, the peritoneal cavity, and the retroperitoneal space

Although it may occur in any species, this problem is chiefly seen in mares. The blood loss may be acute or occasionally more chronic. The condition is more common in older mares and in those suffering from copper deficiency. It occurs more frequently on the right side than on the left. The condition has also been seen in cows after calving.

Etiology   Caused by compression and laceration of the large uterine arteries between the fetus and the maternal pelvis during birth. The problem is more likely to follow the assisted delivery of a large foal. The arteries lie within the broad ligament of the uterus. Damage may result in bleeding being contained within the ligament or, more seriously, unrestricted into the peritoneal cavity.

Clinical signs   These vary with the speed and severity of blood loss. In severe cases the patient may show signs of colicky pain and may collapse and die. *In mares* an extremely unpleasant and terminal rictus of the facial muscles has been described. The animal may show pallor of the mucosae, weakness, and hyperpnea. In less severe cases, colicky pain and discomfort may be present. In mares, swellings may appear in the perineal region caused by pressure from the intrapelvic hematoma. Occasionally, a mild hemorrhage may be followed later by a more severe and possibly fatal one. The extent of the hematoma can be confirmed by rectal examination and defecation may be painful. Ultrasonographic scan of the vaginal wall from within the vaginal lumen will enable a hematoma to be identified, its extent determined, and progress monitored. The hematoma has strands of echogenic material (probably fibrin) crossing the less echogenic areas of clotted blood like a spider's web.

In the cow, evidence of an undiagnosed hematoma may be detected during the rectal examination of routine postnatal checks. The hematoma is in some cases in the caudal part of the pelvis and within the retroperitoneal space. Vaginal pain and dysuria may be seen, together with slight distension of the perineum.

Ultrasonography of the perivaginal tissues is useful to confirm the diagnosis. Occasionally, evidence of earlier arterial damage may be seen by discovery of a pulsating aneurysm in the middle uterine artery (these may become smaller with time and are seldom life threatening).

Treatment   In severe cases little can be done but in less severe cases analgesia, sedation and rest are prescribed. The foal should be protected from injury by his disturbed mother. Blood transfusion might be appropriate in some cases. Antibiotic cover is advisable. In the cow catheterization with a Foley catheter may be required for a few days to assist with the passage of urine until the hematoma has become organized and smaller.

RUPTURE OF THE UTERUS

Incidence   Occurs in all species but is most commonly seen in the cow and ewe.

Etiology   Caused by accidental damage sustained during lay or professional treatment of dystocia. It is more likely to occur in cases of fetopelvic disproportion or if the uterus is damaged by inflammatory changes or compromise of the uterine blood supply. It may rarely be caused by attempts to remove the fetal membranes.

Clinical signs   These are extremely variable. A hole may be detected in the uterine wall during the post-delivery check of the uterus. The fingers or hand may be passed through the defect. If the defect extends through the entire uterine wall, the smooth serosal surfaces of the abdominal organs are palpable.

Loops of maternal small intestine may be found within the uterine lumen, having passed through a defect in the uterine wall. Occasionally these loops may appear at the vulva. It is important to check that the intestine palpated or seen does not belong to a schistosomus calf that is still in the uterus with an exposed abdomen. The size of maternal small intestine is substantially larger than that of a calf.

In other cases, no symptoms of uterine rupture are seen until peritonitis develops within a few hours of birth. This latter symptom is seen especially in cows. The cow appears normal following delivery of her calf. A few hours – or even a day later – she is very depressed, is often pyrexic and toxic, reluctant to rise, grinds her teeth, and groans loudly on expiration. In such cases a peritoneal tap may show signs of an increased neutrophil count and plasma fibrinogen levels rise rapidly.

Treatment   If a very small hole is present and no abdominal contents have passed into the uterus an injection of oxytocin is given. This causes the uterus to contract and involute as quickly as possible. In such cases no further treatment other than antibiotic cover is necessary, although the patient should be carefully monitored.

If a large hole is discovered an attempt should be made to repair it. If the hole is in the greater curvature of the uterus it may be possible – and easier – to repair it via a laparotomy incision. Access to the uterus, especially if it has begun to involute, may be difficult via this approach. Alternatively, it may be possible using long-handled forceps to approach and repair the defect through the vagina.

If peritonitis is present, the condition of the cow must be considered. If she is very toxic and a peritoneal tap suggests severe peritonitis, euthanasia may be the most humane treatment. If the cow is reasonably bright and the defect has been discovered within a few hours of calving, a laparotomy is performed. The uterine wall is explored to identify the position of the hole, which is repaired using a purse string or inversion suture. The peritoneum is lavaged with warm normal saline. Peritoneal lavage can be performed through the laparotomy incision. If laparotomy has not been performed, lavage is carried out through trocars inserted through the abdominal wall. Saline is introduced into the peritoneal cavity through a trocar placed in the right sublumbar fossa. It is drained through another trocar inserted ventrally near the midline. Antibiotic cover and non-steroidal anti-inflammatory drug (NSAID) therapy is prescribed with (in some areas) appropriate tetanus prophylaxis. Treatment must be 'aggressive' if success in this serious condition is to be achieved. Initial doses of antibiotic and NSAID should be given intravenously, supported where necessary by fluid therapy. The antibiotic preparation used must be checked to ensure it can be given intravenously.

LACERATION OF THE CERVIX

Incidence   Uncommon, but if the integrity of the cervical seal is damaged the injury may have an adverse effect upon future fertility. Scar tissue formation may accompany natural repair, which may also compromise cervical dilation at any subsequent parturition.

Etiology   Caused by damage at parturition, especially if the cervix is not fully dilated at the time of birth.

Clinical signs   Laceration is often not observed until a postnatal examination of the genital tract when the cervix has resumed its normal size and shape. A defect in the continuity of the cervical rim may be palpated or observed through a speculum. A duck-billed speculum, which dilates the vagina and allows it to inflate fully with air, is particularly useful at revealing such injuries, which may otherwise be missed.

Treatment   May not be possible in practice because special instruments, including long-handled needle holders are required. Surgery is performed in the standing animal under epidural anesthesia. The cervical defect is cleaned up and the edges of the wound are refreshed with a scalpel. Repair is achieved by placing absorbable sutures through the damaged mucosa and deeply through the submucosa. Long-handled needle-holders and forceps are required to gain access to the cervix. Alternatively, the cervix may be brought back nearer to the vulva using vulsellum forceps. Antibiotic cover is provided. Further breeding is delayed until repair is complete.

LACERATION OF THE VAGINA

Incidence   Occurs in all species but especially in the mare and cow.

Etiology   In the mare laceration may occur spontaneously in cases of malposture such as the foot–nape position where the fetal feet are displaced and are forced into and through the vaginal mucosa by the vigorous straining of the mare. If the displacement of the foot is uncorrected, more severe damage may be sustained by the mare. Intense straining by the mare may force the displaced foot caudally still within the rectum. The ventral part of the anal sphincter and the dorsal commissure of the vulva may be torn, thus creating a rectovaginal fistula with perineal laceration.

The use of excessive force during the correction of a malposture may also result in severe damage especially in cases of fetopelvic disproportion. Vaginal tearing just within the dorsal commissure of the vulva may occur in fat heifers following delivery of the calf. Every effort should be made to avoid this type of injury by generous use of obstetric lubricant, gently stretching the vagina before delivery and only applying moderate force during assisted delivery.

Clinical signs   The severity of these depends on whether the damage is retroperitoneal (when the signs are normally less severe) or whether there is perforation into the peritoneal cavity. In most cases the laceration is retroperitoneal and there are few signs of systemic disturbance. In the mare, perforation into the peritoneal cavity is quickly followed by an increase in the number of white cells in the peritoneal fluid as peritonitis is established. Vaginal damage is encountered at the time of delivery or during the postpartum check routinely performed immediately after fetal delivery. Dorsal wall laceration in heifers or cows is often accompanied by the prolapse of submucosal fat, which is palpable or may be seen just within the vulval lips.

Whenever such an injury is seen a full and careful inspection of the area – under epidural anesthesia if necessary – should follow to establish the extent of the injury and exactly which tissues and structures have been damaged.

Vaginal laceration may involve the mucosa or the whole thickness of the vaginal wall. Occasionally the rectal floor and the anal sphincter may be involved and a rectovaginal fistula is established with a cloaca-like common entrance to rectum and vagina. The perineum may or may not be involved. Such injuries may initially appear to cause few problems and may even be unnoticed. Feces pass into the vagina and the vulval seal is compromised with adverse effects on subsequent fertility.

Treatment   The extent of the damage is carefully established and if peritoneal involvement is suspected in the mare an immediate peritoneal tap should be taken. Signs of peritonitis are treated immediately with 'aggressive' antibiotic and NSAID therapy. Minor lacerations involving the vaginal mucosa only will normally heal quite rapidly without treatment.

Tears in the vaginal wall

These should be repaired immediately, before they become distorted by granulation or scar tissue. An epidural anesthetic is given and stay sutures are placed in both vulval lips to enable them to be held open to permit the obstetrician a good view of and access to the damaged vaginal wall. A continuous suture taking in mucosal and submucosal layers is inserted using absorbable suture material. Antibiotic cover is advised in all cases.

Treatment of rectovaginal fistula

Ideally, repair should take place as soon as the injury occurs in an attempt to ensure first intention healing. In many cases, however, the obstetrician is not called until some time (occasionally some days) after the injury has occurred. It is suggested that repair in such cases

be delayed until 6 weeks after injury is sustained, by which time local swelling and granulation tissue will have settled down.

Surgery is performed in the standing animal under epidural anesthesia. Stay sutures are placed in the vulval lips, which are held open by an assistant to allow good access. The exposed tissues are cleaned with a mild antiseptic solution and any fecal material is removed. The extent of the fistula is now evident and a shelf of normal tissue formed by the vaginal roof and rectal wall is visible at the anterior end of the defect.

Both dorsal edges of the torn vaginal mucosa are dissected away from the submucosal tissue – from the shelf of normal tissue back to the caudal end of the defect. Sufficient vaginal mucosa is freed to enable it to be turned ventrally into the vaginal lumen. The rectal floor is not sutured. Sutures are placed in the dorsal vaginal submucosa – starting at the anterior end – so that the dissected mucosa is pulled together and dead space is eliminated by a series of interrupted sutures using absorbable suture material (Fig. 13.1). Antibiotic cover is provided.

If the anal sphincter is involved it is recommended that this is not repaired at the same time as the fistula. Repair of the sphincter and perineum is delayed until 2 weeks after the original operation (Fig. 13.2) (for a fuller description of this operation, see Aanes (1964) and McKinnon & Voss (1992)).

If the perineum is not involved an alternative approach to a rectovaginal fistula is via an episiotomy incision. The fistula is exposed, the rectal and vaginal walls are dissected free and are repaired.

PROLAPSE OF THE UTERUS

Incidence   Occurs in all the large animal species. It is most common in the cow and ewe, less common in the sow and doe goat, and rare in the mare. Normally the uterus prolapses only after fetal delivery but occasionally in the sow one uterine horn may prolapse while the other – still containing a number of fetuses – remains within the abdomen. In cattle the condition seems to be more common in fat animals with excessive slackening of the pelvic ligaments and perineal tissues. 'Outbreaks' occur on some farms during one calving season and may be associated with diet, possibly with a high estrogen content.

Etiology   Uterine prolapse is essentially an eversion of the organ, which turns inside out as it passes through

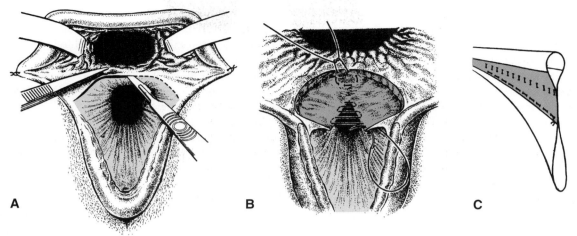

Figure 13.1 Repair of rectovaginal fistula (stage 1) (reproduced, with permission, from McKinnon AO & Voss JL (eds) 1992 Equine reproduction. Lea and Febiger, Philadelphia).

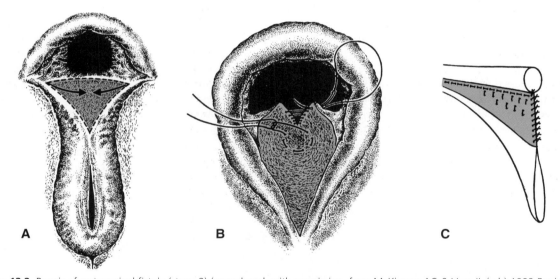

Figure 13.2 Repair of rectovaginal fistula (stage 2) (reproduced, with permission, from McKinnon AO & Voss JL (eds) 1992 Equine reproduction. Lea and Febiger, Philadelphia).

the vagina as a prolapse. Many factors may be involved in the etiology, including:

- Poor uterine tone: uterine inertia – in cattle hypocalcemia (a cause of primary uterine inertia) may predispose. Lack of tone may allow the uterus to fold in and permit part of the wall to move towards the pelvic inlet. Straining then pushes the flaccid organ through the vagina.
- Increased straining, which may be caused by pain or discomfort after parturition.
- Other causes of increased intra-abdominal pressure, including tympany and recumbency.

- Excessive traction at assisted parturition and the weight of retained fetal membranes have been suggested as other predisposing factors.

Clinical signs and treatment   These vary somewhat with the species involved and will be considered separately.

The cow

Clinical signs   The patient is usually found with her uterus already prolapsed. One or both uterine horns may be visible. The mucosal surface of the uterus – with its cotyledons – is visible and part of the chorioallantois may still be attached. The cow may be standing and apparently unconcerned or she may be shocked and recumbent. The uterus may be grossly contaminated with bedding and feces. It may also be lacerated, engorged, and edematous. If recently prolapsed it is warm to the touch but later becomes cold and discolored. Occasionally the cow is found dead. Death is often due to hemorrhage from the ovarian arteries, which may rupture as a result of the excessive tension placed on them by the prolapse.

Prognosis   This depends on: (1) the duration of the problem; (2) the degree of damage and contamination sustained by the uterus; (3) the degree of shock in the cow; (4) the position and accessibility of the patient.

Treatment   On receiving a call, the obstetrician should give advice on first aid care. The uterus should be protected from further damage, wrapped in a clean moist sheet, and, if possible, held above the level of the vulva.

On arrival the following treatment sequence should be followed:

1. Assess the cow's general condition: if she is moribund and severely shocked treatment may not be practical or economical. If there is evidence of hypocalcemia this should be treated.

2. Assess the cow's position: she may be in a most unsuitable position for treatment but it may also be impossible to move her. If her hindquarters are pointing downhill it would be advisable to move her so that her head is lower than her hindquarters. Gravity would thus help rather than hinder replacement.

3. Administer an epidural anesthetic.

4. Position the cow: this is best done by the 'New Zealand method'. The cow is placed in sternal recumbency with her hindlegs pulled out behind her. Two or three assistants are required for this. If the cow is standing she must be cast on her side and the uppermost hindlimb pulled out behind her. She is then rolled on to her other side so that the second hindlimb can be secured and extended caudally. An assistant sits astride her facing backwards and lifting the cow's tail out of the way (Fig. 13.3). See below[*] for an alternative method if sufficient help is not available.

5. Remove gross debris from the prolapsed organ by washing with saline or a very mild antiseptic.

6. Remove the placenta or its remnants from the cotyledons – if it separates easily. If not, leave it attached.

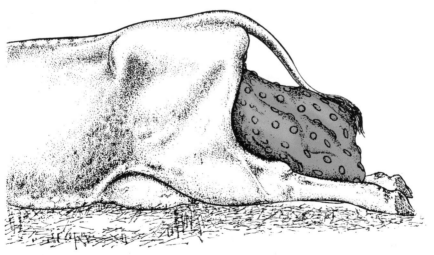

Figure 13.3 Cow – uterine prolapse, patient positioned for replacement.

*On occasion there may be insufficient assistance on the farm to place the cow in position with her hindlegs extended. In such circumstances the obstetrician must use an alternative method of replacement. The cow is given an epidural anesthetic and the uterus is prepared for replacement as in the New Zealand method. The obstetrician, wearing a parturition overall, kneels behind the cow and takes the prolapsed organ on his or her lap. The body of the uterus is first pushed back into the vagina while an assistant, if available, helps by holding the uterine horns above the level of the vulva. Pressure is now directed onto the horns, which are pushed back into their correct position. Replacement is greatly helped if the cow's hindquarters are higher than her forequarters. If raising her hindquarters or lowering her front end is possible this should be done, but only if there is no risk to the prolapsed organ. Postprocedure treatment and care is as before.

7. Repair any gross damage such as tearing using an absorbable suture.
8. Reducing the size of the prolapse – this is not really necessary. Some obstetricians recommend applying sugar or salt to 'draw out the edema'. The use of oxytocin *before* replacement is not advisable. The tightly contracted uterus can be very difficult to replace.
9. The prolapsed uterus is raised above the level of the vulva and eased back through the vagina. The body of the uterus is first pushed into the vagina followed by the horns. Handling the uterus may be aided by wrapping it in clean plastic and also by applying obstetric lubricant. The uterus is often very bulky and the help of an assistant in holding and replacing it is often very useful.
10. The cow is released from the sternal position and, if able, is encouraged to rise. The horns of the uterus are pushed fully back into position aided if necessary by a clean bottle used to fully invert each horn.
11. As soon as the uterus is replaced an injection of oxytocin (20–30 IU) is given by intramuscular injection. This will cause the uterus to involute and reduce the risk of recurrence of the prolapse.
12. Suturing the vulval lips should not be necessary or indeed helpful. Vulval sutures are, however, used by many obstetricians and are expected by many farmers. The suture pattern is as for vaginal prolapse (see Chapter 2).
13. Aftercare: good nursing, a light diet, and moderate exercise are required. Antibiotic cover is recommended. The vulval sutures are removed after 10 days.

If it is impossible to replace the prolapse, amputation may be attempted, although the prognosis for survival must be guarded. The prolapse is opened close to the vulva to reveal the uterine vessels lying within the tense mesometrium. These are each ligated in two places and the mesometrium severed between the ligatures. The vagina is ligated – taking care to avoid the external urethral orifice – and the uterus and cervix are removed.

Note: the general procedures such as cleaning the prolapsed organ are the same in all species.

The mare

Incidence   Uterine prolapse is quite uncommon in the mare.

Etiology   Causes are as in the cow but may be predisposed by a retained placenta in a mare when uterine tone is low. When such mares are examined per vaginam, folds of uterine wall may be found folding inwards towards the cervix.

Clinical signs   The eversion of the uterus is often very sudden. As the equine placenta has no cotyledons and the endometrial surface of the uterus is smooth, care must be taken to ensure that the prolapsed organ is the uterus and not the bladder or the allantoic surface of the placenta.

Treatment   Manual replacement after administration of epidural anesthetic. Replacement is usually achieved much more easily than in the cow.

The ewe and doe goat

Incidence   Uterine prolapse is quite common in sheep and the incidence may be higher during some lambing seasons. The condition appears much less common in goats.

Clinical signs   The ewe is usually discovered with a prolapsed uterus a few hours after lambing (Fig. 13.4). Postparturient discomfort and straining may predispose. The fragile prolapsed uterus is easily damaged and may be contaminated with straw and feces.

Treatment   An epidural anesthetic aids uterine replacement as does slight (and short-term) elevation of the hindquarters. The risk of damage to the uterus during replacement may be reduced by enclosing it in a plastic glove through which it may be manipulated back in greater safety.

The sow

Incidence   It is quite common but the prognosis for successful treatment and survival is guarded unless the case is treated very shortly after the prolapse occurs. One or both horns may be involved. If one horn remains in the abdomen it may contain piglets.

Clinical signs   In many cases the sow is found dead with the uterus prolapsed. One but mostly both uterine horns are involved (Fig. 13.5). The carcass is very pale and the cause of death is hemorrhage from ruptured ovarian or uterine arteries. In very recent cases the sow may appear unconcerned and lies feeding her piglets, but in most cases a degree of shock is present.

Treatment   This is complicated by the length of the uterine horns and the difficulty in replacing them and

Figure 13.4 Ewe – uterine prolapse.

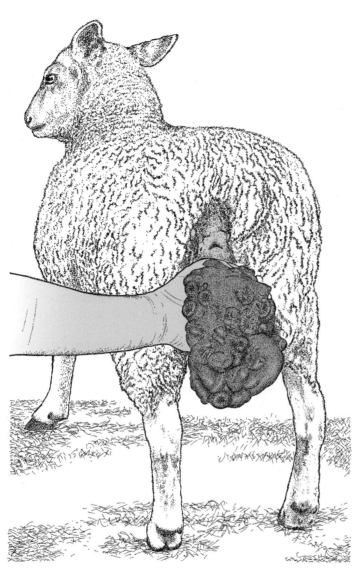

also in ensuring that they are fully inverted. General anesthesia or heavy sedation will be found helpful. The rear end of the sow is raised, taking care not to compromise breathing by allowing the head and neck to be flexed ventrally. The body of the uterus is manually eased back into the vagina. Inversion of the horns is aided by introducing warm water or saline into the lumen of the horns. The weight of fluid will help to pull the horns back into their correct position.

If this method fails the uterus can be pulled back into the abdomen through a flank laparotomy wound. In severely shocked animals euthanasia on welfare and economic grounds may be indicated.

POSTPARTURIENT PROLAPSE OF THE VAGINA

Incidence Occurs in all species but is more common in the ewe and sow, and less common in the cow and rare in the mare. In sows, vaginal prolapse may be accompanied by rectal prolapse. Postparturient vaginal prolapse

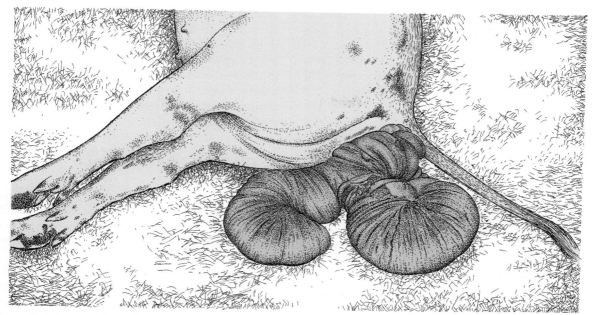

Figure 13.5 Sow – uterine prolapse.

may occur as a recurrence of a preparturient problem or, less commonly, may arise as a new entity. The prognosis is usually reasonably good because the hormone changes that predispose to the preparturient slackening of tissues and the prolapse disappear after birth.

Clinical signs   These are as in the preparturient animal. There is now no longer the problem of anticipated birth but there may be the complication of retained placenta.

Treatment   The prolapse is identified, cleaned, lubricated, and replaced under epidural anesthetic. The addition of xylazine to the epidural injection may prolong its action and reduce the incidence of postreplacement straining. The vulval lips are sutured as in the preparturient animal (see Fig. 2.6). The T-shaped plastic vaginal retainers (see Fig. 2.7) commonly used in preparturient sheep may be less effective because – at least initially – the cervix may be open. Vaginal sutures are removed after 7–10 days.

EVERSION OF THE BLADDER

Incidence   This is seen in the mare, in which the short, wide urethra predisposes to the condition in the postparturient period.

Clinical signs   The everted (prolapsed) organ lies within the vagina or protrudes from the vulva. Close examination will reveal that the inner surface of the bladder is exposed; the trigonum vesicae is seen with urine coming from the ureters. Urine scalding may occur on the mare's thighs.

Treatment   After gentle cleaning the bladder is manually replaced under epidural anesthesia by pushing it back down through the urethra. Antibiotic cover is provided.

HERNIATION OF THE BLADDER

In this condition the bladder passes through a tear in the vaginal floor and its serosal surface appears at the vulva. Thus the peritoneal surface of the bladder and not its inner surface is visible.

Incidence   This uncommon condition may occur in all species as a result of trauma sustained during parturition.

Clinical signs   A fluid-filled viscus appears at the vulva. Great care must be taken to identify the structure accurately. In the cow, for example, it might be mistaken for a portion of fluid-filled amnion. In many cases, obstruction of the urethra occurs as a result of the displacement of the bladder, which fills with urine.

Treatment The bladder is emptied by catheterization or, if this fails, by cystocentesis. Under epidural anesthesia the bladder is replaced in its correct position and the torn vaginal floor is repaired. An indwelling Foley catheter may be left in place for 48 hours to prevent filling of the bladder. Antibiotic cover is provided.

RETROVERSION OF THE BLADDER

Incidence This rare condition is seen chiefly in the sow. The bladder becomes displaced from its normal position beneath the uterus and just in front of the pelvic brim. The bladder moves laterally and caudally and comes to lie beside the vagina. The fundus of the bladder is now directed caudally and the urethra may be partially obstructed.

Clinical signs Straining and discomfort are seen after parturition. The sow postures to urinate but is unable to pass urine. Vaginal and rectal examination reveal a tense and distended viscus lying beside or above the vagina.

Treatment If catheterization of the bladder is possible, an indwelling catheter may be left in place for a few days to allow the sow to live comfortably while her litter become established. After this, unless surgery is contemplated, the sow is euthanized. The condition could be resolved in a valuable sow by retrieving the bladder from the pelvis through a caudal midline laparotomy incision. Cystopexy to the caudal abdominal floor should prevent a recurrence.

INTESTINAL INJURY

Incidence This is uncommon but lesions have been seen in cattle slaughtered after parturition. Signs in life are seldom seen unless severe intestinal damage has been sustained.

Etiology Loops of small or large intestine are trapped and squashed between the fetus and the pelvis. This might occur in cases where dystocia is prolonged, fetal fluids are lost, and excessive traction by laypersons has been used.

Clinical signs Minor intestinal damage will pass unnoticed. If rupture of the bowel has occurred, signs of developing peritonitis will be seen. Within a few hours anorexia, pain, rumenal stasis, intestinal ileus, and pyrexia are evident. A full clinical examination is essential. The presence of peritonitis and its extent is established by rectal examination and a peritoneal tap.

Treatment Intensive antibiotic and supportive therapy including fluids and non-steroidal anti-inflammatory drugs are used. Intraperitoneal antibiotic therapy may also be given. Laparotomy is normally not indicated unless the exact location of the primary injury is known. If signs of peritonitis are seen peritoneal lavage using warmed normal saline may be used. For details of this technique, see p. 211.

RETENTION OF THE FETAL MEMBRANES

The fetal membranes are normally expelled during the third stage of labor. The membranes are said to be retained whenever the third stage of labor is prolonged beyond its normal duration.

Retention of the membranes occurs in all species. It is particularly common in the dairy cow but the consequences of retention may be most serious in the mare. In the polytocus species such as the sow, bitch, and queen retention of the membranes may be associated with retention of one or more fetuses.

The causes of membrane retention are complex. Three main factors are involved:

1. Insufficient expulsive efforts by the myometrium.
2. Failure of the placenta to separate from the endometrium. This may be caused by inflammatory changes, placental immaturity, hormone imbalances, a neutropenia, a lack of polymorph migration to the sites of attachment, and possibly immune deficiencies.
3. Mechanical obstruction – including partial closure of the cervix.

The condition will be considered for each species.

The cow

Incidence The overall incidence among dairy cows is about 4% in the UK, but lower in beef cattle. The incidence is much higher after conditions in which uterine distension and/or poor uterine tone occur. In cases of twin gestation, uterine hydrops, or uterine inertia, the incidence may rise to at least 50% of cases. The incidence is also higher after cases of dystocia due to any cause. Occasionally, the incidence of fetal membrane retention in a herd may rise for a season. The reason for this is often undiagnosed but may include vitamin A, vitamin E/selenium, cobalt, and copper deficiencies. The incidence of retention is also high after premature birth – including induced birth and abortion.

If the fetal membranes are still attached 24 hours after birth they will normally remain – unless removed – until 7 to 10 days later.

Etiology   This was discussed under Incidence, above.

Clinical signs   The membranes are normally visible hanging from the vulva. They become progressively more decomposed, have a fetid odor, and are often contaminated with bedding and feces. Occasionally the membranes are not visible – possibly more frequently after twin calving – and are detected incidentally during a vaginal examination.

The cow usually appears unaffected by fetal membrane retention, although appetite and milk yield may be marginally reduced. If severe uterine infection is superimposed the cow may become dangerously ill.

Subsequent fertility   The incidence of endometritis is higher and return to estrus after calving may be delayed after retention of the fetal membranes. Permanent damage is unlikely and once the cow starts to cycle, fertility should be unaffected.

Treatment   There is some controversy between those who support and those who oppose manual removal. If left untreated, the membranes will eventually separate and be passed by the cow. The odor of the membranes may lead to milk taint and their appearance in a hygienic milking parlor is unpleasant. Physical removal may lead to some minor uterine damage at the point of caruncular attachment but this is unlikely to affect future breeding. On balance, if the membranes are retained it is advisable to try to remove them.

Manual removal of the retained fetal membranes
This is first attempted 72 hours after calving. The obstetrician should set a time limit for removal – if the membranes cannot be removed within 10 minutes they should be left for a further 48 hours before a further attempt at removal is made.

During physical removal of the membranes they are separated at their cotyledonary attachments from the uterine caruncles. There are over 100 caruncles but at the time of removal the membranes are usually only attached to a proportion of them. The points of attachment involve both the pregnant and the non-pregnant horns. In many cases, separation of cotyledons and caruncles has already taken place near the cervix but the placenta is still attached to the caruncles in the uterine fundus.

Strict attention to hygiene is important. A parturition overall and plastic arm-length sleeves should be worn on both arms. Despite the sleeves, the odor of the membranes may gain access to the hands. Two sleeves may be worn on each arm but the sensitivity of the fingers will be reduced.

The perineal area of the cow is washed with mild disinfectant. During the procedure the cow frequently strains and passes feces. Any contamination must be removed and the area washed again before proceeding.

The obstetrician grasps any protruding strands of placenta in one hand and twists them into a 'rope' so that the placenta can be more easily managed. The other lubricated hand is introduced into the uterus. Occasionally at this stage it is found that the membranes are not actually attached at all but are perhaps just trapped by a single cotyledon, which is too large to pass the partially closed cervix. In this case the offending cotyledon is eased through the cervix and the remainder of the placenta is removed by gentle traction.

If the placenta is found to be attached, the hand inside the uterus but outside the placenta searches for the nearest attached caruncle and cotyledon. The chorioallantois is squeezed off the caruncle producing a sensation very similar to that felt when two pieces of Velcro are separated (Fig. 13.6). The obstetrician moves methodically from one cotyledon to the next releasing every one that is still attached to its caruncle. It may be difficult to reach those deep in the fundus of the uterus. Gentle traction on the placenta will normally move these into a position in which they can be reached and separated. Once all the attachments have been released the placenta is gently removed by traction.

If the placenta has not been separated within 10 minutes the attempt should cease – to avoid damage. The case is seen again in 48 hours, when a further attempt at removal is made. If the second attempt is still unsuccessful another is made 48–72 hours later.

After removal of the placenta, antibiotic pessaries may be inserted into the uterus, but it must be remembered that these may have milk withdrawal restrictions. If there is much unpleasant debris in the uterus it may be lavaged with warm saline and the contents siphoned out with a stomach tube. If there is evidence of active infection a parenteral course of antibiotic therapy is prescribed and appropriate milk withdrawal advised.

Occasionally the obstetrician may be unable to get through the partially closed cervix to release the attached cotyledons. In such cases the placenta is

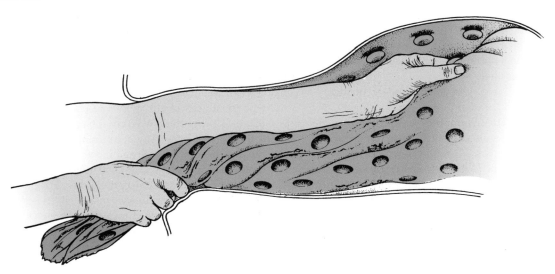

Figure 13.6 Cow manual removal of the placenta (see text).

left to separate naturally. Rarely the cervix may dilate slightly in a few days allowing greater ease of access.
Other methods and aids to placental removal
Weights attached to the placenta and 'cleansing drinks', which usually contain magnesium sulfate, are of no known value in the treatment of retained fetal membranes.

Prevention of placenta retention   If the cow has suffered from any of the predisposing causes of fetal membrane retention mentioned above an attempt may be made to encourage passage of the placenta at the time of delivery. An injection of oxytocin or of prostaglandin F2α or its analogs may be used to encourage uterine involution and placental separation. Oxytocin must be used within 12 hours of calving, after which time myometrial sensitivity to its action is reduced.

The mare

Retention of the fetal membranes in mares is a potentially serious situation and must be handled with care. At one time, especially in heavy horses, placental retention even briefly after foaling was regarded as an emergency. If the placenta was not removed quickly there was a grave risk that the mare would develop an acute form of laminitis known as 'founder'. Modern drug therapy has eliminated some of the risks but many horse owners are still concerned about the dangers of retention.

Incidence   Occurs much less frequently than in cows and may be more common in heavy than in light horses.

Etiology   The causes are in general as in the cow. Low-grade uterine infection may cause placentitis and predispose to retention. Retention is higher following induced birth, dystocia, cesarean section, and abortion.

Clinical signs   The placenta – initially the amnion – is seen hanging from the vulva. The mare may appear unconcerned but nervous horses may be upset by the placenta hanging around their hocks.

Treatment   The placenta is normally passed within 1–3 hours of birth. It is normally passed with its pale gray allantoic surface outermost. The inner velvety and red chorionic surface is innermost.

If the membranes have not been passed within 6 hours of birth   An injection of 10–40 IU of oxytocin is given by intramuscular injection, alternatively, 10–20 IU oxytocin may be given as a bolus intravenously or 20–40 IU oxytocin over a period of an hour in a liter of normal saline by intravenous drip. Before administering oxytocin the obstetrician should carry out a vaginal examination to ensure that no other abnormalities, such as partial uterine prolapse, are present. It is also advisable to commence a course of parenteral antibiotic therapy – a combination of penicillin and streptomycin being suitable. The injection of oxytocin may be repeated 3 hours later if the membranes are still attached. If the mare is upset by her placenta hanging behind her, the membranes can be knotted together so that their length is shortened and they cause less irritation. It is not advisable to add weights to them because this may occasionally predispose to uterine prolapse.

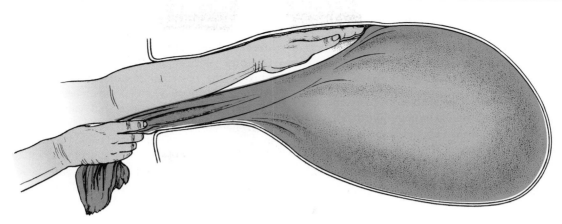

Figure 13.7 Mare manual removal of the placenta (see text).

If the membranes have not been passed within 12 hours of birth An attempt should be made to remove the membranes manually. If they are still tightly attached they should be left for a further 6–12 hours. A further injection of oxytocin is given and antibiotic cover continued.

Manual removal of the fetal membranes Strict attention is paid to hygiene and safety. The mare's tail is bandaged, a leg is held up and the perineal area thoroughly washed with a mild antiseptic solution. The obstetrician should *not* wear a long parturition overall as this may alarm the mare.

The hand is advanced along the dorsal wall of the vagina towards the uterus until the ruptured edge of the chorioallantois is found just anterior to the cervix. The edge may be partially detached from the endometrium or still adherent to it. If attached, the membranes are separated from the endometrium by gently inserting a finger between them and the endometrium. Once a small portion has been separated it is held in one of the obstetrician's hands. Very gentle traction is applied to this part while the other hand is inserted between the chorion and the endometrium. The hand is gently moved from side to side and forwards towards the uterine fundus to separate the two structures (Fig. 13.7). Separation should be achieved without difficulty and resembles separation of two pieces of Velcro attached to each other. The membranes are separated from the entire endometrial surface in both pregnant and non-pregnant horns. The tightest attachments may be at the tips of the uterine horns.

During removal, care must be taken to avoid tearing the placenta or leaving pieces behind. The weight of the placenta should be supported – if not it may drag the tips of the uterine horn towards the cervix and thus predispose to prolapse. After removal, the placenta should be laid out to check that it is all present. It is also advisable to check the chorionic surface for evidence of necrosis or other signs that the fetus may have been compromised in utero. If any large pieces of placenta are missing, the uterus should be searched to locate them. Antibiotic pessaries may be inserted into the uterus and parenteral antibiotic therapy commenced if it has not already been used. Penicillin and streptomycin may be used and ampicillin is one of number of alternatives. Oxytocin (20–40 IU) is given by intramuscular injection to encourage uterine involution.

If the placenta cannot be removed manually within 10 minutes It should be left and the mare given antibiotic and oxytocin treatment. A further attempt is made to remove the placenta manually 12 hours later.

Note: Occasionally, especially after abortion, the placenta remains tightly attached to the endometrium for several days and in rare cases for weeks. In such cases the placenta eventually separates and the mare usually has no residual problems. (Mares that have aborted should always be isolated and the cause of abortion investigated in the appropriate manner.)

Note: An alternative method of placental removal can be attempted if manual removal is proving difficult and it is feared that the mare's health may be deteriorating: The chorioallantois is gently inflated (using a stomach tube and pump) with up to 10 liters of normal saline.

The ends of the chorioallantois are held or tied around the tube to retain the fluid within the distended membranes. The uterine distension usually provokes uterine contractions and straining. Within 10–15 minutes the mare will usually attempt to expel the placenta.

In all cases of retained placenta in the mare, moderate and regular exercise should be maintained. A light diet should be given. The feet should be palpated at least twice daily for evidence of laminitis.

The ewe and doe goat

Retention of the fetal membranes is quite rare in these species. The etiology and predisposing factors are broadly as in the cow. Manual removal may be attempted if the membranes are still present 72 hours after birth. It is often impossible to pass the hand through the cervix but the membranes – if trapped by the closing cervix – can often be retrieved by gentle traction. If access to the cotyledons is possible they are gently separated by squeezing from the uterine caruncles. Antibiotic cover should be provided.

The sow

Fetal membranes are normally passed after each piglet or group of piglets. The last portion of the chorioallantois in each uterine horn has a slightly darker red color than the other portions. Cervical closure does not normally occur until all the piglets have been delivered. If it is suspected that some portions of fetal membrane remain within the uterus a vaginal examination should be performed. A firm grasp should be taken on as much of any placenta encountered as possible to avoid it tearing. Gentle traction should then be applied to the placenta to remove it.

Fetal membrane retention may be an indication that further piglets remain within the birth canal. These should be searched for as described in Chapter 8. An injection of 20 IU oxytocin given by intramuscular injection should be given in an attempt to move any unborn piglets or placenta towards the vagina.

NECROTIC VAGINITIS

Incidence   Seen chiefly in the cow and ewe but occasionally seen in other species. It is especially common in first calf heifers that have suffered dystocia due to fetopelvic disproportion. Although it normally occurs as a separate entity it may be accompanied by a uterine infection or retention of the placenta.

Etiology   Pressure on the walls of the vagina by the fetus or the obstetrician causing mucosal damage (including localized necrosis), which becomes infected.

Clinical signs   There is a foul vaginal discharge accompanied by signs of discomfort, including straining and walking with an arched back. There may occasionally be some depression of appetite and milk yield. The vaginal mucosa is initially very inflamed, quite hard and painful but these signs are followed shortly by the development of green plaques on the surface of the mucosa. Very occasionally the plaques become gangrenous. The plaques are clearly visible just within the vulval lips but may also extend forwards along the vaginal wall. The animal is not normally pyrexic unless uterine infection is present. If uterine infection is suspected a careful rectal examination should be carried out (in the larger species) to investigate the size, state of involution, and consistency of the uterus. Manual vaginal examination is very painful and should be avoided but evidence of a purulent discharge from the uterus may be seen using a well-lubricated vaginal speculum.

Treatment   Application twice daily of soft emollient cream (such as udder cream) to those parts of the vagina that can be reached. If uterine infection is present a course of parenteral antibiotics should be prescribed. Fly repellent should be applied around the perineum to avoid the possibility of blow-fly strike.

POSTPARTURIENT ACUTE SEPTIC METRITIS

Incidence   This condition, sometimes known as puerperal metritis, is a severe life-threatening disease that occurs in all species but has the highest incidence in cattle and sheep. The condition is sporadic but outbreaks of disease may be seen, especially in ewes if standards of hygiene have fallen in the lambing pens.

Etiology   The disease usually, but not always, follows some abnormality of parturition such as a difficult case of dystocia, poor uterine involution, or uterine prolapse. Infection is usually by opportunist organisms such as streptococci, *Arcanobacter pyogenes*, *E. coli*, and occasionally clostridia. A poor immune response locally and parenterally is also probably involved.

Clinical signs and treatment These may vary slightly between species; they are described below.

The cow

Clinical signs The cow is noticed to be ill 24–72 hours after parturition. The animal is dull, pyrexic (usually 1–2°C above normal), and anorexic. Rumenal movements are reduced or absent. There are signs of toxemia and a bloody, fetid vaginal discharge. The animal may strain and walk with her tail elevated. Diarrhea may be present as a result of toxemia and septicemia. The placenta (if present) is tightly attached and has a 'stringy' appearance. Rectal examination reveals that the uterus is poorly involuted and hard to the touch. The vaginal mucosa is inflamed and thickened and the cervix is partially open. If untreated, the cow rapidly becomes recumbent, dehydrated, and comatose. Death may ensue within a few hours.

A full clinical examination must always be performed to ensure that no other problems such as acute mastitis are present.

Prognosis This must always be guarded. The earlier and more effective the treatment and nursing the greater the chances of survival. If recovery is not as good or as speedy as anticipated, the possibility of an underlying metabolic problem such as fatty liver disease must be kept in mind. Clostridial infection of the uterus has a particularly poor prognosis.

Treatment Intravenous antibiotic therapy must be commenced immediately. One of the following antibiotics may be used initially: oxytetracycline, ampicillin, trimethoprim/sulfonamide, or enrofloxacin. Nonsteroidal anti-inflammatory drugs such as flunixin should also be given intravenously. Intravenous (preferably) or oral fluid therapy should also be given to counter dehydration, toxemia, and uremia. Good nursing is essential; the patient must be kept warm and comfortable but also encouraged to move about at regular intervals. Small quantities of good food should be offered and water must always be within easy reach.

It is generally best not to use intrauterine therapy during the acute illness. The pain associated with getting drugs into the uterus and their rapid removal by the circulation makes their use contraindicated until the acute phase of the infection has passed. If the placenta is still attached no attempt should be made to remove it until infection is under control and the animal is starting to show improvement.

The mare

Acute metritis is fortunately rare in horses but when it occurs it tends to be very severe. It may be complicated by laminitis, and, in some areas, by tetanus. Treatment and management are generally as in the cow with special management of the laminitis.

The ewe

Outbreaks of septic metritis are occasionally encountered in flocks where hygiene has suddenly deteriorated because of insufficient staff or other reasons. An overall review of procedures on the farm must be undertaken. Lambing may, if possible, have to be moved to new premises. Any ewe assisted at lambing must receive a full course of prophylactic antibiotics. Clostridial vaccination must be reviewed if infections with this group of organisms are encountered.

Similar problems may be encountered among goats where does are batch-kidded, although individual cases may be encountered on other premises.

Treatment is in general as in the cow. Intravenous fluid therapy should be used with caution in small ruminants, which appear to be particularly susceptible to pulmonary edema if overperfusion of the circulation occurs. Oral fluid replacement therapy can readily be given by nasogastric tube.

The sow

Mild metritis in the sow is quite commonly seen as part of the mastitis–metritis–agalactia syndrome. Acute septic metritis may be associated with the presence of dead pigs in the uterus. The prognosis is very guarded and fatal toxemia readily ensues. The sow is weak, reluctant to rise, and may have purple patches on her skin associated with septicemia. A gentle attempt should be made to remove any piglets discovered in the uterus during the mandatory vaginal examination. For details of the technique for removing dead piglets, see Chapter 8. Intravenous antibiotic and supportive therapy is given, with intensive nursing.

ABNORMALITIES OF THE MILK SUPPLY

A good accessible milk supply is essential to all young animals. The obstetrician should always check that milk is available for the young before leaving a maternity case.

Colostral intake is essential in the immediate postnatal period and a good milk supply later for growth and development. Whenever neonates are ill they must be examined and treated as a matter of urgency. The health and milk supply of their mother must also always be investigated.

Failure of the milk supply

Agalactia can be caused by:

1. *Aplasia of the mammary glands*: total absence of mammary tissue is occasionally seen in goats. Inverted nipples in gilts should be detected when they are selected for breeding. If a number of inverted nipples are present in an animal that has farrowed, some of the litter may be deprived of nourishment. Supplementation with artificial milk may be required.

2. *Failure of milk let-down*: failure of this important reflex can result from a number of causes:
   a. *Nervous inhibition*: the mother who has usually given birth for the first time is too anxious to settle down and feed her young. Providing a quiet environment will help but sedation and an injection of oxytocin may be required.
   b. *Inhibition through pain*: especially common in sows if the piglets' teeth have not been clipped. Also seen in nervous mares with sensitive udders who resent the foal seeking the teat. Teeth in piglets should be clipped. Patient management is usually successful in the mare. Milk let-down can be encouraged by administration of oxytocin.
   c. *Lack of stimulation of the teats by the offspring*: hypothermia, disease, hypoglycemia, and starvation may weaken the litter, who provide insufficient stimulus to cause milk let-down. This problem emphasizes the need to consider both mother *and* offspring in neonatal problems. Treatment of any disease in the neonates should be undertaken and milk let-down encouraged if necessary and appropriate by administration of oxytocin.

3. *Illness in the dam*: who is so debilitated that she is unable to produce milk. This may happen in any severe illness, including septic metritis, especially when the animal is pyrexic and toxemic.

4. *Injury to the udder*: may damage the gland to such an extent that milk production is prevented. Let-down may also be affected through pain.

5. *Diseases of the mammary glands*: in particular mastitis. Mastitis is particularly important in the immediate neonatal period in cattle. Acute environmental mastitis caused chiefly by *E. coli* and *Streptococcus uberis* may be present and life threatening at the time of birth or immediately afterwards. Full details of treatment are beyond the scope of this book. In summary, aggressive parenteral and local antibiotic therapy is required. Inflammatory changes and toxemia may be helped by non-steroidal anti-inflammatory drugs such as flunixin. Intravenous or oral fluid therapy are also very important. Mastitis in the other species mostly occurs a little later after parturition. In the ewe, acute mastitis may be caused by infection with *Staphylococcus aureus* or *Manheimia haemolytica*. Treatment is basically as in the cow. In pigs, severe mastitis caused by *Klebsiella* infection may develop soon after farrowing. Other organisms such as *E. coli* and *S. aureus* may be responsible for similar symptoms. The udder is extremely hard and signs of toxemia develop rapidly, with dark red blotches appearing on the skin of the jowl and caudal aspects of the hind legs. Treatment is by parenteral administration of antibiotics – the choice being aided, where possible, by sensitivity tests. Intramammary therapy is not possible in sows, although in desperate cases an injection can be made into the affected mammary tissues. Immediate supplies of artificial milk are mandatory for the piglets.

Signs of agalactia

The first signs of a failing milk supply may be seen in the young. They may initially seem hyperactive as they persistently search for food but then become dull, weak, dehydrated, and disinterested. They easily fall victim to neonatal disease. As the young become weaker they fail to stimulate let-down of what milk there is and the situation becomes progressively worse. If failure started at or soon after the time of birth the neonatal animals may be colostrum-deprived. The lack of antibody protection renders them especially susceptible to infection.

Apparent sucking can be deceptive. The neonate may appear to be sucking well but is not actually obtaining any milk. It must be watched carefully to ensure that it is swallowing, that milk is found in its mouth after sucking. In some species it may be possible to see an increase in weight after feeding. The udder should be inspected for signs of abnormality or disease. The presence of milk in the teats and their patency must also be checked.

POSTPARTURIENT RECUMBENCY

This important problem can arise in all species but especially in the large farm animals. The condition may be:

- a continuation of preparturient recumbency
- recumbency arising from damage sustained during birth
- a postparturient recumbency.

All cases of postparturient recumbency must be examined with great care. The causes of the abnormality may be obstetric, medical (and rarely unrelated to parturition), or surgical. Every case must be examined methodically and thoroughly to ensure that no abnormality is overlooked. The importance of this detailed examination cannot be overemphasized. The entire animal must be inspected and examined. This can be physically difficult with a heavy recumbent cow or horse but nonetheless must be done. A fractured limb could be overlooked in a recumbent animal unless each limb is examined in as much detail as possible. The main causes of postparturient recumbency in the various species are listed below. Their important clinical features and an outline of their management is summarized below. For further information the reader is advised to consult appropriate books on medicine and surgery.

Although the condition occurs in all species, it is more common in the cow than in the other species. Diagnosis, prognosis, management, and treatment may be particularly difficult in this species. For this reason, postparturient recumbency will be covered in detail in the cow with comparative details in the other species.

The cow

Postparturient recumbency is a major problem in cattle. It may be acute and rapidly responsive to appropriate therapy or more chronic, less responsive and may progress to the downer cow syndrome.

Mineral deficiencies/metabolic problems

Calcium deficiency   This is an important cause of recumbency in the periparturient cow. The highest incidence is in dairy cows beyond their second lactation in the first 48 hours after calving. The condition (commonly known as 'milk fever') can also occur before birth, during birth as a cause of primary uterine inertia, or occasionally later in lactation. Mildly affected cases may appear slightly ataxic and have some difficulty in rising. In severe cases the animal is recumbent, has a low body temperature, dilated pupils with poor light response, reduced rumenal activity, and may lie with its head turned round against its flank. If untreated the condition progresses to coma and death.

Treatment   Four hundred mL calcium borogluconate with added magnesium, phosphorus, and dextrose (CaMgPD) is given by slow intravenous injection with 400 mL 40% calcium borogluconate given subcutaneously. Before treatment it is wise to take and keep a blood sample in heparin to enable plasma assays of Ca^{2+}, Mg^{2+}, and PO_4^{2-} to be estimated if the case does not respond to treatment. A plasma calcium concentration of <1.5 mmol/L is indicative of a deficiency.

Magnesium deficiency   On some farms, periparturient calcium deficiency is accompanied by a magnesium deficiency – plasma levels of <0.8 mmol/L confirming the problem. Low dietary magnesium intake may also depress calcium intake. Cows affected with the double deficiency may be slightly hyperesthetic and in particular show an exaggerated palpebral reflex.

Treatment   CaMgPD solution given intravenously will usually be beneficial to affected animals. If a serious magnesium deficiency is present, 400 mL of 25% magnesium sulfate injection should be given by subcutaneous injection. A blood sample should be taken before treatment for later evaluation of plasma levels of calcium, magnesium, and phosphorus if there is any doubt about the deficiencies involved. The results of sampling may be confusing if the farmer has already instituted treatment. Severe, sudden, and acute magnesium deficiency in the form of 'staggers' ('grass staggers') seldom occurs at calving time. It may do so, however, in especially harsh weather conditions. Affected animals are severely hyperesthetic and frequently collapse in lateral recumbency. Convulsions, coma, and death may follow unless treatment is given quickly. In addition to the treatment described above, some sedation may be required to control the convulsions until the animal has recovered.

Phosphorus deficiency   The role of phosphorus deficiency is not exactly clear. Some authorities consider that a phosphorus deficiency (<1.3 mmol/L) may delay response to treatment and recovery from a calcium deficiency. In some areas, phosphorus deficiency is associated with a postparturient hemoglobinuria.

Treatment   The organic phosphorus preparation toldimphos (10–25 mL) may be given by intravenous, intramuscular, or subcutaneous injection. Alternatively, half the dose may be given intravenously and half by intramuscular or subcutaneous injection.

Ketosis   This is rarely an acute cause of recumbency in the immediate postparturient period. It may occasionally be an ongoing problem from a preparturient pregnancy toxemia, especially when associated with fatty liver disease. The condition is potentially very serious in the immediate postparturient phase, especially if the animal is not eating.

Treatment   Is by intravenous glucose therapy, oral propylene glycol, and steroids given by intramuscular injection. For further details of treatment, see Chapter 2.

Septicemia/toxemia

Acute mastitis   This condition, especially in the form of environmental mastitis associated with *E. coli* or *Streptococcus uberis* infection, may develop immediately before, during, or after calving. These life-threatening problems may be so acute that the animal is already gravely ill and unable to rise before they are recognized. For this reason, the udder of every calving cow should be actively checked to see if mastitis is present. One or more quarters may be affected and become very hard to the touch. The milk is thin, watery, and may be green or brown instead of having the normal creamy appearance of colostrum. In the very early stages, body temperature may be elevated but as toxemia develops it falls rapidly to normal or below. Diarrhea may be present in severe cases and renal failure may also occur.

Treatment   Requires aggressive therapy with intravenous antibiotics, non-steroidal anti-inflammatory drugs, and fluids. Frequent stripping of the affected quarter is also beneficial.

Acute septic metritis   (see above) May cause recumbency but does not normally develop until 2–3 days after calving. Other septicemias, such as blackquarter, may occur in the postparturient cow and their presence should be detected during the careful and methodical clinical examination required for such cases.

Peritonitis   This may develop as a result of uterine rupture (see above) and is likely to reach its greatest severity 72 hours after parturition rather than in the immediate postparturient period.

Neurological diseases

In the UK the possibility of bovine spongiform encephalopathy (BSE) must be considered although the incidence has fallen with control measures. The cow may have shown mild neurological signs, including changes of temperament, which have become markedly worse after calving and may result in recumbency. BSE is a notifiable disease in the UK and suspicious cases must be reported to the local Divisional Veterinary Manager. Other diseases with neurological signs include chronic ketosis that has persisted since before calving and may be associated with fatty liver disease. Listeriosis, which is often associated with silage feeding may show signs of recumbency but more often of localized facial paralysis.

Physical injury or damage

Nerves, muscles, bones, and occasionally other tissues may be involved.

Obturator paralysis   Caused by fetal pressure on the obturator nerves as they pass from the lumbosacral plexus along the medial surface of the ilia and through the obturator foramen on the pelvic floor. There is often a history of dystocia and in particular of the fetus becoming lodged for a period of time within the pelvis as, for example, in stifle lock. The affected cow is unable to adduct her hindlimbs and in severe cases may be unable to rise (Fig. 13.8). Walking is difficult and if the surface is slippery the legs may splay out laterally and the adductor muscles may become stretched and damaged. If the cow is unable to stand she may be found in sternal recumbency with her limbs held in a very abnormal lateral position.

Treatment   Is non-specific. Good nursing care is essential. The cow should be placed on a non-slip surface, which will aid her attempts to rise. The hindlimbs may be tied together just above the fetlocks with soft rope allowing approximately 20 cm space between them. This will prevent them splaying laterally in an uncontrolled manner.

Peroneal paralysis   Paralysis may develop in cases where the cow has been in prolonged lateral recumbency during calving or dystocia and has sustained pressure damage to one, or occasionally both, peroneal nerves. The cow is usually able to rise and stand but is unable to extend her fetlock on the affected side. The fetlock joint knuckles over in a fully flexed position and the anterior surface of the distal limb may become

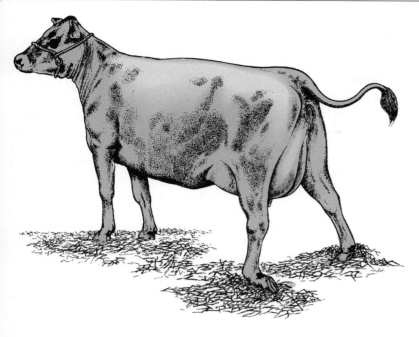

Figure 13.8 Postparturient cow showing signs of obturator and peroneal paralysis.

excoriated (Fig. 13.8). Response to nursing care is usually good and the affected leg returns to normal within a few days to 2 weeks, although a degree of weakness may persist for longer in some animals. Bandaging of the distal limb will reduce damage due to excoriation during the recovery period. Less commonly, the whole of the sciatic nerve (of which the peroneal nerve is a branch) may be affected and the cow's legs are held rigidly forward. This posture may also be adopted if there has been spinal damage involving upper motor neurons.

Fractures/dislocations

Pelvic fracture or fracture of the long bones may occur as a result of the cow falling or being involved in a serious accident before, during or after calving. Pelvic fractures in cattle may be multiple and are detected by demonstrating abnormal movements or crepitus on manipulating the pelvis externally and by rectal palpation. In the case of limb fractures, the affected leg may be grossly swollen with abnormal contours and non-weight-bearing. Gentle manipulation may reveal crepitus detectable by palpation or audible through a stethoscope.

Dislocations of the hip or the sacroiliac articulation are usually accompanied by severe lameness and an unwillingness to rise. Similar signs may be seen in cases where rupture of one or both teres ligaments has occurred. Rectal examination may be helpful in confirming their presence. Other causes of lameness, such as severe laminitis, should also be considered.

Rupture of the gastrocnemius tendon This results in inability to extend the hock and may involve one or both hindlimbs.

Treatment of this group of problems is based, when practical and economical, on surgical principles. Radiographic and other investigations may be useful in confirming diagnoses.

Muscle damage Strain of the longissimus dorsi muscles may be sustained by the patient struggling to get up or occasionally by excessive straining. The back muscles are swollen, warm, and painful to the touch. Treatment is by rest and analgesia.

The compression syndrome Both muscle and nerve damage may develop as a result of recumbency, even for a few hours. The damage is the result of pressure, which may compromise circulation and lead to poor perfusion of the muscles and eventual necrosis. Compression of nerve fibers may have an adverse effect upon motor and sensory function. The longer the compression continues, the greater the likelihood of the damage becoming permanent.

Acute or chronic hemorrhage   This is discussed in detail above; it can weaken the animal to such an extent that she is unable to stand.

Other possible causes of recumbency

A wide range of problems must be considered along with the more common differential diagnoses listed above. Some may not be clearly related to the recent parturition. In some cases, however, the stresses associated with that event and the reduced immune status of the mother at calving may assist the conditions to become established.

Acute enteritis with associated dehydration may cause sufficient weakness and debility to prevent the cow from rising. Causes may include salmonellosis, winter dysentery, mucosal disease, and other enteric pathogens.

Diarrhea may also occur in cases of rumenal acidosis caused by gaining access to a food store and overeating.

Access to heavy metal or plant poisons should be considered and investigated, especially if examination eliminates the more common causes of recumbency.

Starvation – more commonly a cause of preparturient recumbency – may be compounded by the physical effort of calving using residual energy reserves. After calving the animal is simply too weak to rise.

The special problems of the downer cow

The downer cow is an animal that has been recumbent for more than 24 hours after calving. Some definitions have suggested that diagnosis of a downer cow case should refer to those animals in which the common causes of recumbency (mentioned above) have been eliminated. In practice, when the cow is first seen – often after one or more lay treatments – it may not initially be possible to conclude exactly what has caused the recumbency. The case must be investigated fully in the usual way, paying particular attention to the detailed history of the patient and a thorough clinical examination. The clinical impression can be backed up by biochemical and other tests and a plan for treatment is prepared.

Etiology   Most of the causes of recumbency mentioned above can become chronic and the patient suffering from them becomes a downer cow. The chronic nature of the recumbency means that – as a result of damage through compression of muscles and nerves – the condition may become self-perpetuating and often worsen with time.

History   A full evaluation and re-evaluation of the history should always be undertaken. Answers to the following questions should be sought (if the obstetrician attended the original calving case or the recumbency at an earlier stage many of the answers will already be known):

- How long has the cow been recumbent? The longer the recumbency, the poorer the prognosis.
- Has she been up at all since calving and if so for how long? Could she have fallen and suffered more severe injury during an attempt to rise? If she has been up the prognosis is better than if she has never risen after calving.
- Was she assisted at calving and if so what was the nature of this assistance?
- What treatment has the farmer given already? What drugs and what dose or volume was used? Was the treatment appropriate or could further damage have been done? Was the cause of the original recumbency known or diagnosed? If the cow was known to be hypocalcemic and was treated with a correct dose of calcium borogluconate then the persistent recumbency may not be associated with persistent hypocalcemia.
- Has there been any response to treatment so far? Did the animal improve and then deteriorate. Has the cow been milked and how much milk was taken? Excessive milking after milk fever may predispose to a relapse.
- Has the cow attempted to rise? If so can the farmer describe *exactly* what she did? For example, was she able to use one or both limbs, etc.?
- Did she have any problems during pregnancy and if so what were they?
- How was she fed and managed during pregnancy, and especially during the last few weeks? Have any other animals in the group been affected?
- Is the surface on which she is lying suitable for her to stand on if she attempts to rise?
- How much nursing care is and will be available? How valuable is the patient and is the owner prepared to pay for blood tests and other investigations?

Clinical examination   This must be thorough and comprehensive. As in the case of recent recumbency, the list of possible causes (see above) is very large and the clinical examination must therefore cover the whole body and all its systems. Signs of the secondary consequences of recumbency, such as myositis and bed sores, should be carefully sought.

Prognosis   The obstetrician is often under great pressure to give a firm prognosis about the likelihood of recovery. The cow may be very valuable; her future economic performance may be very important; economic considerations and welfare issues must also be borne in mind. The farmer may be happy to pay for continuing treatment if the prognosis is thought to be good. If the prognosis is poor, prolonged and expensive treatment cannot be justified. In some cases the prognosis is very clear. An oblique mid-shaft femoral fracture in an elderly, heavy cow has a poorer prognosis than the cow that has very mild peroneal paralysis in one limb.

The following observations may be, with the case history, of important prognostic and diagnostic value:

- *The nature of the recumbency*: if the cow is flat on her side she may be terminally ill from almost any major disease. If she is on her side despite adequate CaMgPD therapy the prognosis is generally poor. If she is in unsupported sternal recumbency the prognosis is better. The position of the limbs (discussed above) may indicate specific nerve damage.
- *State of alertness*: hyporesponsiveness may indicate a persistent hypocalcemia. Hyperresponsiveness may indicate a persistent hypomagnesemia. In both cases biochemical analysis may confirm whether either element is really deficient. Chronic hyper-responsiveness may suggest the possibility of BSE, which should be considered in the UK.
- *Attempts to rise*: if the cow is almost able to get to her feet and tries to stand frequently the prognosis is better than if she lies passively and makes no attempt to stand even if encouraged to do so. Spontaneous movement around the box or field is also a good sign.
- *Appetite*: an interest in food, a good appetite, and cudding are all good prognostic signs.
- *Biochemical evaluation*: the muscle enzymes creatine kinase (CK) and aspartate aminotransferase (AST) rise rapidly in recumbent animals and to some extent indicate the degree of primary or secondary muscle damage sustained. Serial evaluation of these enzymes, although costly, can be of major prognostic value. Levels of CK and AST that continue to rise rapidly despite good nursing care over a period of 3 days suggest continuing muscle damage caused by pressure. A very poor prognosis is indicated, as it is with rising levels of blood urea.
- *The progress of the case*: the case that shows a daily improvement, albeit a slight one, has a more favorable prognosis than the case whose condition remains unchanged or deteriorates. In many cases it is clear within a few days whether the patient is improving.
- *Help available on the farm*: proper nursing of the recumbent cow (see below) is demanding in terms of time and physical effort. On many farms, nursing is sustainable for perhaps 1 or 2 days but after that, unless obvious and substantial improvement is made, it becomes less feasible. A sole attendant may be quite unable to roll the cow from one side to the other as is required in nursing care.

Treatment   Involves specific treatment for any diagnosed abnormality and non-specific nursing care:

1. If there is doubt concerning the cow's mineral status, more should be given, especially if indicated by reduced blood levels.
2. Specific diseases such as acute mastitis and fatty liver disease should receive a normal, specific course of treatment for that disease.
3. Nursing care should include the following measures:
   a. Provision of appetising food and water within reach. Placing food just beyond the cow's reach may sometimes encourage her to move (if she is able to do so).
   b. The cow should be kept in sternal recumbency but lying on one hindquarter or the other. She should be rolled onto the other quarter four times daily. Pressure points and dependent areas like the ventral abdominal wall must be regularly checked for evidence of impending problems like pressure ulcers, urine scalding, or blowfly strike. At-risk areas should be washed in clean soapy water, rinsed and dried before petroleum jelly (Vaseline™) is applied.
   c. Care of the udder is most important. If the udder is producing milk it should have some milk removed at intervals to prevent an uncomfortable build-up. The udder must be monitored carefully for evidence of mastitis.
   d. The floor surface must not be slippery. A deeply bedded box or a grass field (if the weather is good) may be used. If the animal is able to stand but is unable to adduct her legs it may help to tie them together with soft rope leaving a space of about 20 cm between them.
   e. Lifting the cow is helpful to establish whether she can take her own weight if raised to the standing position. It also enables a detailed examination to be carried out on her legs and the dependent parts of her body. The legs can also be massaged to encourage good circulation. A number of lifting devices are available. The Bagshawe hoist is fixed onto the

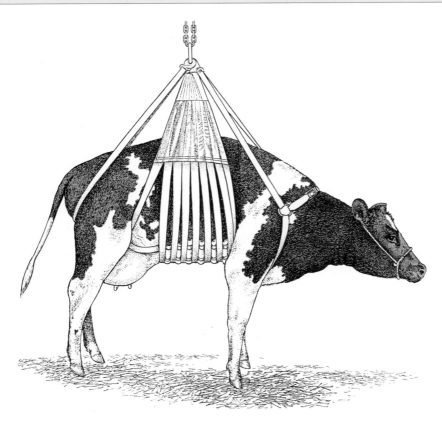

Figure 13.9 Harness for lifting a recumbent cow (Downkow harness; A. Murray Ltd, Chilworthy, UK).

tubera coxae of the cow, which is lifted on a pulley or with the fore-end loader of a tractor or other suitable farm implement. The front of the cow must be controlled and lifted with the aid of a halter on her head. Repeated use of the hoist results in pressure damage to the cow's skin and underlying tissues at the point of attachment. Inflatable cushions can be used to lift the cow but are unstable and the cow cannot attempt to use her legs for walking while supported. Good results have been obtained with the cow harness (Fig. 13.9), which is attached to the cow and lifts her evenly into the standing position. There are a number of other similar devices.

4. *Non-specific drug therapy*: the analeptic action of tripelannamine hydrochloride may stimulate the recumbent cow to rise when given at a dose of 10 mL/450 kg by slow intravenous injection. This drug is not available in some countries.
5. Progress is monitored daily and should be discussed with the owner. Rapid deterioration of the patient or failure to show any improvement despite treatment may require euthanasia on humane grounds. The animal is unlikely to be suitable for human consumption. Transport to a slaughterhouse would be inhumane and the carcass would probably be condemned or rejected on grounds of drug withdrawal periods or the age of the animal.

Many animals who are eating well and not deteriorating physically may spontaneously get to their feet after long periods of recumbency.

The mare

Postparturient recumbency is unusual in mares. Mineral deficiencies such as hypocalcemia are very rare and acute mastitis at foaling is uncommon. Metritis usually develops 2–3 days after foaling and is discussed above. The mare may develop colic after foaling and this is investigated and treated in the usual way. If the mare has survived *hyperlipemia* in late pregnancy she may still be too ill to rise (see Chapter 2).

Some mares become cast at foaling – their vigorous and violent expulsive efforts may leave them with their heads too close to a wall or corner to rise front-end first in the normal equine manner. Treatment is simple: a head collar is placed on the mare and her head is pulled into the center of the box. The mare will normally rise immediately, encouraged if necessary by mild stimulation.

The ewe and doe

Postparturient recumbency is quite common in ewes and is also seen in does. Differential diagnoses include:

- *Mineral deficiency*: calcium deficiency is particularly important but hypomagnesemia is less common at parturition. Initial treatment is by intravenous administration of 100 mL of CaMgPD solution. Pre-treatment blood samples are useful to confirm the diagnosis later, especially if a flock or herd problem is suspected. In sheep flocks a number of animals may be affected at the same time.
- *Septicemia/toxemia*: acute septic metritis or acute mastitis. A very severe metritis may develop shortly after lambing, especially in sheep in which poor lambing hygiene has been practiced. Mastitis seldom occurs at lambing or kidding but the udder should always be carefully checked in recumbent animals.
- *Residual recumbency due to pregnancy toxemia*: mildly affected ewes normally show quite rapid improve-ment after their energy-demanding lambs have been born. In severe cases of grave debility, where secondary complications such as fatty degeneration of the liver and renal dysfunction have occurred, the problem may persist after lambing. Continued nursing care and specific treatment with steroids, intravenous glucose, or oral propylene glycol may help. If rapid improvement within a few days does not ensue, the prognosis is poor.
- *Debility due to starvation*: malnutrition can occur in both lowland and hill flocks. It may be accompanied by the specific signs of pregnancy toxemia but may also result in extremely poor bodily condition and weakness. The additional strain imposed by lambing may cause further deterioration and recumbency despite delivery of the lambs. The prognosis for a return to economic productive status is very poor although good nursing may result in survival.
- *Other causes of recumbency*: these include access to toxic sprays and injuries caused by poor obstetric technique.

The sow

- *The overweight elderly sow*: such animals, which have received little exercise during pregnancy or after farrowing may have great difficulty in getting to their feet, especially in the confines of a farrowing crate. The sow should be encouraged to leave the crate. She should be assisted to her feet by helping take her weight with a careful tail lift. A walk outside especially on grass is very beneficial.
- *Acute mastitis*: *Klebsiella* mastitis may develop rapidly and dangerously in the immediate postparturient period. Clinical signs and suggested treatment regimes are described under Mastitis above. The mammary induration, which is a feature of the mastitis–metritis–agalactia syndrome is unlikely to produce recumbency.
- *Mineral deficiency*: hypocalcemia occurs very rarely in the parturient sow. The signs are similar to those seen in the cow. The sow becomes ataxic and then passes into a comatose state. Intravenous calcium borogluconate at a dose of 80–100 mL of a 20% solution given via an ear vein will often produce a rapid improvement.

REFERENCES

Aanes WA 1964 Surgical repair of third degree laceration and recto-vaginal fistula in the mare. Journal of the American Veterinary Medical Association 144:485–490

McKinnon AO, Voss JL eds 1992 Equine reproduction. Lea and Febiger, Philadelphia, p 423–425

Chapter 14

POSTPARTURIENT PROBLEMS IN THE DOG AND CAT

Any abnormality in the postnatal period must be taken seriously and the animal submitted to a full clinical examination. Whenever illness in the mother is investigated, the health of the offspring should also be evaluated, and vice versa. If the milk supply is compromised by maternal illness, supplementary feeding should be started immediately and continued until no longer needed.

HEMORRHAGE

Some blood loss is inevitable during parturition from minor uterine trauma and some blood is also lost from the placental sites. Apparent but not true maternal hemorrhage may be feared when an umbilical cord ruptures within the birth canal and fetal blood appears at the vulva. True maternal blood loss should never exceed a slow drip from the vulva and any level greater than this must be investigated.

Uterine or vaginal injury resulting from the treatment of dystocia or placental site hemorrhage (the latter being mostly more chronic) are the most likely sources of blood loss. It can be difficult to locate the exact bleeding point because visual access to the mucosal surfaces is limited to the caudal vagina. The anterior vagina can be inspected if a long speculum or pediatric endoscope is available. The possibility of clotting defects must always be remembered and an assessment also made for systemic signs of anemia.

Treatment   An attempt should be made, by visual inspection of the vulval lips and caudal vagina, to locate a bleeding source that can be dealt with by standard hemostatic means.

If necessary, the anterior vagina can be approached surgically by episiotomy and standard methods used to stem hemorrhage. An attempt to control vaginal hemorrhage can also be made by inserting a cotton wool or gauze tampon into the lumen of the vagina. Administration of ecbolics such as oxytocin will cause uterine contraction, which will reduce the size of the uterine lumen and apply some pressure to the uterine walls. Where severe continuing uterine hemorrhage is feared, the organ should be inspected at laparotomy and if necessary removed. Blood transfusion and supportive therapy may be required.

Chronic hemorrhage from the placental sites

This condition, which is sometimes termed subinvolution of the placental sites ('SIPS'), is seen chiefly in the dog but cases in the cat have also been reported. Younger animals are most commonly affected. Some slight blood loss is normally seen for up to 6 weeks postpartum but when the placental sites have not involuted blood loss may continue for up to 15 weeks or even longer. The condition is said to be self-limiting but the blood loss is unslightly and may occasionally be dangerous. Affected animals normally show few systemic signs and a smear of the discharge reveals blood cells only. The exact cause of the condition is not known but it is believed to be associated with invasion of the uterine wall by fetal trophoblast tissues. The tissue resolution and repair that normally follows pregnancy does not occur. Histologically, the affected areas of the uterus show hyperemia, cellular infiltration, and necrosis of the blood vessels. There is a small risk that the uterine mucosa may be more susceptible to endometritis.

Treatment   Many cases will resolve spontaneously but medroxprogesterone acetate at 2 mg/kg is claimed to result in resolution within 24 hours. Such treatment might predispose to the establishment of uterine infection and should be used with care. Hysterectomy may be necessary in cases that fail to resolve.

RETAINED PLACENTA

This is often suspected when in fact the placenta has been eaten by the mother. The condition seldom causes severe problems unless it is accompanied by fetal retention or infection. Clinical signs include a thick, dark vaginal discharge but initially no systemic signs. The uterus may appear distended on palpation and occasionally a portion of placenta can be felt on vaginal examination. Careful abdominal palpation should confirm the presence of a retained fetus. If there is still any doubt about the possibility of fetal retention this should be further investigated by X-ray or ultrasonographic examination. The placenta can be demonstrated in utero by introducing contrast medium into the uterus via the open cervix. Further clarity can be achieved using simultaneous pneumoperitoneum.

Treatment If the placenta can be palpated in the vagina it may be removed by gentle traction using artery or whelping forceps. Oxytocin given by intramuscular injection at a dose of 2–5 IU will aid expulsion provided the uterus is still sensitive to its action. Antibiotic cover is also advisable.

UTERINE PROLAPSE

This is relatively uncommon and occurs more frequently in the cat than the dog. The prolapse may involve both or just one horn, and in the latter case the prolapse may occur before delivery of the litter is complete. Incomplete prolapse may occur in which the partially prolapsed organ can be palpated within the vagina. In toy dogs invagination of one horn within the abdomen has been described. In cats considerable damage can occur rapidly as a result of licking the prolapsed organ.

Treatment In fresh and uncomplicated cases where only a very small portion of the uterus has prolapsed the organ can be cleaned and replaced. It can be encouraged to resume its correct position by introducing warm saline into the lumen under general anesthetic. If this is not possible, or if it is uncertain whether the organ has been fully restored to its correct position, it may be gently pulled back into position via a laparotomy incision. Once the uterus has been returned into the abdomen an injection of 2–5 IU oxytocin will encourage involution. The uterus may be attached to the abdominal wall to prevent further prolapse. If severely damaged the uterus may have to be removed.

UTERINE RUPTURE

Preparturient rupture of the uterus is often the result of external trauma including road accidents. Rupture during or after birth is most likely to occur in cases where the uterine wall is compromised by the presence of infection, a dead fetus, uterine torsion, or careless obstetric procedures. It can also be caused (it is claimed) by excessively large doses of oxytocin.

The clinical signs are greatly influenced by the presence or absence of infection and hemorrhage. Where infection is present, peritonitis, toxemia, and shock develop rapidly. In the absence of infection or hemorrhage, few symptoms may be seen. Hematological parameters may show a rise in fibrinogen levels. Cytological studies of peritoneal fluid may provide useful diagnostic and prognostic information.

Treatment Suspected uterine rupture is treated by intensive care, including antibiotic and fluid replacement therapy. Surgical intervention if the diagnosis is uncertain or severe trauma requiring repair or uterine removal is suspected.

AGALACTIA

Attention may be drawn to this problem initially by hyperactive and vocal, hungry offspring, or later by hypoactive, moribund offspring lapsing into a terminal state. Aplasia of mammary gland tissue is extremely rare in small animals. It should in any case have been spotted during antenatal appraisal of the mother. Milk production can be compromised by mastitis (see below) or by a failure of the milk let-down reflex. The latter is most frequently seen in primiparous patients and is associated with fear, stress, or pain.

Treatment This will depend on the cause but let-down can be helped by administration of 2–5 IU oxytocin given by intramuscular injection, sedation, and patient management. Supplementary feeding should be commenced immediately and continued until maternal supplies are restored.

MASTITIS

Acute mastitis in the cat and dog is relatively uncommon but when it is seen it must be regarded as a potentially life-threatening condition. It must be treated vigorously and with appropriate supplementary care for the offspring.

Etiology   The condition is associated with infection by streptococci, staphylococci, and *E. coli*. It is predisposed by trauma caused by the claws of the offspring or by minor but repeated damage caused when the mother scrapes her udder when she enters and leaves her box. One or more of the mammary glands may be affected and the condition may occur at any time during lactation or occasionally just after weaning and before whelping. Peak occurrence is in the first 2 weeks of lactation.

Clinical signs   The affected glands are hot, swollen, and painful and a degree of pyrexia is evident (Fig. 14.1). Rapid abscessation of one or more of the affected glands may occur. Such abscesses frequently rupture. The subsequent release of large quantities of gray-colored pus leaving a large granulating crater may greatly alarm the owner. In some cases, and especially where there has been delay in seeking help, toxemia and septicemia rapidly ensue. Uterine infection may also be present.

Treatment   Immediate and intense antibotic therapy (e.g. ampicillin or oxytetracycline) given intravenously with non-steroidal anti-inflammatory therapy and fluid therapy if required. Intramammary therapy is not feasible in small animals. Glands about to rupture should be surgically opened. The underlying tissue usually repairs rapidly if kept clean. Local application of antibiotic ointment is often beneficial. Occasionally, gangrenous changes occur in areas of compromised tissue and some sloughing may follow. Severe toxemia is seen in the mother in such cases. In time – if the patient survives the acute phase – good resolution occurs. The offspring

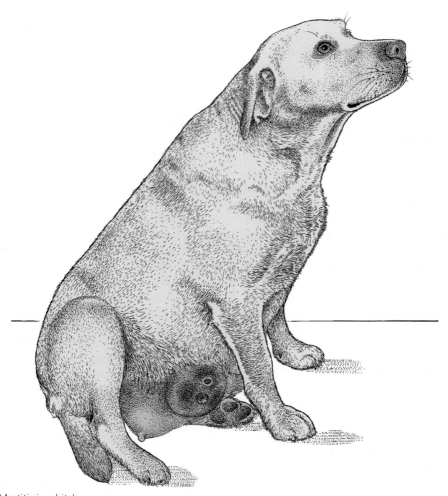

Figure 14.1 Mastitis in a bitch.

may be left on the mother in many cases or at least allowed to suckle at intervals. The affected gland may be protected by strategic bandaging during suckling. Alternatively, a vest may be used, which is adjusted to allow the offspring access to the normal glands only whilst protecting the diseased tissues.

ACUTE METRITIS

Etiology   The condition is associated with invasion of a compromised uterus by opportunist pathogens. The disease can be potentially life threatening. Predisposing factors include retained placenta and a retained fetus. Dystocia, a poor obstetric technique, and delayed uterine involution may also predispose to the condition. Ascending infection from a soiled perineal region has been described in the long-haired cat.

Clinical signs   These include a dark thick sanguino-purulent vaginal discharge with a foul offensive smell. The uterus may be enlarged on palpation and have a doughy consistency. Temperature is usually elevated but in neglected cases toxemia and septicemia are seen and – especially in the cat – rapidly developing dehydration.

Treatment   Intensive broad-spectrum antibiotic and supportive therapy must be commenced without delay. If there is any doubt about fetal retention a radiograph or an ultrasonographic scan should be taken. If a fetus is present, hysterotomy and possibly hysterectomy may be required to save the patient's life (details of surgical technique are discussed in Chapter 11). If surgery is not indicated, uterine lavage with an antibiotic solution or mild antiseptic may be attempted per vaginam. Prostaglandin therapy to produce uterine contraction has been recommended but is contraindicated if the uterine wall is compromised. Even in severely toxemic cases the patient will often make a spectacular recovery following hysterectomy.

VAGINITIS

Occasionally after parturition – and especially when a fetus has been lodged in the vagina for some time – a genital infection involving only the vagina is seen. A vaginal discharge is present but examination reveals no evidence of uterine or urinary tract infection. Systemic illness is rarely seen.

Treatment   Local and parenteral antibiotic therapy with antiseptic lavage if necessary. Occasionally complete resolution of vaginitis does not occur until the animal comes into estrus again.

ECLAMPSIA

Eclampsia is also known as puerperal tetany or lactation tetany.

Etiology   The condition is mostly caused by hypocalcemia. In some cases there is evidence of hypoglycemia and hypomagnesemia either alone or with hypocalcemia. Hypophosphatemia may also be present in some cases. Eclampsia is seen chiefly during lactation in both the dog and cat. The condition is seen more commonly in the dog than the cat but in both species occurs rarely during pregnancy. Eclampsia is most frequently seen in heavily lactating animals with a large, demanding litter. Animals that are reluctant to leave their litter even for short periods in which to feed themselves are particularly prone to the disease. The condition may be predisposed by parathyroid hypofunction, which may in turn be influenced by a dietary calcium:phosphorus imbalance during pregnancy. It has also been suggested that hyperventilation may develop in hyperactive, nervous bitches. The resulting respiratory alkalosis may lead to calcium ions becoming bound to protein and resultant hypocalcemia.

Clinical signs   In the bitch, early signs include unexpected nervousness, panting, whining, and excess salivation. Stiffness of gait may also be seen and in unrecognized or untreated cases temperature rises to 41–42°C. The pupils are dilated, the gait becomes increasingly unsteady and the use of the legs is compromised (Fig. 14.2) Unconsciousness and death may follow.

In the cat, symptoms including restlessness, ataxia, vomiting, and convulsions are seen. Temperature rises up to 42°C but shock and hypothermia may follow in untreated cases.

Treatment   An intravenous injection of a 10% solution of calcium borogluconate solution is given slowly over a period of 10 minutes. The dose for the bitch is 5–20 mL and for the queen cat 2–5 mL. During administration of intravenous calcium the heart rate and rhythm of the patient is carefully monitored. (*Note*: solutions of either 20% or 40% calcium borogluconate are commercially available for large animal treatment. Such solutions must be carefully diluted to a 10% strength with sterile water for injection before use in small animals.) In non-responsive cases additional glucose may be given, but with the preparation recommended this should not be

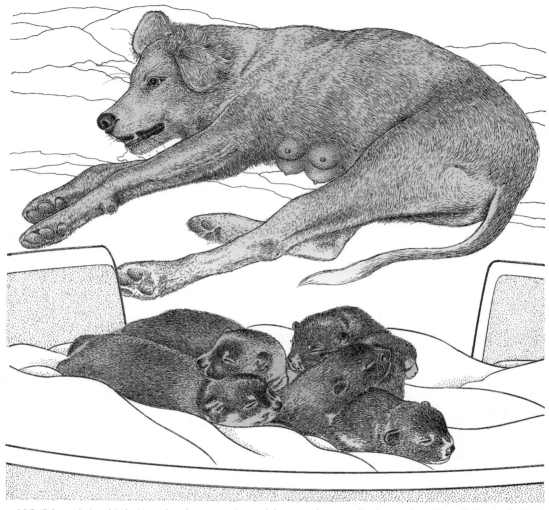

Figure 14.2 Eclampsia in a bitch. Note the plump puppies and the recumbency, salivation, and pupillary dilation in the bitch.

necessary. The incidence of hypoglycemia, hypomagnesemia, and hypophosphatemia is quite low but ideally a blood sample should be taken in heparin before treatment with calcium is commenced. This will enable a retrospective assay to be performed after emergency treatment and confirmation that calcium deficiency was present or, if response to treatment has been poor, blood glucose, magnesium, and phosphorus levels can be obtained. If there is a deficiency of substances other than calcium then a diluted CaMgPD solution should be used.

The patient's diet during lactation may require daily supplementation with 300–500 mg calcium lactate and vitamin D therapy. In the immediate post-treatment period the litter should be temporarily removed. Supplementary feeding of the offspring or occasionally early weaning may be necessary. Affected animals may suffer a relapse requiring further treatment. A chronic form of the eclampsia has been reported, which responds to treatment with prednisolone. Acute eclampsia may recur in affected animals at subsequent lactations.

Prevention   It is now thought that both high- and low-calcium diets are contraindicated during pregnancy. The ideal gestational diet should contain 1.0–1.8% calcium and 0.8–1.6% phosphorus. During lactation the diet should contain at least 1.4% calcium and the calcium : phosphorus ratio should be 1 : 1.

Chapter 15

PREVENTION OF DYSTOCIA

'Dystocia should be avoided whenever possible. The condition has many adverse effects – financial and otherwise. Specifically, the losses that may occur include:

- Compromising the patient's welfare: if a case of dystocia is treated by a veterinary obstetrician it is hoped that any pain and suffering will be kept to a minimum. Regrettably, some cases of dystocia – especially in cattle – are badly handled by owners and attendants and in many cases excessive force may be used inadvertently. Severe damage may be sustained by both the cow and her calf. The cow might, for example, suffer from a severe vaginal laceration. The calf – if it lives – might sustain limb fracture and other damage.
- The distress of the considerate owner at seeing their animal suffering from dystocia is perhaps less easily quantified but is nonetheless very important. The fetus(es) may die during a difficult delivery. This will by itself have inevitable financial consequences. In addition will be the loss of genetic material such as the progeny of a particular blood-line or of a much loved pet.
- If dystocia is prolonged the fetus may become acidotic and this may predispose it to other diseases. There is evidence in a number of species that a fetus born following dystocia has a poorer chance of survival and may show greater morbidity than a fetus delivered by a normal uncomplicated birth. Poor growth of the neonate may result in it attracting a smaller price if and when it is eventually sold.
- In some cases the mother may die, with the financial consequences of her death and the losses of her production potential.
- Considerable aftercare may be required for the mother who has suffered dystocia, especially if this has been complicated by tissue damage and infection. The veterinary costs of these complications may be high.
- Production of milk from a cow that has suffered dystocia may not be as good as anticipated. She may require longer to become pregnant again. The target of producing one calf per year may be missed. The financial consequences of this increase with every day during which she fails to conceive.

CAN DYSTOCIA AND THE ASSOCIATED LOSSES BE AVOIDED?

It is probably impossible to avoid all cases of dystocia. For example, the cause of fetal malposture is not really known; it appears to arise spontaneously. Thus it is probably impossible to avoid a case of dystocia in the mare caused by lateral deviation of the fetal head. It is unlikely that the next time the mare foals her fetus will again suffer from maldisposition, although it might by chance do so. The fact that the mare has a history of dystocia may increase the amount of supervision her next foaling receives. Should dystocia arise again it may be detected and hopefully corrected at an early stage, with less serious consequences.

Some cases of dystocia occur as a result of a breeding policy that predisposes to them. The most important cause of bovine dystocia is fetopelvic disproportion. The incidence of this form of dystocia has increased with the increasing numbers of so-called continental breeds. Many of these breeds have excellent beef potential and their calves are large and of high value. Indiscriminate crossing of indigenous cattle with the continental breeds in the 1960s undoubtedly led to an increase in the incidence of fetopelvic disproportion. Many calves were lost during delivery and an unacceptable number of cows and heifers sustained damage – sometimes irreparable – when attempts were made to deliver their calves. The problem could be avoided by not using the continental breeds for crossing, but the value of the calves produced would be smaller. This would probably be commercially unacceptable.

Studies have shown that fetal size in cattle is influenced by many factors and that careful selection of these factors can allow the continental breeds to be used but with a lower and acceptable level of dystocia. Selection of individual factors can be difficult and time consuming but the incidence of dystocia can be reduced by breeding from selected strains of cattle. The incidence of dystocia in some strains of Charolais cattle is much lower than in others, even though carcass quality is as good. By selecting breeding animals for ease of calving without loss of carcass quality the overall incidence of dystocia can be lowered within a breed.

In nature, a process of self-selection by which the incidence of dystocia is reduced has occurred. The incidence of dystocia in some feral breeds of animals is lower than in the more specialized modern breeds. Fetopelvic disproportion at birth is almost unknown in the Shetland cow. It has been suggested that this is because during the many centuries of its development strains of the species with small pelvises would die out if they suffered dystocia. Thus any disadvantageous tendency would tend eventually to die out and successful strains would not suffer problems with fetopelvic disproportion.

Uterine inertia is one of the most common causes of dystocia in the bitch. The problem may arise without warning but some bitches may suffer from the condition every time they whelp. There is some evidence that a tendency to uterine inertia may possibly be hereditary. The problem could be avoided in such animals by deciding not to breed from them or their progeny. A high rate of stillbirth can occur if uterine inertia is not treated promptly and effectively. However, if a bitch with a tendency to uterine inertia is bred from then action can be taken to diagnose and deal with the problem at an early stage. Prompt treatment should enable the level of stillbirth among the puppies to be kept to a minimum.

Brachycephalic breeds of bitch, such as the bulldog, tend to suffer from a greater incidence of dystocia than breeds with longer, more pointed fetal heads. This is because the large, round, shortnosed head of the brachycephalic puppy is more readily deviated away from entering the maternal pelvis. Cesarean section is frequently required to deliver the puppies. However, some strains known as 'self-whelping' have been developed and selected in which the incidence of dystocia is lower. Members of these strains have been shown to have a lower incidence of dystocia while not compromising

the breed standards. Strains in which the incidence of dystocia is high should not be used for breeding. Some veterinarians strongly discourage owners to breed again from a bitch who has required a cesarean section to deliver her litter.

Artificial breeding techniques, especially artificial insemination (AI) and embryo transfer (ET) are widely used in some species, especially farm animals. AI and ET have great potential for rapid improvement of livestock but also – unless carefully controlled – for increasing the incidence of dystocia. An AI bull may sire many thousands of calves during and after his lifetime. The incidence of dystocia among the progeny of such bulls is carefully monitored to avoid the risk that large numbers of animals with problems such as small pelvises or large calves might be produced.

When ET became popular embryos were placed in any recipient almost regardless of her ability to physically give birth to the fetus placed in her uterus. The incidence of dystocia in such cases was high and legislation has been introduced prohibiting implantation of embryos into recipients unless they are considered capable of giving birth per vaginam.

ROLE OF THE VETERINARY OBSTETRICIAN IN REDUCING THE INCIDENCE OF DYSTOCIA

The obstetrician rarely has contact with a dystocia case until problems at birth occur and are possibly at an advanced stage. At this stage of contact it is too late to prevent the dystocia that has already occurred. Advice may be given, however, on how the risks of dystocia in the patient or members of its group might be reduced on future occasions.

Antenatal care is widely practiced in human obstetrics but is still relatively uncommon in veterinary obstetrics. It can be argued that antenatal care and guidance should be practiced in all the domestic species. Ideally it should be, and a considerable amount of information is available concerning pregnancy and parturition, both normal and abnormal, in the domestic animals. There are various ways in which such information can be disseminated and it helps if owners seek such information from the veterinary profession. Advice is sought by clients and especially by novice breeders. In small animal practice, in particular, opportunities for antenatal advice arise quite frequently and the nature of this advice is discussed in Chapter 9. Antenatal care is also now being practiced with valuable horses, and this is discussed in Chapter 5.

Ideally, the veterinary obstetrician should take every opportunity to offer guidance on the prevention of dystocia. The importance of early professional diagnosis and treatment when it does occur should also be stressed at every opportunity. Such advice can be imparted during an individual consultation either directly or assisted by the use of prepared information sheets. It can also be offered at farmers' or dog breeders' and other similar meetings or discussions.

Although dystocia cannot be totally prevented, there are many ways in which its incidence and the severity of its effects and consequences can and should be reduced.

SPECIFIC METHODS FOR REDUCING THE INCIDENCE OF DYSTOCIA AND ITS DEFECTS

These include:

Monitoring the plans for breeding

- Selecting strains of a species for breeding that have a low incidence of dystocia while maintaining good breed standards.
- Ensuring that the mother is in good health and is physically large enough and fit enough to breed. Attainment of minimum weight before breeding may help ensure the animal has also achieved sufficient body size to give birth without difficulty. In cattle, for example, dairy heifers should ideally not be served until they weigh 400 kg. Pelvic size can also be measured – externally and internally. Pelvic area in cattle should ideally exceed 200 cm^2. To achieve this pelvic area, it is suggested that heifers should be retained for breeding only if the distance between their coxal tuberosities is greater than 40 cm. More detailed pelvimetry will enable other important pelvic diameters to be evaluated.
- Avoidance, whenever possible, of breeding from animals with a history of dystocia. Taking special care of such animals that have accidentally or purposefully been bred from again.

Monitoring the pregnancy

- *Accurate diagnosis of pregnancy*: so that the date of birth of the offspring is known. The variation in

pregnancy length in the horse causes difficulty in accurately predicting the birth date in advance.
- *Diagnosing litter size*: in some species, such as the sheep, diagnosing the litter size is helpful in the prevention of pregnancy toxemia, which may predispose to fetal loss and dystocia. Careful nutritional management of those animals with multiple fetuses will help reduce the risk of pregnancy toxemia. Regular checking of plasma β-hydroxybutyrate levels in ruminants provides a useful early warning sign of impending energy deficiency during pregnancy. In the mare, early diagnosis of unwanted twin pregnancy enables prompt action to be taken to terminate it or destroy one of the two fetuses.
- *Careful investigation and treatment of any maternal illness or abnormal signs during pregnancy*: occasionally the fetus or the uterus may be found to be slightly abnormal during routine pregnancy diagnosis. These findings should be followed up and the patient re-examined at a later stage. The use of ultrasonographic monitoring is extremely useful in such cases.
- *Supervision of pregnancy*: to ensure that the mother is as free as possible from stress. Early warnings of possible problems should be given if an individual or a group of pregnant animals is believed to be at risk from disease, nutritional, or environmental stress.
- *Monitoring the fetus during pregnancy*: in human obstetrics this is done as a matter of routine at regular intervals throughout pregnancy. Special attention is paid to the at-risk fetus. This is already possible in animals with a history of fetal loss or when maternal illness may affect fetal health. Routine fetal monitoring is not currently practiced. External signs of fetal health – normal abdominal enlargement, fetal movement, and the absence of any adverse signs such as a foul vaginal discharge – can be evaluated without the need for special equipment. More detailed assessment of fetal health is possible, especially with the aid of ultrasonography. Using the ultrasonographic probe (either externally or per rectum, depending on species) the fetus and its surrounding fluids can be assessed in considerable detail.
- *Monitoring the hormonal support of pregnancy*: regular assay of plasma progesterone in animals with a history of habitual abortion may provide useful information concerning the security of their current pregnancy. This has been used in both the mare and the bitch with a history of repeated abortion not associated with an infectious cause. Animals

whose plasma progesterone has fallen below normal levels have been given progesterone or progestagen supplementation. There is currently no scientific proof that such supplements are effective.

- *Rectal examination in cattle*: an additional important but simple examination in cattle might include a rectal examination 10–14 days before birth is due. It should be possible – although sometimes difficult – to estimate the size of the calf and its presentation. If the calf is particularly large, induction of birth might be considered. If the calf was in posterior presentation special care could be taken at birth to ensure that delivery was not prolonged.

- *Using technology*: the well-being of the fetal foal has been studied in detail experimentally and some techniques, including ultrasonographic evaluation and the monitoring of fetal electrocardiographs, have been found most useful. Some techniques can be used routinely in practice but others, such as amniocentesis, require hospital facilities. For further discussion of this topic see Schott (1992).

Monitoring the birth process

- *Ensuring that proper facilities are available for the animal to give birth*: the facilities should allow sufficient space, protection, and comfort for the patient. They should also permit unobtrusive observation of the patient by her attendants, who should be able to monitor her progress without disturbing her. Facilities for catching and restraining the patient with ease for a more detailed obstetrical examination to be performed with minimum disturbance to the patient should be available.

- *Supervision*: the degree of supervision should increase as the anticipated time of birth approaches. In all species the external signs of approaching birth, although well documented, are variable, as are the lengths of the stages of normal parturition. In the mare, daily evaluation of various cations in the milk (if it is present in the udder) can be used to assess fetal maturity and the proximity of impending birth. These changes are discussed in detail on p. 244.

- *Observing the birth process*: when birth is underway its progress should be monitored unobtrusively to ensure that proper progress is being made. Inexperienced owners should be advised about the progress of normal birth and the variations that can occur.

- *Investigating abnormalities*: any apparent abnormality should be investigated and professional help sought without delay. Excessive interference should be avoided but in general it is better to examine a case prematurely than when it is too late.

- *Managing prolonged gestation*: the management of prolonged gestation is discussed in detail in the chapters on dystocia in the various domestic species. In some circumstances it may be necessary to induce birth and the methods for achieving this in each species are discussed below.

INDUCTION OF BIRTH IN ANIMALS

Induction of birth is regularly used in pigs, cattle, and less commonly in horses and goats for management reasons. It is also used in all species when the health of the pregnant mother or her offspring is at risk if pregnancy is allowed to continue. A number of drugs may be used but in general they mimic the effect of fetal stress on the pituitary–adrenal axis, which has been shown to precede birth in many domestic species. The exact pathway of hormone change has not been worked out for all species. In cattle it is believed that fetal steroids – or their substitutes – may aid the conversion of placental progesterone into estrogen. Rising estrogen and falling progesterone levels in the maternal circulation aid the production of oxytocin receptors and allow ecbolic action of oxytocin and prostaglandin F2α on the uterine muscles.

Not every technique is appropriate or effective in each species and we will consider the reasons for induction and the techniques available for each of the domestic animals in turn.

Some techniques are effective only at certain stages of pregnancy. Induction of birth is not a natural process and problems may occur from time to time.

Supervision of induced birth must always be as good if not better than the supervision needed with natural birth. The induced fetus may need special care if it is immature and planning to ensure the availability of colostrum is important.

Cattle

Indications

- To terminate pregnancy in an animal mated 'by mistake', e.g. in a postpubertal heifer calf served by her father. Also in cases of mummified fetus.

- To avoid prolonged gestation and the probability of an oversized calf causing dystocia.

- To terminate an abnormal pregnancy, e.g. hydrops allantois or in cases of maternal illness such as pregnancy toxemia (quite rare in cattle) or threatened damage such as a ventral hernia or rupture of the prepubic tendon.

- To tighten the calving pattern in a herd.
- To time calving to coincide with grass availability (this happens in New Zealand).

Methods available

These are dependent on the stage of pregnancy and the speed with which it is required to induce calving or abortion.

Induction of parturition of up to 120 days gestation

Until 120 (range 100–150) days of pregnancy, maintenance of bovine pregnancy depends solely on the corpus luteum, after this stage the placenta is the main source of progesterone.

Treatment   Prostaglandin F2α: cloprostenol 500 μg or dinoprost 25 mg both by intramuscular injection. Abortion is expected in about 3 days – the fetus may need to be removed from the vagina after it has been expelled from the uterus.

Induction of parturition of up to 120–250 days gestation

At this stage of pregnancy, induction is normally carried out to terminate an undesired pregnancy or to induce lactation at a time when good supplies of grass are available for the dairy herd.

Treatment   Long-acting corticosteroid: e.g. 25 mg dexamethasone trimethyl acetate given by intramuscular injection. Abortion is expected in 14–16 days. Treatment is effective in 80–90% of animals. Dystocia due to fetal malpresentation may occur and the aborted fetus may require assistance to allow it to be delivered.

Although calves may survive after only 8 months gestation they may not do so unless they are at least 275 days gestation. Placental retention is less common following the use of the long-acting corticosteroids than after prostaglandins or the short-acting steroids. Colostrum production is often very reduced and antibody absorption by the calf is poor.

Induction of parturition at 250–275 days gestation

Treatment

Medium-acting corticosteroid: e.g. 20–30 mg betamethasone given by intramuscular injection. Fetal delivery is expected in 5–11 days. If calving has not occurred by 5 days a further injection of either prostaglandin F2α or short-acting steroid, e.g. 20 mg dexamethasone phosphate, may be given.

Induction of parturition at, near, or after term

Treatment

Medium-acting or short-acting corticosteroid and/or prostaglandin F2α: e.g. 20–30 mg betamethasone or 500 μg cloprostenol given by intramuscular injection. Fetal delivery is expected within 3 days. Some claim that prostaglandin used alone may increase the risk of retained fetal membranes or even uterine rupture. At Cambridge, the author has successfully used a combination of 20 mg betamethasone and 500 μg cloprostenol (a prostaglandin F2α analog) given at the same time by intramuscular injection. The cow would normally be expected to calve in about 26 hours. In general, the closer to the calving date, the quicker the onset of induction.

Preparations for induced calving in late pregnancy

- Ensure the farmer can maintain a close watch on induced animals in case calving difficulties arise.
- Ensure the farmer has supplies of colostrum, as some induced cows calve with little.
- Ensure good facilities for any premature calves, which are very susceptible to cold and to the risk of neonatal infection.
- Warn the farmer of the high incidence of retained fetal membranes, which will need veterinary attention, and that the next conception may be delayed as a result.

Horses

Indications

- Scheduling foaling for medical reasons so that the veterinary surgeon can be in attendance at a predicted time if either the mare's or foal's life is at risk.
- Teaching or research purposes, e.g. in the production of gnotobiotic foals.

Notes

- Prolonged gestation is *not* a reason for induction of birth in mares because gestational length is very variable in this species. Although the average gestational length in mares is 330 days, a normal range may be 320–365 days. The 'window of viability' in foals is narrow and the chances of survival are severely reduced for any animal born in a dysmature state. The foal is often small in cases of prolonged gestation compared with the calf, which tends to be oversized in similar circumstances.

- Fetal maturity in the foal cannot be predicted by gestational length. If – as is usually the case – a living foal is the target at induction, every effort must be made to ensure the foal is mature.
- Udder development and the filling of the teats with a thick, sticky colostrum ('waxing') is probably the best external indication of imminent foaling. It is also sometimes an indication of threatened abortion in horses much earlier on, e.g. 7 months gestation. Relaxation of the pelvic ligaments, especially in primiparous mares, is an unreliable indication of imminent foaling. The cervix mostly slackens as parturition approaches but in some mares it remains tightly closed until first-stage labor is underway. In other animals, the cervix may be soft and partially open for several days before birth commences.
- Analysis of cations in mares' milk as an indication of approaching parturition and fetal maturity can be helpful. Calcium levels of over 40 mg/dL are indicative of fetal maturity, whereas levels below 12 mg/dL are not indicative of fetal immaturity. The results are less reliable in maiden mares.
- Changes in sodium and potassium levels are also useful if assayed daily. Sodium levels are around 120 mg/dL a few days before foaling but fall to 10 mg less than 24 hours before foaling. Conversely, potassium levels rise from 5 mg to nearly 20 mg/dL as birth approaches. If plotted graphically, the cross-over point of falling sodium and rising potassium occurs just before the fetus is mature and birth is due. Once this cross-over point is detected, safe induction of birth should be possible. Whenever induction is planned in mares, a quiet and clean environment is essential.

Termination of early pregnancy (<35 days)

This may be indicated in some cases of twin conception or misalliance.

Treatment   Prostaglandin F2α injection: e.g. 5 mg dinoprost given by intramuscular injection. This is only effective until 35 days, at which time endometrial cups are formed. Their presence, and hormone secretions, will prevent termination of pregnancy using prostaglandin injection until the cups disappear at approximately 120 days gestation. Hence the importance of early and accurate pregnancy diagnosis in mares.

Termination of pregnancy after 35 days

After 35 days, termination of pregnancy can be achieved by manual dilation of the cervix and irrigation of the uterus with warm normal saline; 5–10 mg dinoprost is given 12–24 hours before cervical dilation is attempted. Return to estrus may not occur until after 120 days from the initial service and covering during the same breeding season may not be possible.

Induction of parturition at or near term

This is subject to fetal maturity.

Treatment   Oxytocin, prostaglandin F2α, and corticosteroids can all be used but most agree that *oxytocin is the drug of choice*. Corticosteroids are somewhat unreliable and are seldom used in practice. Oxytocin has the major advantage that it works very quickly, so that birth can be induced often within 1 hour of administration. Prostaglandins can produce somewhat capricious results and may act within 1 hour or over 5 hours. Birth is less smooth than with oxytocin.

Induction using oxytocin

Oxytocin can be used in a number of ways:

- *Injection of oxytocin in a saline drip*: an intravenous catheter is placed in the jugular vein and a liter of sterile normal saline connected; 60–100 IU oxytocin is injected into the saline and the solution is run-in slowly – the rate being adjusted to ensure the liter will run in during a period of 1 hour. If the mare is restless, this method can be difficult to manage but birth should commence within 30 minutes. Once birth is underway the drip can be stopped. This method has been superseded by the bolus method (see below).
- *Bolus injection of oxytocin*: 2.5–15 IU oxytocin are given intravenously. The lower dose is often very effective. Some authors suggest that the bolus should be repeated at 20-minute intervals but work at Cambridge with pony mares suggests that a single small dose is often highly effective. In some cases a 'priming' dose of oxytocin is given by intramuscular injection, but this does not seem to be essential.

With both methods the mare must be monitored carefully in an unobtrusive way to ensure that nothing goes wrong. It may be wise to check the mare per vaginam after about 30 minutes to ensure that the foal's presentation is normal. Occasionally, premature placental separation occurs and the red, intact chorion may suddenly appear at the vagina. In natural birth this is sometimes described as a 'red bag' foaling. If this happens, the chorion must be carefully and quickly ruptured to release the foal and allow it to be born. This problem is said to be particularly likely to occur if the mare is unwell or if the higher levels of oxytocin have been given.

Induction using prostaglandin F2α

An injection of prostaglandin F2α (e.g. 5 mg dinoprost) is given intramuscularly after the mare has been assessed for fetal maturity as described above. Considerable sweating may occur and the exact timing of fetal delivery is unpredictable. The foal may be born within the range of 1–6 hours after injection.

Induction using corticosteroids

Corticosteroids are seldom used to induce birth in horses because oxytocin works so well. There are few indications for the use of corticosteroids but the following regime has been suggested: 100 mg dexamethasone daily by intramuscular injection for 4 days. Birth should occur within 7 days.

Sheep
Indications

- To induce birth in cases of pregnancy toxemia.
- To induce birth where parturition is believed to have been delayed.

Drugs available

Corticosteroids and estradiol benzoate are effective. Prostaglandin F2α and its analog may be used alone or in combination with corticosteroids.

Induction using corticosteroid   16 mg of either betamethasone or dexamethasone are given by intramuscular injection. Lambing normally follows within 72 hours.

Induction using corticosteroids and prostaglandin F2α   16 mg of either betamethasone or dexamethasone, and 125 μg of cloprostenol are given by intramuscular injection. Lambing normally follows in 24–72 hours.

Induction using estradiol benzoate   5 mg given by intramuscular injection. Birth normally follows about 48 hours later.

Goats
Indications

- To enable better supervision of birth to reduce kid mortality.
- To reduce doe mortality.
- To enable kids to be collected before they have taken colostrum, e.g. in diseases like caprice arthritis encephalitis syndrome (CAE).

Drugs available

Prostaglandin F2α and corticosteroids may be used, the former being particularly effective.

Induction using prostaglandin F2α   5 to 10 mg of dinoprost or 62.5–125 μg of cloprostenol is given by intramuscular injection. In one herd, goats were dosed at 144 days of gestation. If injected at 7–8 a.m. they were expected to kid by the afternoon of the following day. Most will kid 30–36 hours after induction. In another study, cloprostenol was given in divided doses – the first of 100 μg followed 10 hours later by a further dose of 50 μg. Time to birth was 34–39 hours and subsequent milk yield was reported to be better than that following a single dose of cloprostenol.

Induction using corticosteroids   20 mg dexamethasone may be given by intramuscular injection within 10 days of birth. Kidding should follow in 24–48 hours. Prostaglandin F2α is more predictable in its action and is probably the drug of choice in goats.

Pigs
Indications

- To initiate farrowing in a sow that is overdue or suffering from primary uterine inertia.
- To allow planned farrowing on pig farms. This is widely practiced on many pig farms and has a number of advantages. These include: (1) reduction of piglet mortality by ensuring that attendants are present during farrowing – losses through injury from the sow or stillbirth should be reduced; (2) saving on staff time; (3) enabling fostering between litters to be carried out more easily; (4) facilitating batch farrowing; (5) making full and effective use of farrowing facilities; (6) avoiding farrowing out of hours, at weekends, and on bank holidays.

Induction using oxytocin

This technique is only appropriate when the sow is actually ready to farrow and the uterus is sensitive to oxytocin. It cannot be used for general induction of birth. If a sow appears ready to farrow, has milk, and the cervix appears relaxed or is easily dilated then oxytocin may be used. A dose of 20 IU is given by intramuscular injection. Oxytocin is painful when given by intramuscular injection but the sow's attention may be distracted by rubbing her udder gently. If the uterus is sensitive to oxytocin, farrowing should commence within half an hour. Further oxytocin injections may be required later. Oxytocin has also been used to 'speed up' farrowing in sows. The same dose is employed for this. If employed for this last purpose it should be used with great care. It should not be used unless there is clear evidence that there is no obstruction within the birth canal.

Induction using prostaglandin

Sows are normally injected 2 days before their expected farrowing date. It helps to know the average gestation length of each farm. In farms where gestation length averages 116 days the sows may be induced at 114 days. On some farms injecting of the sows at 11.00 a.m. on one day may be followed by farrowing the following afternoon. Two drugs are in common use: dinoprost, which is synthetic prostaglandin F2α, dose 2 mL (10 mg) or cloprostenol, a synthetic prostaglandin F2α analog, dose 125 µg. Both drugs are given by intramuscular injection.

Dogs

Methods available

Induction of birth can be achieved by the use of a number of drugs. These include oxytocin, which is effective if the bitch is ready to whelp. The effectiveness of other drug therapy to induce parturition during pregnancy depends on the special features of the canine corpora lutea (CLs). Until 20 days after ovulation, the CLs are autonomous. After this time they are prolactin-dependent and thus at this stage luteolysis can be induced by the antiprolactin drug cabergoline. The canine CLs are somewhat resistant to prostaglandin F2α and repeated injections of this drug are required to cause luteolysis. Prostaglandin F2α can also be used in combination with cabergoline to terminate canine pregnancy. The antiprogesterone drug aglepristone induces luteolysis and termination of pregnancy at any stage of metestrus. It is also an effective treatment for misalliance in the bitch.

The dosage and mode of administration drugs mentioned here is discussed below. They have been used to induce parturition at various stages of pregnancy in the bitch. They have not all been licensed for use at all stages of pregnancy. The time of onset of the induced parturition is not always predictable. In some cases, part of the litter may be retained in the uterus, necessitating cesarean section or hysterectomy to complete removal of all the fetuses. The drugs should be used with great caution in late pregnancy until they have been further and fully evaluated. If induction of parturition in an overdue bitch using oxytocin is unsuccessful, an elective cesarean section is probably the safest alternative. The management of the overdue bitch is discussed in detail in Chapter 9.

Induction at term using oxytocin

This technique has been used by the author in bitches that had passed their expected whelping date. As in other species, the drug is effective only in cases where the uterus is responsive to oxytocin; at other times it is ineffective. Depending on the size of the bitch, 2–5 IU oxytocin are given by intramuscular injection. Before using oxytocin the bitch must be examined carefully to ensure that she is ready to whelp. It is not possible to palpate the cervix in most bitches but the state of relaxation of the anterior vagina may mirror the state of the cervix (see Fig. 9.7). It is essential to ensure that no obstructive dystocia is present. Oxytocin is painful in bitches and care must be taken to ensure that the obstetrician and owner are not bitten.

Management of the overdue bitch is discussed in further detail in Chapter 9.

Termination of pregnancy in the bitch

Termination of pregnancy using aglepristone
Aglepristone can be used to terminate pregnancy in bitches up to 45 days from mating. Two doses (10 mg/kg body weight) are given 24 hours apart by subcutaneous injection. Injection sites should be massaged thoroughly after administration of aglepristone to reduce transient pain. Animals treated after the 20th day of pregnancy may show visible signs of parturition, including fetal expulsion and mammary congestion. Treated bitches should be given an ultrasonographic scan 10 days after treatment to ensure that pregnancy has been completely terminated.

Aglepristone has also been used to induce birth in late pregnancy. A single dose of aglepristone (15 mg/kg) has been followed 24 hours later by two hourly injections of oxytocin at a dose of 0.15 IU/kg. Parturition follows within 21 to 38 hours. The speed of induction by this method would be too slow in cases where urgent termination of pregnancy was required to preserve fetal or maternal life. In such cases cesarean section would be indicated.

Termination of pregnancy using cabergoline and prostaglandin F2α   Cabergoline and prostaglandin F2α can be used to terminate pregnancy at 28–35 days. Cabergoline (5 μg/kg) is given daily by mouth for 10 days. Cloprostenol (5 μg/kg) is given by subcutaneous injection every second day for 10 days. Fetal resorption or abortion may occur. Treated bitches should be given an ultrasonographic scan 10 days after treatment to ensure that the pregnancy has been terminated. Cabergoline and prostaglandin F2α are not currently licensed to be used to terminate pregnancy in the bitch.

Surgical termination of pregnancy

Ovarohysterectomy can be performed to terminate pregnancy in the bitch at any stage of pregnancy. The earlier it is performed in pregnancy the better. There is a small but distinct risk of prolonged lactation occurring in bitches that are spayed during metestrus when progesterone production is high.

Cats

Termination of pregnancy by drug therapy

Feline pregnancy can be terminated by using cabergoline and prostaglandin F2α, as in the bitch. Aglepristone has also been used for this purpose in early and late pregnancy at a dose of 15 mg/kg body weight. None of these products is licensed for use in the cat. Surgical termination may be preferable.

Surgical termination of pregnancy

Ovarohysterectomy may be carried out safely at any stage of pregnancy in the queen cat. The earlier in pregnancy it is performed the better.

REFERENCE

Schott HC 1992 In: McKinnan AO, Voss JL (eds) Equine reproduction. Lea & Febiger, Philadelphia, p 964–975

INDEX

Note: Page numbers in **bold** indicate the main pages where the subject is discussed.